Artificial Intelligence and Pet Imaging, Part I

Editors

BABAK SABOURY
ARMAN RAHMIM
ELIOT SIEGELL

PET CLINICS

www.pet.theclinics.com

Consulting Editor
ABASS ALAVI

October 2021 • Volume 16 • Number 4

ELSEVIER

1600 John F. Kennedy Boulevard • Suite 1800 • Philadelphia, Pennsylvania, 19103-2899

http://www.pet.theclinics.com

PET CLINICS Volume 16, Number 4
October 2021 ISSN 1556-8598, ISBN-13: 978-0-323-83560-2

Editor: John Vassallo (j.vassallo@elsevier.com)
Developmental Editor: Karen Solomon

PET Clinics (ISSN 1556-8598) is published quarterly by Elsevier Inc., 360 Park Avenue South, New York, NY 10010-1710. Months of issue are January, April, July, and October. Periodicals postage paid at New York, NY, and additional mailing offices. Subscription prices per year are $254.00 (US individuals), $501.00 (US institutions), $100.00 (US students), $282.00 (Canadian individuals), $514.00 (Canadian institutions), $100.00 (Canadian students), $275.00 (foreign individuals), $514.00 (foreign institutions), and $140.00 (foreign students). To receive student and resident rate, orders must be accompanied by name of affiliated institution, date of term, and the signature of program/residency coordinator on institution letterhead. Orders will be billed at individual rate until proof of status is received. Foreign air speed delivery is included in all Clinics subscription prices. All prices are subject to change without notice. POSTMASTER: Send address changes to PET Clinics, Elsevier Health Sciences Division, Subscription Customer Service, 3251 Riverport Lane, Maryland Heights, MO 63043. **Customer Service: 1-800-654-2452 (U.S. and Canada); 314-447-8871 (outside U.S. and Canada). Fax: 314-447-8029. E-mail: journalscustomerservice-usa@elsevier.com (for print support); journalsonlinesupport-usa@elsevier.com (for online support).**

Reprints. For copies of 100 or more of articles in this publication, please contact the Commercial Reprints Department, Elsevier Inc., 360 Park Avenue South, New York, NY 10010-1710. Tel.: 212-633-3874; Fax: 212-633-3820; E-mail: reprints@elsevier.com.

PET Clinics is covered in MEDLINE/PubMed (Index Medicus).

Contributors

CONSULTING EDITOR

ABASS ALAVI, MD, MD (Hon), PhD (Hon), DSc (Hon)
Professor of Radiology, Division of Nuclear Medicine, Department of Radiology, Hospital of the University of Pennsylvania, University of Pennsylvania Perelman School of Medicine, Philadelphia, Pennsylvania, USA

EDITORS

BABAK SABOURY, MD, MPH, DABR, DABNM
Chief Clinical Data Science Officer, Oncoradiologist and Nuclear Medicine Physician, Director-Center for Precision Dosimetry and Radiopharmaceutical Treatment Planning, Department of Radiology and Imaging Sciences, Clinical Center, National Institutes of Health, Bethesda, Maryland, USA; Adjunct Professor, Department of Computer Science and Electrical Engineering, University of Maryland Baltimore County, Baltimore, Maryland, USA; Department of Radiology, Hospital of the University of Pennsylvania, Philadelphia, Pennsylvania, USA

ARMAN RAHMIM, PhD, DABSNM
Professor, Departments of Radiology and Physics, University of British Columbia, Senior Scientist and Provincial Medical Imaging Physicist, BC Cancer, BC Cancer Research Institute, Vancouver, British Columbia, Canada

ELIOT SIEGEL, MD
Professor, Department of Radiology, University of Maryland School of Medicine, Baltimore, Maryland, USA

AUTHORS

ANA A. BAUMANN, PhD
Brown School of Social Work, Washington University in St. Louis, St Louis, Missouri, USA

BARRY A. SIEGEL, MD
Professor of Radiology, Division of Nuclear Medicine, Mallinckrodt Institute of Radiology, Alvin J. Siteman Cancer Center, Washington University School of Medicine, St Louis, Missouri, USA

JEAN-MATHIEU, BEAUREGARD, MD, MSc, FRCPC
Assistant Professor, Department of Radiology and Nuclear Medicine, Cancer Research Centre, Université Laval, Department of Medical Imaging, Research Center (Oncology Axis), CHU de Québec - Université Laval, Québec City, Quebec, Canada

PATRICK G. LYONS, MD, MSc
Department of Medicine, Division of Pulmonary and Critical Care Medicine, Washington University School of Medicine in St Louis, Healthcare Innovation Lab, BJC HealthCare, St Louis, Missouri, USA

SANGTAE AHN, PhD
Senior Engineer, GE Research, Niskayuna, New York, USA

TZU-AN SONG, MS
Graduate Student, Department of Electrical and Computer Engineering, University of Massachusetts Lowell, Lowell, Massachusetts, USA

EVREN ASMA, PhD
Manager, PET Image Reconstruction and Physics, Canon Medical Research, Vernon Hills, Illinois, USA

BAHAR ATAEINIA, MD, MPH
Department of Radiology, Massachusetts General Hospital, Boston, Massachusetts, USA

ANDREA G. BOTTINO, PhD
Associate Professor, Department of Computer and Control Engineering, Polytechnic University of Turin, Turin, Italy

TYLER J. BRADSHAW, PhD
Associate Scientist, Department of Radiology, University of Wisconsin-Madison, Madison, Wisconsin, USA

JULIA BROSCH-LENZ, PhD
Research Fellow, Department of Integrative Oncology, BC Cancer Research Institute, Vancouver, British Columbia, Canada

IRÈNE BUVAT, PhD
Institut Curie, Université PSL, Inserm, Orsay, France

ADAM CHANDLER, PhD
Lead Collaboration Scientist, Global Scientific Collaborations Group, United Imaging Healthcare, America, Houston, Texas, USA

SIMON R. CHERRY, PhD
Department of Biomedical Engineering, University of California, Davis, Davis, California, USA; Department of Radiology, UC Davis Medical Center, Sacramento, California, USA

JIANAN CUI, PhD
Department of Radiology, Center for Advanced Medical Computing and Analysis, Gordon Center for Medical Imaging, Massachusetts General Hospital, Harvard Medical School, Boston, Massachusetts, USA

JOYITA DUTTA, PhD
Associate Professor, Department of Electrical and Computer Engineering, University of Massachusetts Lowell, Lowell, Massachusetts, USA; Instructor, Radiology, Gordon Center for Medical Imaging, Massachusetts General Hospital, Harvard Medical School, Boston, Massachusetts, USA

VINCENT GAUDET, PhD, PEng
Professor, Department of Electrical and Computer Engineering, University of Waterloo, Waterloo, Ontario, Canada

KUANG GONG, PhD
Department of Radiology, Center for Advanced Medical Computing and Analysis, Gordon Center for Medical Imaging, Massachusetts General Hospital, Harvard Medical School, Boston, Massachusetts, USA

PEDRAM HEIDARI, MD
Department of Radiology, Massachusetts General Hospital, Boston, Massachusetts, USA

ALVIN IHSANI, PhD
Senior Software Systems Engineer, NVIDIA, Westford, Massachusetts, USA

ABHINAV K. JHA, PhD
Assistant Professor, Department of Biomedical Engineering, Mallinckrodt Institute of Radiology, Alvin J. Siteman Cancer Center, Washington University in St. Louis, St Louis, Missouri, USA

KYUNGSANG KIM, PhD
Department of Radiology, Center for Advanced Medical Computing and Analysis, Gordon Center for Medical Imaging, Massachusetts General Hospital, Harvard Medical School, Boston, Massachusetts, USA

IVAN KLYUZHIN, PhD
Department of Integrative Oncology, BC Cancer Research Institute, Department of Radiology, University of British Columbia, Vancouver, British Columbia, Canada

ELIZABETH LI
Department of Biomedical Engineering, University of California, Davis, California, USA

QUANZHENG LI, PhD
Associate Professor, Department of Radiology, Center for Advanced Medical Computing and Analysis, Gordon Center for Medical Imaging,

Massachusetts General Hospital, Harvard Medical School, Boston, Massachusetts, USA

CHI LIU, PhD
Associate Professor, Department of Radiology and Biomedical Imaging, Yale School of Medicine, New Haven, Connecticut, USA

JUAN LIU, PhD
Postdoctoral Associate, Department of Radiology and Biomedical Imaging, Yale School of Medicine, New Haven, Connecticut, USA

ZIPING LIU, BS
Department of Biomedical Engineering, Washington University in St. Louis, St Louis, Missouri, USA

MASOUD MALEKZADEH, MS
Graduate Student, Department of Electrical and Computer Engineering, University of Massachusetts Lowell, Lowell, Massachusetts, USA

ALAN B. McMILLAN, PhD
Associate Professor, Department of Radiology, University of Wisconsin-Madison, Madison, Wisconsin, USA

NILOUFAR MIRIAN, MSc
Graduate Student, Department of Radiology and Biomedical Imaging, Yale School of Medicine, New Haven, Connecticut, USA

KYLE J. MYERS, PhD
Senior Advisor, Division of Imaging, Diagnostics, and Software Reliability, Office of Science and Engineering Laboratories, Center for Devices and Radiological Health, Food and Drug Administration (FDA)

CHRISTOPHE NIOCHE, PhD
Institut Curie, Université PSL, Inserm, Orsay, France

REZA YOUSEFI NOORAIE, PhD, MD
Department of Public Health Sciences, University of Rochester School of Medicine and Dentistry, New York, New York, USA

NANCY A. OBUCHOWSKI, PhD
Quantitative Health Sciences, Cleveland Clinic Foundation, Cleveland, Ohio, USA

FANNY ORLHAC, PhD
Institut Curie, Université PSL, Inserm, Orsay, France

SVEN PREVRHAL, PhD
Senior Scientist, Philips Research Europe, Hamburg, Germany

MD ASHEQUR RAHMAN, BS
Department of Biomedical Engineering, Washington University in St. Louis, St Louis, Missouri, USA

ARMAN RAHMIM, PhD, DABSNM
Professor, Departments of Radiology and Physics, University of British Columbia, Senior Scientist and Provincial Medical Imaging Physicist, BC Cancer, BC Cancer Research Institute, Vancouver, British Columbia, Canada

BABAK SABOURY, MD, MPH, DABR, DABNM
Chief Clinical Data Science Officer, Oncoradiologist and Nuclear Medicine Physician, Director-Center for Precision Dosimetry and Radiopharmaceutical Treatment Planning, Department of Radiology and Imaging Sciences, Clinical Center, National Institutes of Health, Bethesda, Maryland, USA; Adjunct Professor, Department of Computer Science and Electrical Engineering, University of Maryland Baltimore County, Baltimore, Maryland, USA; Department of Radiology, Hospital of the University of Pennsylvania, Philadelphia, Pennsylvania, USA

PETER J.H. SCOTT, PhD
Department of Radiology, University of Michigan, Ann Arbor, Michigan, USA

ELIOT SIEGEL, MD
Professor, Department of Radiology, University of Maryland School of Medicine, Baltimore, Maryland, USA

ARKADIUSZ SITEK, PhD
Director, Sano Centre for Computational Medicine, Kraków, Poland

KRIS THIELEMANS, PhD
Professor, Institute of Nuclear Medicine, UCL, Director, Algorithms and Software Consulting Ltd, London, United Kingdom

AMIRHOSEIN TOOSI, PhD
Post-Doc Research Fellow, Department of
Integrative Oncology, BC Cancer Research
Institute, Vancouver, British Columbia, Canada

CARLOS URIBE, PhD, MCCPM
Medical Imaging Physicist, Department of
Functional Imaging, BC Cancer, Department of
Radiology, University of British Columbia,
Vancouver, British Columbia, Canada

GUOBAO WANG, PhD
Department of Radiology, University of
California, Davis Medical Center, Sacramento,
California, USA

YIRAN WANG
Department of Biomedical Engineering,
University of California, Davis, Davis,
California, USA; Department of Radiology,
University of California, Davis Medical Center,
Sacramento, California, USA

E. WILLIAM WEBB, PhD
Department of Radiology, University of
Michigan, Ann Arbor, Michigan, USA

DUFAN WU, PhD
Department of Radiology, Center for Advanced
Medical Computing and Analysis, Gordon
Center for Medical Imaging, Massachusetts
General Hospital, Harvard Medical School,
Boston, Massachusetts, USA

FERESHTEH YOUSEFIRIZI, PhD
Post-Doctoral Fellow, Department of
Integrative Oncology, BC Cancer Research
Institute, Vancouver, British Columbia, Canada

**KATHERINE ZUKOTYNSKI, MD, PhD,
FRCPC**
Associate Professor, Department of Medicine
and Radiology, McMaster University, Hamilton,
Ontario, Canada

Contents

Artificial intelligence has witnessed exponential growth in the past decade. Advances in computing power and the design of sophisticated artificial intelligence algorithms have enabled computers to outperform humans in a variety of tasks. Yet, artificial intelligence's path has never been smooth, having essentially fallen apart twice in its lifetime after periods of popular success. We provide a brief rundown of artificial intelligence's evolution, highlighting its crucial moments and major turning points from inception to the present. In doing so, we attempt to learn, anticipate the future, and discuss what steps may be taken to prevent another winter.

Artificial intelligence (AI) has seen an explosion in interest within nuclear medicine. This interest is driven by the rapid progress and eye-catching achievements of machine learning algorithms. The growing foothold of AI in molecular imaging is exposing nuclear medicine personnel to new technology and terminology. Clinicians and researchers can be easily overwhelmed by numerous architectures and algorithms that have been published. This article dissects the backbone of most AI algorithms: the convolutional neural network. The algorithm training workflow and the key ingredients and operations of a convolutional neural network are described in detail. Finally, the ubiquitous U-Net is explained step-by-step.

Artificial intelligence (AI) has significant potential to positively impact and advance medical imaging, including positron emission tomography (PET) imaging applications. AI has the ability to enhance and optimize all aspects of the PET imaging chain from patient scheduling, patient setup, protocoling, data acquisition, detector signal processing, reconstruction, image processing, and interpretation. AI poses industry-specific challenges which will need to be addressed and overcome to maximize the future potentials of AI in PET. This article provides an overview of these industry-specific challenges for the development, standardization, commercialization, and clinical adoption of AI and explores the potential enhancements to PET imaging brought on by AI in the near future. In particular, the combination of on-demand image reconstruction, AI, and custom-designed data-processing workflows may open new possibilities for innovation which would positively impact the industry and ultimately patients.

> Artificial intelligence-based methods are showing promise in medical imaging applications. There is substantial interest in clinical translation of these methods, requiring that they be evaluated rigorously. We lay out a framework for objective task-based evaluation of artificial intelligence methods. We provide a list of available tools to conduct this evaluation. We outline the important role of physicians in conducting these evaluation studies. The examples in this article are proposed in the context of PET scans with a focus on evaluating neural network-based methods. However, the framework is also applicable to evaluate other medical imaging modalities and other types of artificial intelligence methods.

> Novel diagnostic and therapeutic radiopharmaceuticals are increasingly becoming a central part of personalized medicine. Continued innovation in the development of new radiopharmaceuticals is key to sustained growth and advancement of precision medicine. Artificial intelligence has been used in multiple fields of medicine to develop and validate better tools for patient diagnosis and therapy, including in radiopharmaceutical design. In this review, we first discuss common in silico approaches and focus on their usefulness and challenges in radiopharmaceutical development. Next, we discuss the practical applications of in silico modeling in design of radiopharmaceuticals in various diseases.

> Artificial intelligence and machine learning are poised to disrupt PET imaging from bench to clinic. In this perspective, the authors offer insights into how the technology could be applied to improve the radiosynthesis of new radiopharmaceuticals for PET imaging, including identification of an optimal labeling approach as well as strategies for radiolabeling reaction optimization.

> PET can provide functional images revealing physiologic processes in vivo. The precision of PET imaging is compromised by physical degradation factors as well as scan-time and dose limits. The collected raw data are transformed to PET images through image reconstruction, which is an essential step for PET. The early image reconstruction methods are analytical approaches based on idealized mathematical models. Iterative approaches were developed to consider physical factors during image reconstruction. Nowadays, deep learning methods have injected new vitality into PET image reconstruction. In this article, we provide a review of the evolution of image reconstruction in PET.

Recent developments in artificial intelligence (AI) technology have enabled new developments that can improve attenuation and scatter correction in PET and single-photon emission computed tomography (SPECT). These technologies will enable the use of accurate and quantitative imaging without the need to acquire a computed tomography image, greatly expanding the capability of PET/MR imaging, PET-only, and SPECT-only scanners. The use of AI to aid in scatter correction will lead to improvements in image reconstruction speed, and improve patient throughput. This article outlines the use of these new tools, surveys contemporary implementation, and discusses their limitations.

High noise and low spatial resolution are two key confounding factors that limit the qualitative and quantitative accuracy of PET images. Artificial intelligence models for image denoising and deblurring are becoming increasingly popular for the postreconstruction enhancement of PET images. We present a detailed review of recent efforts for artificial intelligence-based PET image enhancement with a focus on network architectures, data types, loss functions, and evaluation metrics. We also highlight emerging areas in this field that are quickly gaining popularity, identify barriers to large-scale adoption of artificial intelligence models for PET image enhancement, and discuss future directions.

Artificial intelligence (AI) techniques for image-based segmentation have garnered much attention in recent years. Convolutional neural networks have shown impressive results and potential toward fully automated segmentation in medical imaging, and particularly PET imaging. To cope with the limited access to annotated data needed in supervised AI methods, given tedious and prone-to-error manual delineations, semi-supervised and unsupervised AI techniques have also been explored for segmentation of tumors or normal organs in single- and bimodality scans. This work reviews existing AI techniques for segmentation tasks and the evaluation criteria for translational AI-based segmentation efforts toward routine adoption in clinical workflows.

Radiomics has undergone considerable development in recent years. In PET imaging, very promising results concerning the ability of handcrafted features to predict the biological characteristics of lesions and to assess patient prognosis or response to treatment have been reported in the literature. This article presents a checklist for designing a reliable radiomic study, gives an overview of the steps of the pipeline, and outlines approaches for data harmonization. Tips are provided for critical reading of the content of articles. The advantages and limitations of handcrafted radiomics compared with deep-learning approaches for the characterization of PET images are also discussed.

The uEXPLORER total-body PET/CT system provides a very high level of detection sensitivity and simultaneous coverage of the entire body for dynamic imaging for quantification of tracer kinetics. This article describes the fundamentals and potential benefits of total-body kinetic modeling and parametric imaging focusing on the noninvasive derivation of blood input function, multiparametric imaging, and high-temporal resolution kinetic modeling. Along with its attractive properties, total-body kinetic modeling also brings significant challenges, such as the large scale of total-body dynamic PET data, the need for organ and tissue appropriate input functions and kinetic models, and total-body motion correction. These challenges, and the opportunities using deep learning, are discussed.

We highlight emerging uses of artificial intelligence (AI) in the field of theranostics, focusing on its significant potential to enable routine and reliable personalization of radiopharmaceutical therapies (RPTs). Personalized RPTs require patient-specific dosimetry calculations accompanying therapy. Additionally we discuss the potential to exploit biological information from diagnostic and therapeutic molecular images to derive biomarkers for absorbed dose and outcome prediction; toward personalization of therapies. We try to motivate the nuclear medicine community to expand and align efforts into making routine and reliable personalization of RPTs a reality.

Artificial intelligence (AI) has been rapidly adopted in various health care domains. Molecular imaging, accordingly, has demonstrated growing academic and commercial interest in AI. Unprepared and inequitable implementation and scale-up of AI in health care may pose challenges. Implementation of AI, as a complex intervention, may face various barriers, at individual, interindividual, organizational, health system, and community levels. To address these barriers, recommendations have been developed to consider health equity as a critical lens to sensitize implementation, engage stakeholders in implementation and evaluation, recognize and incorporate the iterative nature of implementation, and integrate equity and implementation in early-stage AI research.

PET CLINICS

SERIES OF RELATED INTEREST

Advances in Clinical Radiology
Available at: Advancesinclinicalradiology.com
MRI Clinics of North America
Available at: MRI.theclinics.com
Neuroimaging Clinics of North America
Available at: Neuroimaging.theclinics.com
Radiologic Clinics of North America
Available at: Radiologic.theclinics.com

THE CLINICS ARE AVAILABLE ONLINE!
Access your subscription at:
www.theclinics.com

PET CLINICS

PROGRAM OBJECTIVE
The goal of the *PET Clinics* is to keep practicing radiologists and radiology residents up to date with current clinical practice in positron emission tomography by providing timely articles reviewing the state of the art in patient care.

TARGET AUDIENCE
Practicing radiologists, radiology residents, and other health care professionals who provide patient care utilizing radiologic findings.

LEARNING OBJECTIVES
Upon completion of this activity, participants will be able to:
1. Review existing AI techniques and potentials uses for PET imaging.
2. Discuss the benefits and challenges of total-body kinetic modeling.
3. Recognize how AI technology could be applied to improve the design and synthesis of new radiopharmaceuticals for PET imaging.

ACCREDITATION
The Elsevier Office of Continuing Medical Education (EOCME) is accredited by the Accreditation Council for Continuing Medical Education (ACCME) to provide continuing medical education for physicians.

The EOCME designates this journal-based CME activity for a maximum of 14 *AMA PRA Category 1 Credit*(s)™. Physicians should claim only the credit commensurate with the extent of their participation in the activity.

All other health care professionals requesting continuing education credit for this enduring material will be issued a certificate of participation.

DISCLOSURE OF CONFLICTS OF INTEREST
The EOCME assesses conflict of interest with its instructors, faculty, planners, and other individuals who are in a position to control the content of CME activities. All relevant conflicts of interest that are identified are thoroughly vetted by EOCME for fair balance, scientific objectivity, and patient care recommendations. EOCME is committed to providing its learners with CME activities that promote improvements or quality in healthcare and not a specific proprietary business or a commercial interest.

The planning committee, staff, authors, and editors listed below have identified no financial relationships or relationships to products or devices they or their spouse/life partner have with commercial interest related to the content of this CME activity:
Bahar Ataeinia, MD, MPH; Ana A. Baumann, PhD; Jean-Mathieu Beauregard, MD, MSc, FRCPC; Andrea G. Bottino, PhD; Julia Brosch-Lenz, MSc; Irène Buvat, PhD; Regina Chavous-Gibson, MSN, RN; Jianan Cui, PhD; Joyita Dutta, PhD; Vincent Gaudet, PhD, Peng; Kuang Gong, PhD; Pedram Heidari, MD; Abhinav K. Jha, PhD; Kyungsang Kim, PhD; Ivan Klyuzhin, PhD; Quanzheng Li, PhD; Chi Liu, PhD; Juan Liu, PhD; Ziping Liu, BS; Patrick G. Lyons, MD, MSc; Masoud Malekzadeh, MS; Niloufar Mirian, MSc; Kyle J. Myers, PhD; Christophe Nioche, PhD; Reza Yousefi Nooraie, PhD, MD; Nancy A. Obuchowski, PhD; Fanny Orlhac, PhD; Md Ashequr Rahman, BS; Arman Rahmim, PhD, DABSNM; Babak Saboury, MD, MPH, DABR, DABNM; Peter J.H. Scott, PhD; Eliot Siegel, MD; Barry A. Siegel, MD; Arkadiusz Sitek, PhD; Tzu-An Song, MS; Reni Thomas; Amirhosein Toosi, PhD; Carlos Uribe, PhD, MCCPM; John Vassallo; Vignesh Viswanathan; E. William Webb, PhD; Dufan Wu, PhD; Fereshteh Yousefirizi, PhD; Katherine Zukotynski, MD, PhD, FRCPC

The planning committee, staff, authors, and editors listed below have identified financial relationships or relationships to products or devices they or their spouse/life partner have with commercial interest related to the content of this CME activity:
Sangtae Ahn, PhD: Employment: GE Healthcare

Evren Asma, PhD: Employment: Canon Medical Research USA, Inc.

Tyler J. Bradshaw, PhD: Research Support: GE Healthcare

Adam Chandler, PhD: Employment: United Imaging Healthcare Co., Ltd.

Simon R. Cherry, PhD: Research Support: United Imaging Healthcare Co., Ltd.

Alvin Ihsani, PhD: Emplyment: NVIDIA Corporation

Elizabeth Li: Research Support: United Imaging Healthcare Co., Ltd.

Alan B. McMillan, PhD: Research Support: GE Healthcare

Sven Prevrhal, PhD: Employment: Philips

Kris Thielemans, PhD: Owner: Algorithms and Software Consulting Ltd

Yiran Wang: Research Support: United Imaging Healthcare Co., Ltd.

Guobao Wang, PhD: Research Support: United Imaging Healthcare Co., Ltd.

UNAPPROVED/OFF-LABEL USE DISCLOSURE

The EOCME requires CME faculty to disclose to the participants:

1. When products or procedures being discussed are off-label, unlabelled, experimental, and/or investigational (not US Food and Drug Administration [FDA] approved); and

2. Any limitations on the information presented, such as data that are preliminary or that represent ongoing research, interim analyses, and/or unsupported opinions. Faculty may discuss information about pharmaceutical agents that is outside of FDA-approved labelling. This information is intended solely for CME and is not intended to promote off-label use of these medications. If you have any questions, contact the medical affairs department of the manufacturer for the most recent pre-scribing information.

TO ENROLL

To enroll in the *PET Clinics* Continuing Medical Education program, call customer service at 1-800-654-2452 or sign up online at http://www.theclinics.com/home/cme. The CME program is available to subscribers for an additional annual fee of USD 254.00

METHOD OF PARTICIPATION

In order to claim credit, participants must complete the following:

1. Complete enrolment as indicated above.

2. Read the activity.

3. Complete the CME Test and Evaluation. Participants must achieve a score of 70% on the test. All CME Tests and Evaluations must be completed online.

CME INQUIRIES/SPECIAL NEEDS

For all CME inquiries or special needs, please contact elsevierCME@elsevier.com.

Preface
PET and AI Trajectories Finally Coming into Alignment

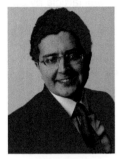

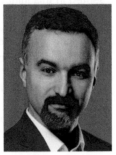

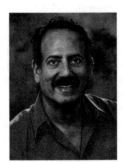

Babak Saboury, MD, MPH, DABR, DABNM

Arman Rahmim, PhD, DABSNM

Eliot Siegel, MD

Editors

As two of the "hottest" and rapidly evolving areas of research and development in medicine, both with tremendous future potential and accelerating clinical applications in patient care, PET and AI (Artificial Intelligence) have been on a collision path for the past several years, but only recently have these fields begun to form a synergistic partnership. This first issue and a subsequent second issue in *PET Clinics* are planned to make up for lost time in the medical literature and address the emerging opportunities, challenges, and practical clinical implications of AI for PET. Like PET, the basic technologies underlying AI have existed for decades but have only recently been made practical by advances in hardware, specifically, the utilization of graphics-processing units during the past decade. These were applied with tremendous success to a challenge in computer vision resulting in a major leap forward that has enabled a new era of practical applications in image and speech recognition, near autonomous self-driving cars, language translation, advanced predictive modeling in a wide variety of disciplines, and high-profile success in board games, such as Chess and Go, Poker, and a variety of video games, all of which were previously thought to be within the sole domain of humans. The term AI has become synonymous with deep learning or convolutional neural networks within the past several years, while it continues to be also used in its original definition as the use of computer systems using algorithms to perform tasks that typically require human intelligence. The use of deep learning represents a fundamental paradigm shift from previous approaches in the detection and diagnosis of disease, as these algorithms are generated directly from large, annotated data sets without requiring the many handcrafted, painstaking steps typically required in the development of computer-aided detection and diagnosis algorithms. This generation of "computer code" directly from the data represents a means of rapidly turning large PET annotated data sets into a wide variety of different potentially useful clinically useful tools.

A variety of medical AI applications have recently emerged, most notably in medical imaging, such as detection of early signs of stroke on computed tomographic (CT) scans, assessment of delays in pediatric bone development, detection and assessment of lung nodules, and hundreds of other applications. Ironically, despite the early and successful adoption of computerized techniques and analytics in nuclear medicine, deep learning (AI) advances have focused much more on mammography, CT, MR imaging, and conventional radiography. This may in large part be due to greater availability to computer scientists and other AI researchers of large public databases with those modalities and relatively sparse availability of readily accessible nuclear medicine data sets. As an inherently multimodality imaging specialty, PET/CT offers an intriguing, inherent breadth of data from the combination of pixel data representing electron density (and in some cases dynamic contrast enhancement) with

PET Clin 16 (2021) xv–xvi
https://doi.org/10.1016/j.cpet.2021.07.003
1556-8598/21/© 2021 Published by Elsevier Inc.

molecular activity, which can be assessed at a single or multiple time points. While CT scans have served as a common source of data for deep learning, neither PET-only images nor CT plus PET have been as widely utilized for AI applications (though there is a significant upward trend which this special issue covers).

The first issue of this special AI issue (consisting of 14 articles) has a technical focus, spanning the wide range of steps and aspects wherein AI can have significant presence. It will first delve into the history as well as "anatomy and physiology" underpinnings of AI (articles by Toosi and colleagues; Bradshaw and McMillan). AI has profound potential for in silico radiopharmaceutical development (article by Ataeinia and Heidari) as well as radiochemistry and radiochemical engineering (article by Webb and Scott). One of the fascinating things about deep learning is the ability to use it not only to analyze images but also to generate images using a sample database, enabling its application in image reconstruction, which is perhaps a "killer application" at the present time, offering the potential for decreased imaging times and patient doses and improved image quality (article by Gong and colleagues). In addition, AI application in improved attenuation and scatter correction (article by McMillan and Bradshaw), postreconstruction image enhancement (noise reduction and/or resolution enhancement; article by Liu and colleagues), and high-throughput segmentation (eg, tumors or normal organs; article by Yousefirizi and colleagues) are covered. Furthermore, both handcrafted and deep radiomics methods and applications have been on the rise (article by Orlhac and colleagues). An innovative application of AI is in total body kinetic modeling (article by Wang and colleagues). Similarly, AI has potential in refining and optimizing personalized radiopharmaceutical therapies (Theranostics; article by Brosch-Lenz and colleagues). Techniques for objectively evaluating AI-based imaging methods and for implementing them equitably using evidence-based practice are also discussed in two of the articles

in this issue (articles by Jha and colleagues; Nooraie and colleagues). In addition to the technology being explored and discussed from a research and clinical practice perspective, the industry perspective which is, of course, critically important to practical implementation, is presented in this initial issue as well (article by Sitek and colleagues).

We wish to especially acknowledge the members of the SNMMI AI task force who both directly, through their contributions to this issue, and indirectly, through their insightful discussions, played a major role in crafting this two-part series.

Babak Saboury, MD, MPH, DABR, DABNM
Department of Radiology and Imaging Sciences
Clinical Center
National Institutes of Health (NIH)
9000 Rockville Pike
Bethesda, MD 20892, USA

Department of Radiology
Hospital of the University of Pennsylvania

Department of Computer Science & Electrical
Engineering
University of Maryland, Baltimore County

Arman Rahmim, PhD, DABSNM
Departments of Radiology and Physics
University of British Columbia
BC Cancer Research Institute
675 West 10th Avenue
Office 6-112
Vancouver, BC V5Z 1L3, Canada

Eliot Siegel, MD
Department of Radiology
University of Maryland School of Medicine
655 West Baltimore Street
Baltimore, MD 21201, USA

E-mail addresses:
babak.saboury@nih.gov (B. Saboury)
arman.rahmim@ubc.ca (A. Rahmim)
esiegel@umaryland.edu (E. Siegel)

A Brief History of AI: How to Prevent Another Winter (A Critical Review)

Amirhosein Toosi, PhD[a],*, Andrea G. Bottino, PhD[b],
Babak Saboury, MD, MPH, DABR, DABNM[c,d,e], Eliot Siegel, MD[f],
Arman Rahmim, PhD, DABSNM[g,h]

KEYWORDS

- Artificial intelligence • Machine learning • Deep learning • Artificial neural networks • Perceptron

KEY POINTS

- The area of artificial intelligence (AI), regarded as one of the most mystifying fields of science, has seen exponential growth in the last decade, with a remarkably wide range of applications that have already influenced our daily lives.
- Computers may already surpass humans in a variety of tasks thanks to the advancements in processing power and the development of advanced AI algorithms, specifically in the areas of computer vision and speech recognition.
- However, the path of AI has never been smooth, having nearly come apart twice in its lifetime ('winters' of AI), both following periods of popular glory ('summers' of AI).
- We provide a condensed rundown of AI's evolution across decades, highlighting key moments and crucial turning points from its inception to the present.
- By doing so, we attempt to learn, foresee the future, and explore possible preventative action to avoid another 'winter'.

INTRODUCTION

Artificial intelligence (AI) technology is sweeping the globe, leading to bold statements by notable figures: "[AI] is going to change the world more than anything in the history of mankind,"[1] "it is more profound than even electricity or fire",[2] and "just as electricity transformed almost everything 100 years ago, today I actually have a hard time thinking of an industry that I don't think AI will transform in the next several years."[3] Every few weeks there is news about AI breakthroughs. Deep-fake videos are becoming harder and harder to tell apart from real ones.[4,5] Intelligent algorithms are beating humans in a greater variety of games more easily. For the first time in history, in arguably the most complex board game (named "Go"), DeepMind's AlphaGo has beaten the world champion.

[a] Department of Integrative Oncology, BC Cancer Research Institute, 675 West 10th Avenue, Vancouver, British Columbia V5Z 1L3, Canada; [b] Department of Computer and Control Eng., Polytechnic University of Turin, Corso Duca degli Abruzzi, 24, Turin 10129, Italy; [c] Department of Radiology and Imaging Sciences, Clinical Center, National Institutes of Health, 9000 Rockville Pike, Bethesda, MD 20892, USA; [d] Department of Computer Science and Electrical Engineering, University of Maryland Baltimore County, Baltimore, MD, USA; [e] Department of Radiology, Hospital of the University of Pennsylvania, 3400 Spruce St, Philadelphia, PA 19104, USA; [f] Department of Radiology, University of Maryland School of Medicine, 655 W. Baltimore Street, Baltimore, MD 21201, USA; [g] Department of Radiology, University of British Columbia, Senior Scientist & Provincial Medical Imaging Physicist, BC Cancer, BC Cancer Research Institute, 675 West 10th Avenue, Office 6-112, Vancouver, British Columbia V5Z 1L3, Canada; [h] Department of Physics, University of British Columbia, Senior Scientist & Provincial Medical Imaging Physicist, BC Cancer, BC Cancer Research Institute, 675 West 10th Avenue, Office 6-112, Vancouver, British Columbia V5Z 1L3, Canada
* Corresponding author.
E-mail address: atoosi@bccrc.ca

PET Clin 16 (2021) 449–469
https://doi.org/10.1016/j.cpet.2021.07.001

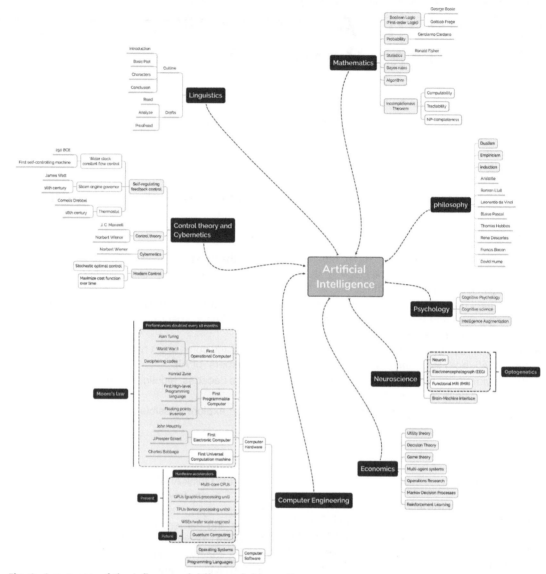

Fig. 1. A summary of the influence of different fields on AI.

AI has been around for decades, enduring "hot and cold" seasons and, like any other field in science, AI developments indeed stand on the shoulders of giants (**Fig. 1**). With these ideas in mind, this article aims to provide a picture of what AI essentially is and the story behind this rapidly evolving and globally engaged technology.

WHAT IS ARTIFICIAL INTELLIGENCE?

AI is "the theory and development of computer systems able to perform tasks normally requiring human intelligence, such as visual perception, speech recognition, decision-making, and translation between languages."[6] Marvin Minsky, an American mathematician, computer scientist,

and famous practitioner of AI defines AI as "the science of making machines do things that would require intelligence if done by men."[7] John McCarthy who coined the term "artificial intelligence" in 1956, described it as "the science and engineering of making intelligent machines. IBM suggests that "Artificial intelligence enables computers and machines to mimic the perception, problem-solving, and decision-making capabilities of the human mind."[8] McKinsey & Company explains it as a "machine's ability to mimic human cognitive functions, including perception, reasoning, learning, and problem-solving."[9]

Russel and Norvig[10] proposed 4 conceivable approaches to AI: acting humanly, thinking humanly, acting rationally, and thinking rationally

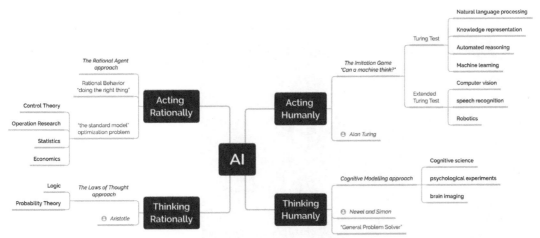

Fig. 2. Summary of 2-dimensional AI approaches as proposed by Russel and Norvig. (*Data from* Norvig, Peter, and Russell, Stuart. Artificial Intelligence: A Modern Approach, EBook, Global Edition. United Kingdom, Pearson Education, 2021.)

(Fig. 2). The British mathematician Alan Turing published an article in 1950 ("Computers and intelligence"[11]) in which he proposed a tool to determine the difference between a task performed by a person and a machine. This test, known as the Turing test, consists of a series of questions to be answered. A computer can pass the test if a human interrogator cannot tell whether the answers to the questions come from a person or a computer. As such, to pass the test, the computer is required to have a number of essential capabilities such as:

- Natural language processing, to manage a natural and effective communication with human beings;
- Knowledge representation, to store the information it receives;

- Automated reasoning, to perform question answering and update the conclusion; and
- Machine learning, to adjust to new situations and recognize new patterns.

In Turing's view, a physical simulation of a human is totally irrelevant to demonstrate intelligence. Other researchers, however, have suggested a complete Turing test[12–14] that involves interaction with real-world objects and people. Hence, the machine should be equipped with 2 additional (and vital) capabilities to pass the "extended" version of the Turing test:

- Computer vision and speech recognition, to see and hear the environment; and
- Robotics, to move around and interact with the environment.[15]

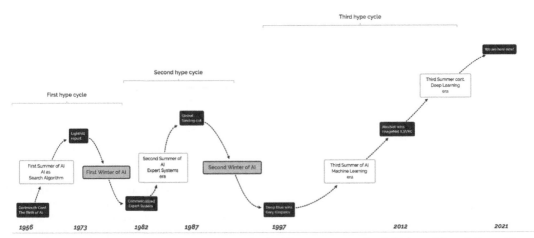

Fig. 3. Dividing the history of AI into 3 recurring cycles (public excitements/time). (*Adapted from* T. Noguchi et al., "A practical use of expert system "AI-Q" focused on creating training data," 2018 5th International Conference on Business and Industrial Research (ICBIR), 2018, pp. 73-76; With permission. (Figure 1 in original).)

A

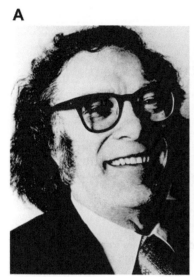

B

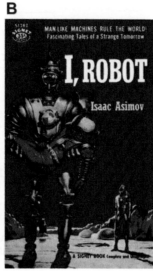

Fig. 4. (*A*) Isaac Asimov, the well-known sci-fi writer. (*B*) I, Robot, Asimov's sci-fi book series.[22]

HISTORY OF ARTIFICIAL INTELLIGENCE

The field of AI has experienced extreme ascends and descends over the last 7 decades. These recurring ridges of great promise and valleys of disappointment referred to as AI's summers and winters, have divided the history of AI into 3 distinct cycles (**Fig. 3**). These different cycles and seasons will be discussed in this article.

Prehistoric Events

When science fiction writer Isaac Asimov wrote his timeless book *I, Robot* in 1942, he likely did not imagine that this work, 80 years later, would become a primary source for defining the laws governing human–robot interactions in modern AI ethics. Although Asimov's novels (**Fig. 4**) are often considered as the birthplace of the ideas of intelligent machines,[16] McCulloch and Pitts' article, "A Logical Calculus of the Ideas Immanent in Nervous Activity" published in 1943,[17] was the first step toward the implementation of AI.[18–21]

Based on Alan Turing's "On Computable Numbers,[23]" their model provided a way to describe brain functions abstractly and demonstrated that simple elements connected in a neural network can have enormous computational power. The article received little attention until John von Neumann, Norbert Wiener, and others applied its concepts. The "McCulloch–Pitts" neuron, was the first mathematical model of an artificial neural network. This model, inspired by the basic physiology and function of the brain's neurons, showed that essentially any computable function could be

modeled as a connected network of such neurons.[15] Based on this work, 6 years later, Donald Hebb proposed a simple learning rule to tune the strength of the neuron connections.[24] His learning method, namely, Hebbian learning,[25] is considered as the inspiring model for neural networks learning.

Building on these works, 1 year later, in the summer of 1950, 2 Harvard undergrad students, Marvin Minsky and Dean Edmonds, built the first analog neural net machine called SNARC.[26] SNARC stands for "stochastic neural-analog reinforcement calculator" and was based on a network of 40 interconnected artificial hardware neurons built using 3000 vacuum tubes and the remains of a B-24 bomber's automatic pilot mechanism. SNARC was successfully applied to find the way out from a maze (**Fig. 5**).

AI developed significantly from the studies of Alan Turing (**Fig. 6**) during his short life, considered in all respects as one of the fathers of AI. Although Turing owes much of his fame to the work he did at the Bletchley Park center to decode German communications during World War II, his remarkable work toward the theory of computation dates back to his article published when he was only 24.[23] Turing demonstrated that his universal computing machine could perform any imaginable mathematical computation if it could be represented as an algorithm. John von Neumann stated that Turing's article laid the groundwork for the central concept of modern computers. A few years later, in 1950, in his article entitled "Computing machinery and intelligence,"[11] Turing raised the fundamental question of "Can a machine think?"

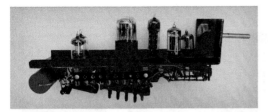

Fig. 5. One node of 40 nodes constructing the stochastic neural–analog reinforcement calculator (SNARC).[27]

The imitation game or the Turing test evaluates the ability of a machine to think. In this test, a human was asked to distinguish between a machine's written answers and those of a human (see **Fig. 6**). A machine is considered as being intelligent if the human interrogator could not tell if the answer is given by a human or a machine.[28]

Before the term AI was coined, many works were pursued that were later recognized as AI, including 2 checkers-playing games, developed almost at the same time by Arthur Samuel at IBM and Christopher Strachey at the University of Manchester in 1952.

The First Summer of Artificial Intelligence

The term AI was coined around 6 years after Turing's article,[11] in the summer of 1956, when John McCarthy, Marvin Minsky, Claude Shannon, and Nathaniel Rochester gathered common interest in automata theory, neural networks, and cognitive science (a 2-month workshop at Dartmouth College). There, the term artificial intelligence was coined by McCarthy. McCarthy defined AI as "the science and engineering of making intelligent machines," emphasizing the parallel growth between computers and AI. The conference is sometimes referred to as the birthplace

of AI, because it coordinated and energized the field,[15] and this time is considered as the beginning of an era called the first summer of AI.

One of the consequent results of the Dartmouth Conference was the work of Newell and Simon. They presented a mathematics-based system for proving symbolic logic theories, called the logic theorist, along with a list processing language for writing them called an information processing language.[29] Soon after the conference, their program was able to prove most of theorems (38 out of 52 of them) in the second chapter of Whitehead & Russell's *Principia Mathematica*. In fact, the program was able to give a solution for one of the theorems that was shorter than the one in the text. Newell and Simon later released their general problem solver, which was designed to mimic the problem-solving protocols of the human brain.[30] The general problem solver is counted as the first work in the reasoning humanly framework of AI.

Using reinforcement learning, Arthur Samuel's 1956 checker player quickly learned to play at an intermediate level, better than its own developer.[31] Reinforcement learning is a type of AI algorithm where an AI agent learns how to interact with its surrounding environment to achieve its goal through a reward-based system. He demonstrated his checker player program on television, making a great impression.[32] His work is considered to be the first reinforcement learning-based AI program, and indeed the forefather of later systems such as TD-GAMMON in 1992, one of the world's best backgammon players,[33] and AlphaGo in 2016, which shocked the world by defeating the human world champion of Go.[34] A turning point in AI, and specifically in neural networks, occurred in 1957 when the psychologist researcher Frank Rosenblatt (considered a father of deep learning[35]) built the Mark I Perceptron at

A   **B**

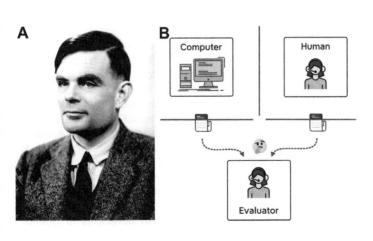

Fig. 6. (*A*) Alan Turing. (*B*) Schematic of the Turing test (the imitation game).

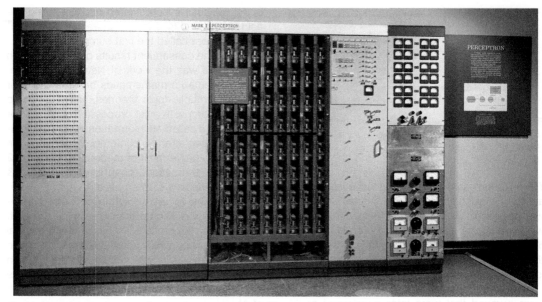

Fig. 7. Mark I Perceptron at the Smithsonian museum.[38]

Cornell.[36] He built an analog neural network with the ability to learn through trial and error. More precisely, the perceptron was a single-layer neural network being able to classify the input data into 2 potential categories. The neural network produces a prediction, say left or right, and if it is incorrect, it attempts to get more accurate the next time. Accuracy increases with each iteration. A 5-ton IBM 704 computer the size of a room was fed by a large stack of punch cards (**Fig. 7**). The computer learned to identify cards on the left and cards on the right in 50 attempts. Mark I Perceptron is considered as one of the forefathers of modern neural networks.[37]

In 1958, John McCarthy introduced the AI-specific programming language named LISP, which became the prevailing AI programming language for the next 3 decades. In his article entitled "Programs with Common Sense," he proposed a conceptual approach for AI systems based on knowledge representation and reasoning.[39] LISP is the first high-level AI programming language. In addition, 1958 is an important year because the first experimental work involving evolutionary algorithms in AI[40] was conducted by Freidberg toward automatic programming.[41] Nathaniel Rochester and Herbert Gelernter of IBM developed a geometry theorem–proving program in 1959. Their AI-based program called the "geometry machine" was able to provide proofs for geometry theorems, which many math students had found quite tricky.[42] Written in FORTRAN, their geometry machine program

is regarded as one of the first AI programs that could perform a task as well as a human. Another important event during the early 1960s is the emergence of the first industrial robot. Named "Unimate," the robotic arm was used on an assembly line in General Motors in 1961 for welding and other metalworks.[43]

In 1962, Widrow and Frank Rosenblatt revisited Hebb's learning method. Widrow enhanced the Hebbian learning method in his network called Adaline[44] and Rosenblatt in his well-known Perceptrons.[36] Marvin Minsky in 1963 proposed a simplification approach for AI use cases.[45] Marvin Minsky and Seymour Papert suggested that AI studies concentrate on designing programs capable of intelligent behavior in smaller artificial environments. The so-called blocks universe, which consists of colored blocks of different shapes and sizes arranged on a flat surface, has been the subject of many studies. The framework called Microworld became a backbone for subsequent works. Instances are James Slagle's SAINT program for solving closed-form calculus integration problems in 1963,[46] Tom Evans's ANALOGY in 1964 for solving an IQ test's geometric problems,[47] and the STUDENT program, written in LISP by Daniel Bobrow in 1967, for solving algebra problems.[48] ELIZA, the first chatbot in the history of AI, was developed by Joseph Weizenbaum at MIT in 1966. ELIZA was designed to serve as a virtual therapist to ask questions and provide follow-ups in response to the patient.[49] SHAKEY, the first omni-purpose mobile platform robot, was also developed at Stanford

Research Institute in 1966 with reasoning about its surrounding environment.[50]

The First Winter of Artificial Intelligence

The hype and high expectations caused by the media and the public from one side, and the false predictions and exaggerations by the experts in the field about their outcome from the other side, led to major funding cuts in AI research in the late 1960s. Governmental organizations like the Defense Advanced Research Projects Agency (DARPA) had already granted enormous funds for AI research projects during the 1960s. Two reports brought about major halts in supporting the research: the US government report, namely ALPAC in 1966,[51] and the Lighthill report of the British government in 1973.[52] These reports mainly targeted the research pursued in AI, mostly the research works done on artificial neural networks and came up with a grim prediction for the technology's prospects. As a result, both the US and the UK governments started to decrease support for AI research at universities. DARPA, which had previously funded various research projects in the 1960s, now needed specific timelines and concise explanations of each proposal's deliverables. These events slowed the advancement of AI and ushered in the first AI winter, which lasted until the 1980s.

It is crucial to recognize the 3 key factors that caused this major halt in AI research for that era. First, many early AI systems pursued the thinking humanly approach to solve the problems. In other words, instead of taking a bottom-up approach and starting from thoroughly analyzing the task, providing a possible solution, and turning it into an implementable algorithm, they took the opposite direction, merely relying on replicating the way humans perform the task. Second, there was a failure to recognize the complexity of many of the problems. Resulting from the oversimplification of the AI frameworks proposed by Marvin Minsky, most early problem solving systems succeeded mainly on toy (simplistic) problems, by combining simple steps to come up with a solution. However, many of the real-world problems that AI was attempting to solve were in fact intractable. It was commonly assumed that scaling up to bigger problems was merely a matter of faster hardware and greater memory capacity. However, developments in computational complexity theory proved it wrong. The third factor was related to the negative conceptions about neural networks and the limitations of their fundamental structures. In 1969, Minsky pointed out the limited representational abilities of a perceptron (to be exact, a single-layer perceptron cannot implement the classic XOR logical function) and, despite not being a general critique about neural networks, this factor also contributed to global funding cuts in neural networks research.

Expert Systems, the Revival of Artificial Intelligence, and the Second Summer

Mainstream AI research efforts during the previous 2 decades were generally based on so-called weak AI, that is, providing general solutions based on search algorithms in a space of all possible states built on basic reasoning steps. Despite being general purpose, these approaches suffered from a lack of scalability to larger or more complex domains. To address these drawbacks, in the early 1980s, researchers decided to take a more robust approach using domain-specific information for stronger reasoning but in narrower areas of expertise. The new approach, so-called expert systems, originated at Carnegie Mellon University and was quickly able to find its way to corporations. DENDRAL, created at Stanford by Ed Feigenbaum, Bruce Buchanan, and Joshua Lederberg in the late 1960s and early 1970s, and inferred molecular structure from mass spectrometry data, was an early success story. DENDRAL was the first effective knowledge-intensive system, relying on a vast range of special purpose laws, to provide expertise rather than basic knowledge.

In 1971 at Stanford University, Feigenbaum started the Heuristic Programming Project aimed at extending the area in which expert systems could be applied. The MYCIN system was one of the successful consequent results of the new wave, developed in the mid 1970s for the purpose of blood infection diagnosis by Edward Shortliffe under the supervision of Bruce Buchanan and Stanley Cohen. MYCIN could perform identification of bacteria causing sepsis and recommend antibiotics dosage based on patient weight. It could perform diagnosis on par with the human experts in the field, and significantly better than medical interns, benefiting from around 600 deduced rules in the form of a knowledge base, from extensive interviews with the experts, by means of integrating uncertainty calculations.[53] Meanwhile, one of the most important moves toward deep convolutional neural networks happened in 1980. The "neocognitron," the first convolutional neural network architecture, was proposed by Fukushima in 1980.[54] Several learning algorithms were suggested by Fukushima to train the parameters of a deep neocognitron so that it could learn internal representations of input data. This work is in fact regarded as the origin of today's deep convolutional neural networks.

R1, developed by McDermott in 1982, was the first successful commercial expert system used in the digital equipment industry, for the configuration of new computer systems' orders.[55] In nearly 4 years, the firm added $40 million of revenue using R1. By 1988, most corporations in the United States benefited from expert systems, either by being a user of the system or doing research in the field.[56] The application of expert systems to real-world problems resulted in the development of a wide range of representations and reasoning tools. The Prolog language gained popularity in Europe and Japan, whereas the PLANNER language family thrived more in the United States. In Japan, the government started a 10-year plan to keep up with the new wave by investing more than $1.3 billion in intelligent systems. The US government, by establishing the Microelectronics and Computer Technology Corporation in 1982, revived AI research in hardware, chip design, and software research. The same change happened in the UK as well, resulting in reassignment of funds previously cut. All these events during the 1980s led to a period of summer for AI. The AI industry thrived from billions of dollars invested in the field, and various activities emerged from expert systems developer companies to domain-specific hardware, computer vision, and robotic systems. Overall, the AI industry boomed from a few million dollars in 1980 to billions of dollars in the late 1980s, including hundreds of companies building expert systems, vision systems, robots, and software and hardware specialized for these purposes.

The Second Winter of Artificial Intelligence

Despite all efforts and investments made during the early 1980s, many companies could not fulfill their ambitious promises. Hardware manufacturers declined to keep up with the requirements of specialized needs of the expert systems. Hence, the thriving industry of expert systems in the early 1980s declined tremendously and inevitably collapsed by the end of the 1990s and the AI industry faced another winter that lasted until the mid 1990s. This second period of so-called winter in the history of AI had been so harsh that AI researchers subsequently tended to avoid even the term AI by choosing other titles such as informatics or analytics. Despite the big shutdown of AI-based research works, the second winter was the time when the very well-known backpropagation algorithm was revisited by many research groups.[57,58] Backpropagation, which is a primary learning mechanism for artificial neural networks, was vastly used in learning problems during these years and eventually led to a new wave of interest in neural networks. The lesson learned during the periods of AI's winter made researchers more conservative. As a result, during the late 1980s and the 1990s, the field of AI research witnessed a major conservative shift toward more established theories like statistics-based methods. Among these theories finding their way to the field were hidden Markov models.[59] Being strictly mathematics based and resulting from extensive training on large real-world datasets, hidden Markov models became a trustable framework for AI research, especially in handwriting recognition and speech processing, helping them to make their way back to the industry.

Another important outcome of this conservative shift in the field of AI was the development of public benchmark datasets and related competitions in its various subfields. Instances include the Letter Dataset,[60] Yale face database,[61] MNIST dataset,[62] Spambase Dataset,[63] ISOLET Dataset,[64] TIMIT,[65] JARtool experiment Dataset,[66] Solar Flare Dataset,[67] EEG Database,[68] Breast Cancer Wisconsin (Diagnostic) Dataset,[69] Lung Cancer Dataset,[70] Liver Disorders Dataset,[71] Thyroid Disease Dataset,[72] Abalone Dataset,[73] UCI Mushroom Dataset,[74] and other datasets that have been gathered during the 1990s. The availability of these public benchmarks became an important means for rigorous measurement of AI research advancements.

Man versus Machine

The gradual public interest in AI during the early 1990s opened doors to other emerging or established fields such as control theory, operational research, and statistics. Decision theory and probabilistic reasoning started being adopted by AI researchers. Uncertainty was represented more effectively by introducing Bayesian networks to the field.[75] Rich Sutton in 1998 revisited reinforcement learning after around 30 years by adopting Markov decision processes.[76] This step led to a growth in applying reinforcement learning on various problems, such as planning research, robotics, and process control. The vast amount of available data in different areas on the one hand, and the influences of statistical methods such as machine learning and optimization on AI research methods, on the other, resulted in significant readoption of AI in subfields, including multiagent models, natural language processing, robotics, and computer vision. As such, new hopes for AI shaped again in the early 1990s. Eventually, in 1997, AI-equipped machines showed off their power against Man to the public.[77] Chess-playing AI software developed in IBM, called Deep Blue, eventually won over the great maestro chess world champion, Garry Kasparov. Broadcasted live, Deep Blue captured the public's imagination once again toward AI systems of the future. The news was so breathtaking that IBM's share values rose up to all-time highs.[78]

Information Age: Enter Big Data

Massive advances in microchip manufacturing technologies in the late 1990s led to emerging powerful computers, concurrent to the growth of the global Internet that generated massive amounts of data. This information included enormous unprocessed text, video, voice, and images, along with semiprocessed data such as geographic tracking, social media-related data, and electronic medical records, ushering in the era of big data.[79] In the computer vision area in 2009, the ImageNet dataset was created gathering millions of labeled images, significantly contributing to the field.[80] There was a new beginning of wide interests in AI from the industry. Notable steps were taken in 2011 when IBM's Watson defeated human champions in the highly popular TV quiz show *Jeopardy*,[81] significantly boosting public impression of the state-of-the-art in AI, and with the introduction of Apple's Siri intelligent assistant.

Return of Neural Networks

In 1989, Yann LeCun revisited convolutional neural networks and, using gradient descend in their training mechanism, demonstrated the ability to perform well in computer vision problems, specifically in handwritten digit recognition.[82] Yet, it was in 2012 that these networks came to the forefront. A deep convolutional neural network developed in Geoffrey Hinton's research group at the University of Toronto surpassed the ImageNet Large Scale Visual Recognition Challenge (ILSVRC) competitors by significantly enhancing all ImageNet classification benchmarks.[83] Before the use of deep neural networks, all best-performing methods were mostly so-called classical machine learning methods using hand-crafted features. By 2011, the computing power of graphics processing units had grown enough to help the researchers train deep networks with higher dimensions both in terms of width and depth in a shorter time. Since the earlier implementation of Convolutional Neural Networks on graphics processing units in 2006,[84] which resulted in 4 times faster performance compared with central processing units, Schmidhuber's team at IDSIA could achieve a 60 times

faster performance on graphics processing units in 2011.[85] Meanwhile, the availability of huge amounts of labeled data such as millions of labeled images in the ImageNet dataset helped researchers to overcome the problem of overfitting. Eventually, in 2012 Hinton's team proposed a deep convolutional neural network architecture, named AlexNet (after the team's leading author Alex Krizhevsky), which was able to train more layers of neurons. Using many mechanisms and techniques such as rectified linear unit activation functions and the dropout technique, AlexNet could achieve higher discriminative power in an end-to-end fashion, that is, to feed the network with merely the pure images of the dataset.[86] This event is regarded as the birth of the third boom in AI. Since then, deep learning-based methods have continued to achieve outstanding feats, including outperforming or performing on par with human experts in certain tasks. Instances include AI-related fields such as computer vision, natural language processing, medical image diagnosis,[87] and natural language translation. The progress of deep neural networks gained public attention in 2016 at the time when Deep Mind's AlphaGo beat the world champion of Go.[34] AI became again the target of the media, public, governments, industries, scholars, and investor's interests. Deep learning methods have nowadays entirely dominated AI-related research, creating entirely new lines of research and industries. In 2018, Yoshua Bengio, Geoffrey Hinton, and Yann LeCun won the Turing award for their pioneering efforts in deep learning. **Fig. 8** summarizes the timeline of AI from the time it was born up to now.

Where Do We Stand Now?

The previous section presented a brief story of AI's journey, with all its ups and downs over the decades. This journey has not been easy, with multiple waves and seasons. Specifically, AI has faced 2 main breakdowns (so-called winters) and 3 main breakthroughs (so-called AI summers or booms). Thanks to the convergence of parallel processing, higher memory capacity, and more massive data collection (eg, big data), AI has enjoyed a steady upward climb since the early 2020s. With all these pieces in place, much better algorithms have been developed, assisting this steady progression.

Computers are becoming faster. Computing power has continued to double nearly every 2 years (Moore's law). Advancements in technology occur 10 times faster, that is, what used to take years, now may happen in the course of weeks or even days.[88]

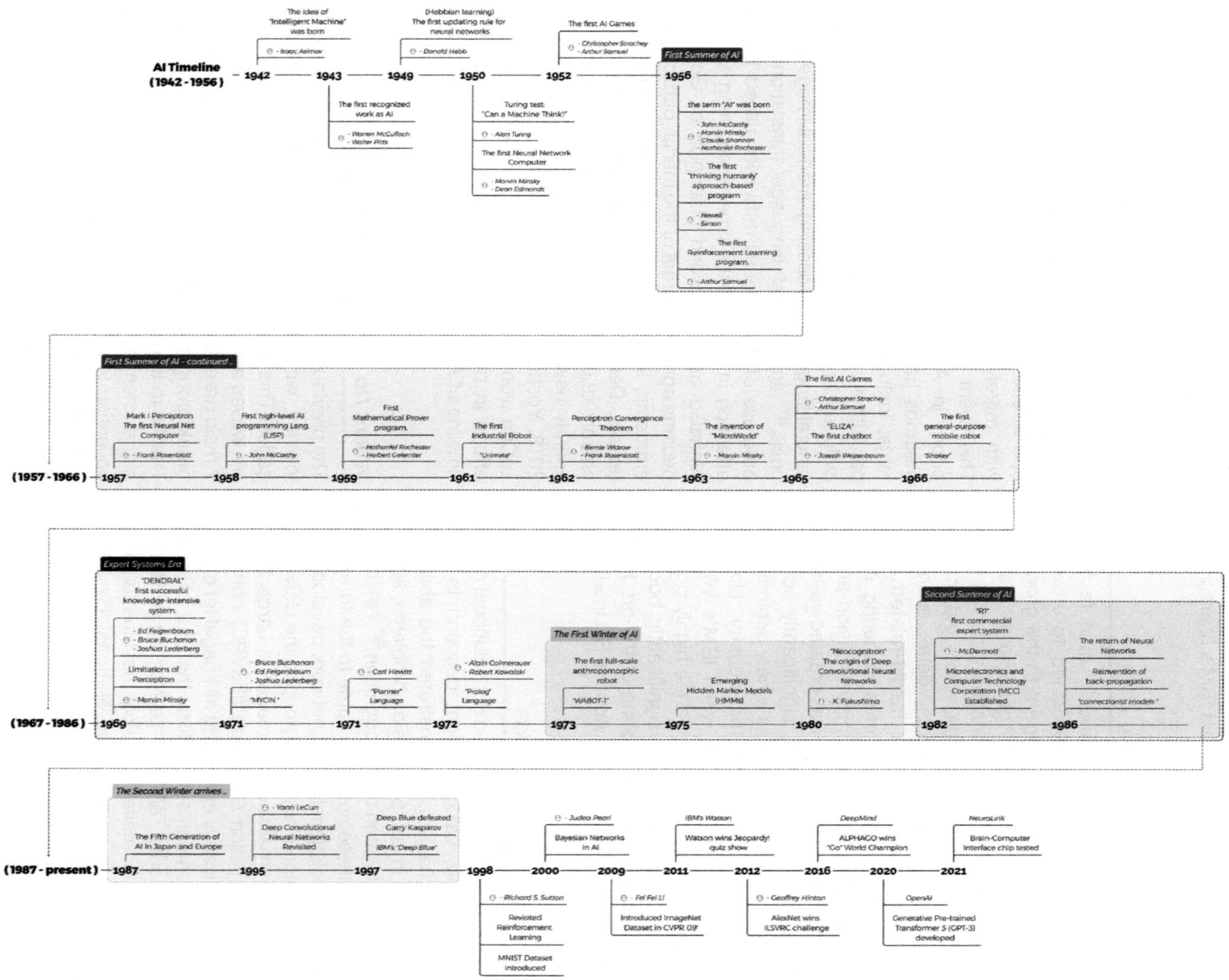

Fig. 8. The timeline of developments in AI.

On a global scale, AI is becoming an attractive target for investors, producing billions of dollars of profit per annum. From 2010 to 2020, global investment in AI-based startup companies has steadily grown from $1.3 billion to more than $40 billion, with an average annual growth rate of nearly 50%, whereas in 2020 only, corporate investment in AI is reported to be nearly $70 billion globally.[89]

In the academic sector, from 2000 up until 2020, the number of peer-reviewed AI articles per year has grown roughly 12 times worldwide. AI conferences have witnessed similar significant increases in terms of the number of attendants. In 2020, NeurIPS accepted 22,000 attendees, more than 40% growth over 2018, and 10-fold more compared with 2012.

Concurrently, AI has become the most popular specialization among computer science PhD students in North America, nearly 3 times the next rival (theory and algorithms).[90] In 2019, more than 22% of PhD candidates in computer science majored in AI and machine learning.

With the introduction of machine learning, the environment of the health care and biology sectors has changed dramatically. AlphaFold, developed by DeepMind, used deep learning to make a major advance in the decades-long biology problem of protein folding. Scientists use machine learning algorithms to learn representations of chemical molecules to plan more efficient chemical synthesis. ML-based approaches were used by PostEra, an AI startup, to speed up coronavirus disease 2019–related drug development during the pandemic.[90]

This progress suggests that we are in the midst of the next hype cycle. And this new hype is focused on applications with life-or-death implications, such as autonomous vehicles, medical applications, and so on, making it critical that AI algorithms be trustworthy.

The Future of Artificial Intelligence

Numerous AI-related startups have been founded in recent years, with both companies and governments investing heavily in the sector. If another AI winter occurs, many will lose their jobs, and many startups will be forced to close, as has occurred in the past. According to McKinsey & Company, the economic gap between an approaching winter period and continued prosperity by 2025 would be in the tens of billions of dollars.[9]

A recurrent pattern in previous AI winters has been the promises that sparked initial optimism yet turned out to be exaggerated. During both AI winters, budget cuts had a major effect on AI research. The Lighthill report resulted in funding cuts in the UK during the first AI winter, as well as cuts in Europe and the United States. DARPA support was cut, resulting in the second AI winter. Significant attention needs to be paid to technical challenges and limitations. Let us recall what was faced by the perceptron in the 1960s in being noted as unable to solve the so-called XOR problem, or limitations faced by expert systems in the 1980s. AI has appeared particularly vulnerable to overestimations coupled to technical limitations. Overall, the hype and fear that comes with reaching human-level intelligence have quickly contributed to exaggerations and public coverage that is not common in other innovative tech sectors. To avoid a next winter of AI, a number of important considerations may need to be made.

i. It is extremely important to be aware of philosophic arguments about the utter sublimeness of what it means to be human, and to not make exaggerated claims about ascension of AI systems to being human (see very illustrating documentary[91]). In addition, these philosophic arguments (eg, by Hubert Dreyfus based on the philosophy of Martin Heidegger), had they been more extensively and interactively considered, could have likely contributed to further success by AI in early years (eg, earlier attention to 'connectionist' approaches to AI).

ii. Neglects regarding above point, as well as exciting early successes, contribute to exaggerated claims that AI will solve any important problem soon. This is what happened that contributed to the first winter of AI, where AI researchers made overconfident and overoptimistic predictions about upcoming successes, given the early promising performances of AI on simpler examples.[92] A lack of appreciation for the computational complexity theory was another reason for AI scientists to believe that scaling up of simple solutions to larger tasks is just a matter of using faster hardware and larger memories.

iii. According to a recently released report,[93] 40% of startups established in Europe that claim to use AI in their provided services do not actually do so, largely because the definition of AI is ambiguous for the majority of the public and the media. Therefore, given recent excitement around AI and the resulting hype and investment growth in the field, some businesses try to benefit from this ambiguity by misusing terms such as AI, machine learning, and deep learning. Thus, it is crucial to define these terms more clearly with respect to other related concepts and define what they have in common and what they do not.

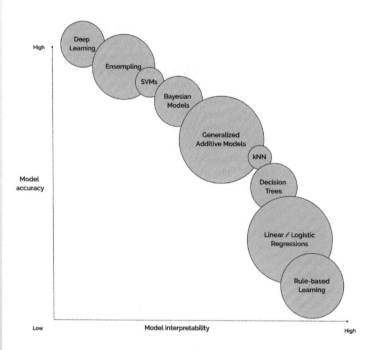

Fig. 9. Trade-off between interpretability and performance for AI models. kNN, k-nearest neighbor. (*Adapted from* Arrieta, Alejandro Barredo, et al. "Explainable Artificial Intelligence (XAI): Concepts, taxonomies, opportunities and challenges toward responsible AI." Information Fusion 58 (2020): 82-115. With permission. (Figure 12 in original).)

iv. There is significantly troubled trends in scientific methodology and dissemination by AI researchers, contributing to the hype and confusion: these trends include failure to distinguish between explanation and speculation, failure to identify real sources of performance gains, confusing/misleading use of math, and misuse of language.[94] According to a recent study[95] reviewing a spectrum of machine learning approaches for detecting and prognosticating coronavirus disease 2019 from standard-of-care chest radiographs and computed tomography images, none of the more than 400 studies were found suitable

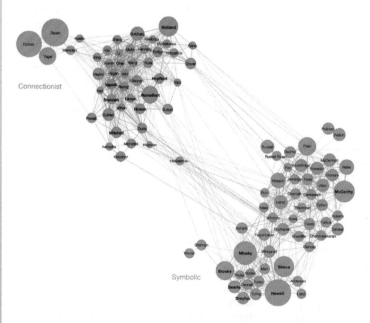

Fig. 10. Co-citation network of the 100 most cited authors with "artificial intelligence" in the title. The names of some important authors, clearly distributed by the community, are presented. At the heart of the connectionists, some core figures in deep learning appear. On the symbolic side, some core figures are laid out in a way that represents their proximities and divergences, surrounded by primary contributors to the construction of cognitive modeling, expert systems, and even those critical of symbolic AI (Dreyfus, Searle, Brooks). This figure is not comprehensive and misses some key contributors; it is intended to demonstrate existing dichotomies in connectionist and symbolic frameworks. (*From* Cardon, Dominique, Jean-Philippe Cointet, and Antoine Mazières. "Neurons spike back. The invention of inductive machines and the artificial intelligence controversy", Réseaux, vol. 211, no. 5, 2018, pp. 173-220. Available at: https://neurovenge.antonomase.fr/. Accessed May 18 2021; with permission.).)

for clinical application! The studies suffered from one or multiple issues including use of poor-quality data, poor application of machine learning methodology, poor reproducibility, and biases in study design.

v. AI, in its essence, is vague and covers a broad scope. As observed by Andrew Moore,[96] "Artificial intelligence is the science and engineering of making computers behave in ways that, until recently, we thought only human intelligence is able to perform." The critical point in this definition lies in the phrase "until recently," which points to the moving target of AI through time. In other words, ideas and methods are being referred to as AI as long as they have not been completely discovered. Once they are figured out, they may be no longer associated with AI and receive their own tag. This phenomenon is known as the AI effect,[97] which contributes to the fast decline in public excitement about groundbreaking achievements in AI.

vi. An important challenge with AI technologies, more specifically deep learning-based AI, is its so-called black box, opaque nature of decision-making. That is, when a deep learning algorithm makes a decision, the process of its inference or the logic behind it may not be representable. Although in some tasks such as playing board games, for example, "Go," where the objective is merely winning the game, this concern does not reveal itself, in critical tasks; for example, in health care, where a decision impacts humans lives, this issue can lead to trustworthiness challenges (other examples of critical tasks include transportation and mobility systems, and social or financial systems).

vii. One very specific concern is issue of bias. As an example, soon after Google introduced bidirectional encoder representations from transformers (BERT), one of the most sophisticated AI technologies in language models, scientists learned an essential flaw in that system. BERT and its peers (GPT-2, GPT-3, t5, etc) were more likely to equate males with computer programming and, in general, failed to give females adequate respect. BERT, which is now being used in critical services such as Google's Internet search engine, is one of a number of AI systems (so-called transformers) that learn from massive amounts of digitized data, such as old books, Wikipedia pages, tweets, forums, and news stories. The main problem with BERT or generative pretrained transformers (GPT-3), BERT's rival introduced by OpenAI, and similar universal language models is that they are too complex even for their own designers (GPT-3's full version has 175 billion parameters[98]); in fact, scientists are still learning how these models work. One certain fact about these systems is that they pick up biases as they learn through human-generated data. Because these mechanisms can be used in a variety of sensitive contexts to make critical and life-changing choices, it is critical to ensure that the decisions do not represent biased attitudes against particular communities or cultures. Thus, builders of AI systems have a duty to steer the design and use of AI in ways that serve society.

Overall, the future of AI seems to be promising. AI eventually will drive our automobiles, aid physicians in making more precise diagnoses, assist judges in making more consistent judgments, help employers in hiring more qualified applicants, and much more. We are aware, however, that these AI systems may be fragile and unjust. By adding graffiti to a stop sign, the classifier may believe it is no longer a stop sign. By adding subtle noise or signal to a benign skin lesion image, the classifier may be fooled into believing it is malignant (eg, adversarial attacks). Risk management instruments used in US courts have been shown to be racially discriminatory. Corporate recruitment tools have been shown to be sexist.

Toward trustworthy AI, organizations around the world are coming together to establish consistent standards for evaluating responsible implementation of AI systems and to encourage international support for AI technologies that benefit humanity and the environment. Among these tries is the European Commission's report on Ethics guidelines for trustworthy AI[99] and DARPA's XAI (eXplainable AI) roadmap.[100]

According to Arrieta and colleagues,[101] a trade-off between interpretability of AI models and their accuracy (performance) can be observed, given fair comparison conditions (**Fig. 9**). Simpler AI approaches, such as linear regression and decision trees, are self-explanatory (interpretable) because the classification decision border may be depicted in a few dimensions using model parameters. However, for tasks such as categorization of medical images in health care, these may lack the necessary complexity, yet to acquire the trust of physicians, regulators, and patients, a medical diagnostic system needs to be visible, intelligible, and explainable; it should be able to explain the logic of making a certain decision to stakeholders engaged in the process. Newer rules, such as the European General Data Protection Regulation, are making the use of black box models more difficult in different industries because retraceability of judgments is increasingly required. An AI system designed to assist professionals should be explainable and allow the human expert to retrace their steps and use their judgment. Some academics point out that humans are not always competent or willing to explain their choices. However, explainability is a fundamental enabler for AI deployment in the real world because it ensures that technology is used in a safe, ethical, fair, and trustworthy manner. Breaking AI misconceptions by demonstrating what a model primarily looked at while making a judgment can help end-users to trust the technology (eg, via use of heat maps/activation maps). For non–deep learning users, such as most medical professionals, it is even more vital to show such domain-specific attributes used in the decision.

For further enhanced AI, a way forward seems to be the convergence of symbolic and connectionist methods, which would incorporate the former's higher interpretability with the latter's significant recent success (more on these next). For instance, the use of hybrid distributional models, which combine sparse graph-based representations with dense vector representations and connect those to lexical tools and knowledge bases, appears to be promising toward explainable AI in the medical domain.[102] However, the main

Abbreviations List and Glossary	
Term	**Definition**
AAAI	The Association for the Advancement of AI, an international scientific society devoted to promoting research in, and responsible use of, AI.
Artificial intelligence (AI)	The study and development of computer systems capable of imitating intelligent human behaviour.
AI4ALL	AI4ALL is a not-for-profit organization dedicated to advancing diversity and inclusion in the field of AI.
AI Index Report	The AI Index is a public-facing annual study on the state of AI in all relevant fields.
AlphaFold	AlphaFold is a machine learning algorithm built by Google's DeepMind that predicts the structure of proteins.
Artificial neural networks (ANN)	A type of computer system that is, supposed to operate in a manner comparable with the human brain and nervous system.
Backpropagation	Most popular method for training feedforward neural networks.
Bayesian networks	A probabilistic graphical model that utilizes a directed acyclic graph (DAG) to describe a set of variables and their conditional dependencies.
BERT	Bidirectional Encoder Representations from Transformers (BERT) is a Google-developed machine learning methodology for pre-training in natural language processing (NLP).
Big data	A branch of study that focuses on methods for analyzing, extracting information from, or otherwise dealing with data volumes that are too vast or complicated for typical data-processing application software to handle.
Cognitive science	The scientific study of the mind and its processes on an interdisciplinary level.
Computer vision	Computer vision is an interdisciplinary scientific topic that examines how computers can extract

(continued on next page)

(continued)

Term	Definition
	information from digital images or video streams at a high degree of understanding.
Convolutional neural networks (CNN)	A type of feed-forward neural network that consists of a large number of convolutional layers stacked on top of one another. It is primarily used for computer vision tasks.
CVPR	The Conference on Computer Vision and Pattern Recognition (CVPR), is an annual conference on computer vision and pattern recognition.
Data science	An interdisciplinary field that uses scientific methods, procedures, algorithms, and systems to mine organized and unstructured data for information and insights.
Decision theory	The study of an agent's decisions is called decision theory. It is closely related to the discipline of game theory and is researched by economists, statisticians, data scientists, psychologists, biologists, social scientists, philosophers, and computer scientists.
Deep learning (DL)	An area of machine learning that focuses on algorithms inspired by the brain's structure and function.
Deep Mind	Deep Mind is an AI company and research laboratory of Alphabet Inc., based in the UK. It was created in September 2010 and was bought by Google in 2014.
Expert systems	A computer program that simulates the decision-making abilities of a human expert. It is supposed to handle difficult problems through the use of bodies of knowledge, which are mostly represented as if–then rules.
General problem solver (GPS)	A computer software designed in 1959 to act as a universal problem solver.
GPT-3	Generative Pre-trained Transformer 3 (GPT-3) is a deep learning-based autoregressive language model that generates human-like writing.
GPU	A graphics processing unit (GPU) is a specialized electronic circuit that is, capable of swiftly manipulating and altering memory to expedite the production of images in a frame buffer for output to a display device.
Hidden Markov model (HMM)	A type of Markov model in which the represented system is considered to be a Markov process.
ILSVRC	The ImageNet Large Scale Visual Recognition Challenge is an annual software competition in which participants compete to classify and recognize objects and scenes properly.
ImageNet	A big visual database that was created for the purpose of doing research on visual object recognition software.

(continued on next page)

(continued)

Term	Definition
Logical notation	Refers to a collection of symbols that are frequently used to convey logical representations.
Machine learning (ML)	A subset of AI in which computers learn how to do tasks through the use of massive amounts of data rather than being programmed.
Markov decision processes	A discrete-time stochastic control process that provides a mathematical framework for modeling decision-making in situations where outcomes are partly random and partly under control.
Microelectronics and Computer Technology Corporation (MCC)	One of the largest computer industry research and development consortia in the United States.
MNIST dataset	The Modified National Institute of Standards and Technology database (MNIST) is a massive collection of handwritten digits that is, frequently used to train image processing systems.
Moore's law	Moore's law is a historical observation and projection of a pattern in which the number of transistors in a dense integrated circuit doubles approximately every 2 years.
Natural language processing (NLP)	Series of methods for processing of natural languages, such as translating.
NeurIPS	NeurIPS, The Conference and Workshop on Neural Information Processing Systems, is an annual conference on machine learning and computational neuroscience held in December.
Perceptron	A supervised learning approach for binary classifiers in machine learning.
Reinforcement learning (RL)	A subfield of machine learning that studies how intelligent entities should behave to optimize the concept of cumulative reward.
ReLU (rectified linear unit)	The rectifier, or ReLU (Rectified Linear Unit), is an activation function whose positive portion is specified as the argument's positive component.
Speech recognition	Refers to the technology that enables computers to comprehend spoken language.
Strong AI	A machine described as being capable of applying intelligence to any challenge.
Turing test	A test of a machine's ability to demonstrate intelligent behavior that is, comparable to, or indistinguishable from, human behavior.
XOR function	A logical "exclusive OR" operator that returns TRUE if one of the logical propositions is true and FALSE if both statements are true. It also returns FALSE if neither of the statements is true.
Vanishing gradients	When backpropagation is used to train artificial neural networks, the gradient can become

(continued on next page)

Term	Definition
(continued)	
	vanishingly small in some situations, thereby preventing the weight from changing its value.
Weak AI	Used in contrast with "strong AI," which is described as a machine capable of applying intelligence to any problem, rather than just one specific problem.
WiML Workshop	The annual WiML Workshop is a technical event where women can share their machine learning research.
XAI	XAI is a type of AI in which the solution's outcomes are understandable by humans. It contrasts with the concept of the "black box" in machine learning, in which even the designers of the AI are unable to explain why it made a certain decision.

obstacle toward this solution is the historical division between these 2 paradigms.

The deep neural network approach is not novel. Today, it is fulfilling the promise stated at the beginning of cybernetics by benefitting from developments in computer processing and the existence of massive datasets. These techniques, however, have not always been deemed to constitute AI. Machine-learning approaches based on neural networks (connectionist AI) have been historically scorned and ostracized by the symbolic school of thinking. The rise of AI, which was clearly distinct from early cybernetics, amplified the friction between these 2 approaches. The cocitation network of the top-cited authors in articles mentioning AI demonstrates the drift between researchers who have used the symbolic or connectionist paradigms (**Fig. 10**).

Despite the obvious separation that existed among the intellectuals from these 2 schools, a third subfield of AI has been emerging, namely neuro-symbolic AI, which focuses on combining the neural and symbolic traditions in AI for additional benefit.[103] The promise of neuro-symbolic AI is largely based on the aim of achieving a best of both worlds scenario in which the complementary strengths of neural and symbolic techniques can be advantageously merged. On the neural side, desirable strengths include trainability from raw data and robustness against errors in the underlying data, whereas on the symbolic side, one would like to retain these systems' inherent high explainability and provable correctness, as well as the ease with which they can be designed and function using deep human expert knowledge. In terms of functional features, using symbolic approaches in conjunction with machine learning—particularly deep learning, which is currently the subject of the majority of research—one would hope to outperform systems that rely entirely on deep learning on issues such as out-of-vocabulary handling, generalizable training from small datasets, error recovery, and, in general, explainability.[103]

SUMMARY

Rapid developments in AI are changing different aspects of human life. Advances both in computational power and AI algorithm design have enabled AI methods to outperform humans in an increasing number of tasks. AI has experienced decades of praise and criticism; its path has never been smooth. With the 2 winters that the field has experienced, after 2 waves of great growth and high expectations, as well as the costs that the community of researchers, corporations, start-ups, and governments have paid, it is critical for us to recognize that the current wave of high hopes and high expectations should not be taken for granted.

DISCLOSURE

This work was in part supported by the Canadian Institutes of Health Research (CIHR) Project Grant PJT-162216. The authors also wish to acknowledge valuable feedback from Ian Janzen of BC Cancer Research Institute.

REFERENCES

1. Catherine Clifford. Kai Fu lee. 2019. Available at: https://www.cnbc.com/2019/01/14/the-oracle-of-ai-these-kinds-of-jobs-will-not-be-replaced-by-robots-.html. Accessed on February 13, 2021.
2. Catherine Clifford. Sundar Pichai. 2018. Available at: https://www.cnbc.com/2018/02/01/google-ceo-sundar-pichai-ai-is-more-important-than-fire-electricity.html. Accessed on April 28, 2021.
3. Lynch S. Andrew Ng: why AI is the new electricity. Insights by Stanford business. 2017;11. Available at: https://www.gsb.stanford.edu/insights/andrew-ng-why-ai-new-electricity. Accessed on April 27, 2021.
4. BBC news. Deepfake queen to deliver channel 4 Christmas message. BBC. 23 Dec 2020. Available at: https://www.bbc.com/news/technology-55424730. Accessed May 17, 2021.
5. Vincent J. Tom Cruise deepfake creator says public shouldn't be worried about 'one-click fakes.' In: the Verge [Internet]. 2021. Available at: https://www.theverge.com/2021/3/5/22314980/tom-cruise-deepfake-tiktok-videos-ai-impersonator-chris-ume-miles-fisher. Accessed May 25, 2021.
6. Oxford languages and Google - English. 20 may 2020. Available at: https://languages.oup.com/google-dictionary-en/. Accessed April 14, 2021.
7. Dennis MA. Marvin Minsky. Encyclopedia Britannica 2021. Available at: https://www.britannica.com/biography/Marvin-Lee-Minsky. Accessed on May 10, 2021.
8. IBM Cloud Education. What is artificial intelligence (AI)?. Available at: https://www.ibm.com/cloud/learn/what-is-artificial-intelligence. Accessed April 14, 2021.
9. Chui M, Harrysson M, Manyika J, et al. Applying AI for social good | Mc Kinsey et al. Available at: https://www.mckinsey.com/featured-insights/artificial-intelligence/applying-artificial-intelligence-for-social-good. Accessed on May 15, 2021.
10. Russell SJ, Norvig P. Artificial intelligence: a modern approach. Prentice Hall; 1995. p. 932.
11. Turing AM. I.—computing machinery and intelligence. Mind 1950;LIX:433–60.
12. Hernandez-Orallo J. Beyond the Turing test. J Log Lang Inf 2000;9:447–66.
13. Dowe DL, Hajek AR. A computational extension to the Turing Test. Proceedings of the 4th conference of the Australasian cognitive science society. NSW, Australia: University of Newcastle; 1997. Citeseer. Available at: https://citeseerx.ist.psu.edu/viewdoc/download?doi=10.1.1.133.4643&rep=rep1&type=pdf.
14. Hayes, Patrick, and Kenneth Ford. "Turing test considered harmful." In IJCAI (1), pp. 972-977. 1995.
15. Russell SJ (stuart J, Norvig P. Artificial Intelligence A Modern Approach - Fourth Edition. 2020.
16. Haenlein M, Kaplan A. A brief history of artificial intelligence: on the past, present, and future of artificial intelligence. Calif Manage Rev 2019;61:5–14.
17. McCulloch WS, Pitts W. A logical calculus of the ideas immanent in nervous activity. Bull Math Biophys 1943;5:115–33.
18. McCulloch & Pitts publish the first mathematical model of a neural network. Available at: https://www.historyofinformation.com/detail.php?entryid=782. Accessed June 7, 2021.
19. History of the perceptron. Available at: https://web.csulb.edu/~cwallis/artificialn/History.htm. Accessed June 7, 2021.
20. Neural networks - history. Available at: https://cs.stanford.edu/people/eroberts/courses/soco/projects/neural-networks/History/history1.html. Accessed June 7, 2021.
21. Piccinini G. The first computational theory of mind and brain: a close Look at Mcculloch and Pitts's "logical calculus of ideas immanent in nervous activity". Synthese. 2004;141:175–215.
22. Someday R. May save or destroy us all—for now, they're still kinda dumb. Available at: https://www.collectorsweekly.com/articles/robots-are-still-kinda-dumb/. Accessed April 29, 2021.
23. Turing AM. On computable numbers, with an application to the entscheidungsproblem. Proc Lond Math Soc 1937;s2-42:230–65.
24. Hebb DO. The organization of behavior; a neuropsychological theory. pdfs.semanticscholar.org. Available at: https://pdfs.semanticscholar.org/efee/3a0d3e8b34e45188dca4e19c15e6b6029edd.pdf%3C/eref. Accessed on April 15, 2021.
25. Song S, Miller KD, Abbott LF. Competitive Hebbian learning through spike-timing-dependent synaptic plasticity. Nat Neurosci 2000;3:919–26.
26. Bernstein J. Marvin Minsky's vision of the future. The new Yorker. 1981. Available at: https://www.newyorker.com/magazine/1981/12/14/a-i. Accessed May 17, 2021.
27. Akst J. Machine, learning, 1951. The scientist Magazine. 2019. https://www.the-scientist.com/foundations/machine–learning–1951-65792. Accessed April 25, 2021.
28. Singh P. A Must-Read history of artificial intelligence 2020. Available at: https://cyfuture.com/blog/history-of-artificial-intelligence/. Accessed on February 10, 2021.
29. Crevier D. Ai: The Tumultuous History Of The Search For Artificial Intelligence. Basic Books; 1993.
30. Newell A, Shaw JC, Simon HA. Report on a general problem solving program. Pittsburgh, PA: IFIP congress; 1959. p. 64.

31. Samuel AL. Some studies in machine learning using the game of checkers. IBM J Res Dev 2000; 44:206–26.

32. Bleakley C. Poems that solve puzzles: the history and science of algorithms. Oxford University Press; 2020. p. 86.

33. Tesauro G. Temporal difference learning and TD-Gammon. Commun ACM 1995;38:58–68.

34. Silver D, Huang A, Maddison CJ, et al. Mastering the game of Go with deep neural networks and tree search. Nature 2016;529: 484–9.

35. Tappert CC. Who Is the Father of Deep Learning? 2019 International Conference on Computational Science and Computational Intelligence (CSCI). ieeexplore.ieee.org; 2019. pp. 343–348.

36. Rosenblatt F. The perceptron, a perceiving and recognizing automaton Project Para. Cornell Aeronautical Laboratory; 1957.

37. Professor's perceptron paved the way for AI – 60 years too soon. Available at: https://news.cornell.edu/stories/2019/09/professors-perceptron-paved-way-ai-60-years-too-soon. Accessed April, 26 2021.

38. One-page Schoolhouse. Available at: https://ronkowitz.blogspot.com/2017/11/perceptron.html. Accessed April 29, 2021.

39. McCarthy J, Others. Programs with common sense. RLE and MIT computation center; 1960. Available at: http://jmc.stanford.edu/articles/mcc59.html. Accessed on April 18, 2021.

40. De Jong K, Fogel DB, Schwefel H-P. A2. 3 A history of evolutionary computation. A1 1 Introduction. Available at: http://citeseerx.ist.psu.edu/viewdoc/download?doi=10.1.1.375.6494&rep=rep1&type=pdf#page=28. Accessed on April 14, 2021.

41. Friedberg RM. A learning machine: part I. IBM J Res Dev 1958;2:2–13.

42. Gelernter H, Hansen JR, Loveland DW. Empirical explorations of the geometry theorem machine. Papers presented at the May 3-5, 1960, western joint IRE-AIEE-ACM computer conference. New York, NY, USA: Association for Computing Machinery; 1960. pp. 143–149.

43. Nof SY. Handbook of industrial robotics. John Wiley & Sons; 1999.

44. Widrow B, Others. Adaptive "adaline" Neuron Using Chemical "memistors." 1960.

45. Minsky M. Society of mind. Simon and Schuster; 1988.

46. Slagle JR. A Heuristic program that solves symbolic integration problems in Freshman calculus. J ACM 1963;10:507–20.

47. Evans TG. A heuristic program to solve geometric-analogy problems. Proceedings of the April 21-23, 1964, spring joint computer conference. New York, NY, USA: Association for Computing Machinery; 1964. pp. 327–338.

48. Mathematics Genealogy project. Available at: https://mathgenealogy.org/id.php?id=13379. Accessed May 4, 2021.

49. Salecha M. Story of ELIZA, the first chatbot developed in 1966. 5 Oct 2016. Available at: https://analyticsindiamag.com/story-eliza-first-chatbot-developed-1966/. Accessed April 26, 2021.

50. Shakey. Available at: http://www.ai.sri.com/shakey/. Accessed May 4, 2021.

51. Hutchins J. ALPAC: the (in) famous report. Readings in Machine Translation 2003;14:131–5.

52. Lighthill report. Available at: http://www.chilton-computing.org.uk/inf/literature/reports/lighthill_report/p001.htm. Accessed May 3, 2021.

53. Shortliffe EH, Buchanan BG. A model of inexact reasoning in medicine. Math Biosci 1975;23:351–79.

54. Fukushima K. Neocognitron: a self-organizing neural network model for a mechanism of pattern recognition unaffected by shift in position. Biol Cybern 1980;36:193–202.

55. McDermott J. R1: a rule-based configurer of computer systems. Artif Intell 1982;19:39–88.

56. Olsen K, Anderson H. Digital equipment corporation. First People; 1983. p. 25. Available at: https://microsoft.fandom.com/wiki/Digital_Equipment_Corporation.

57. Rumelhart DE, Hinton GE, Williams RJ. Learning representations by back-propagating errors. Nature 1986;323:533–6.

58. Ian G, Yoshua B, Aaron C. Deep learning. MIT Press; 2016.

59. Baum LE, Petrie T. Statistical inference for Probabilistic functions of finite state Markov chains. aoms 1966;37:1554–63.

60. Frey PW, Slate DJ. Letter recognition using Holland-style adaptive classifiers. Mach Learn 1991;6:161–82.

61. Georghiades A, Belhumeur P, Kriegman D. Yale face database, vol. 2. Center for computational Vision and Control at Yale University; 1997. p. 33. Available at: http://cvc.cs.yale.edu/cvc/projects/yalefaces/yalefaces.html. Accessed on 21 May, 2021.

62. Lecun Y, Bottou L, Bengio Y, et al. Gradient-based learning applied to document recognition. Proc IEEE 1998;86:2278–324.

63. Dimitrakakis C, Bengio S. Online policy adaptation for ensemble algorithms. IDIAP; 2002. Available at: https://infoscience.epfl.ch/record/82788/files/rr02-28.pdf.

64. Fanty M, Cole R. Spoken letter recognition. Adv Neural Inf Process Syst 1990;3:220–6.

65. Zue V, Seneff S, Glass J. Speech database development at MIT: Timit and beyond. Speech Commun 1990;9:351–6.

66. Pettengill GH, Ford PG, Johnson WT, et al. Magellan: radar performance and data products. Science 1991;252:260–5.

67. Li J, Dong G, Ramamohanarao K, et al. DeEPs: a new instance-based lazy discovery and classification system. Mach Learn 2004;54:99–124.

68. Ingber L. Statistical mechanics of neocortical interactions: canonical momenta indicators of electroencephalography. Phys Rev E 1997;55: 4578–93.

69. Nick Street W, Wolberg WH, Mangasarian OL. Nuclear feature extraction for breast tumor diagnosis. Biomedical Image Processing and Biomedical Visualization. International Society for Optics and Photonics; 1993. p. 861–70.

70. Hong Z-Q, Yang J-Y. Optimal discriminant plane for a small number of samples and design method of classifier on the plane. Pattern Recognit 1991;24: 317–24.

71. Bagirov AM, Rubinov AM, Soukhoroukova NV, et al. Unsupervised and supervised data classification via nonsmooth and global optimization. TOP 2003;11:1–75.

72. Quinlan JR, Compton PJ, Horn KA, Lazarus L. Inductive knowledge acquisition: a case study. Proceedings of the Second Australian Conference on Applications of expert systems. USA: Addison-Wesley Longman Publishing Co., Inc.; 1987. pp. 137–156.

73. Clark D, Schreter Z, Adams A. A quantitative comparison of dystal and backpropagation. Australian conference on neural networks. 1996.

74. Iba W, Wogulis J, Langley P. Trading off Simplicity and coverage in Incremental concept learning. In: Laird J, editor. Machine learning Proceedings 1988. San Francisco (CA): Morgan Kaufmann; 1988. p. 73–9.

75. Pearl J. Causality. Cambridge University Press; 2009.

76. Sutton & Barto book: reinforcement learning: an introduction. Available at: http://incompleteideas. net/book/first/the-book.html. Accessed May 3, 2021.

77. Weber B. Computer Defeats Kasparov, Stunning the chess experts. The New York Times; 5 May 1997. Available at: https://www.nytimes.com/1997/05/05/ nyregion/computer-defeats-kasparov-stunning-the-chess-experts.html. Accessed May 3, 2021.

78. Higgins C. A brief history of deep Blue, IBM's chess computer. 29 Jul 2017. Available at: https:// www.mentalfloss.com/article/503178/brief-history-deep-blue-ibms-chess-computer. Accessed May 3, 2021.

79. Morris MA, Saboury B, Burkett B, et al. Reinventing Radiology: big data and the future of medical imaging. J Thorac Imaging 2018;33:4–16.

80. Gershgorn D. The data that transformed AI research—and possibly the world. In: Quartz [Internet]. 26 Jul 2017. Available at: https://qz.com/ 1034972/the-data-that-changed-the-direction-of-ai-research-and-possibly-the-world/. Accessed May 4, 2021.

81. Gabbatt A. IBM computer Watson wins Jeopardy clash. The Guardian 2011. Available at: http://www. theguardian.com/technology/2011/feb/17/ibm-computer-watson-wins-jeopardy. Accessed May 16, 2021.

82. LeCun Y, Boser B, Denker JS, et al. Back-propagation applied to handwritten zip code recognition. Neural. 1989. Available at: https:// www.mitpressjournals.org/doi/abs/10.1162/neco. 1989.1.4.541. Accessed on May 27, 2021.

83. ImageNet large scale visual recognition competition 2012 (ILSVRC2012). Available at: https://image-net. org/challenges/LSVRC/2012/results.html. Accessed May 4, 2021.

84. Chellapilla K, Puri S, Simard P. High performance convolutional neural networks for document processing. Tenth International Workshop on Frontiers in Handwriting Recognition. Suvisoft; 2006. Available at: https://hal.inria.fr/inria-00112631/. Accessed on May 27, 2021.

85. Ciresan DC, Meier U, Masci J, et al. Flexible, high performance convolutional neural networks for image classification. Twenty-second international joint conference on artificial intelligence. people.idsia.ch; 2011. Available at: http://people.idsia.ch/~juergen/ ijcai2011.pdf. Accessed on May 27, 2021.

86. Krizhevsky A, Sutskever I, Hinton GE. Imagenet classification with deep convolutional neural networks. Adv Neural Inf Process Syst 2012;25:1097–105.

87. Liu X, Faes L, Kale AU, et al. A comparison of deep learning performance against health-care professionals in detecting diseases from medical imaging: a systematic review and meta-analysis. Lancet Digit Health 2019;1:e271–97.

88. Manson M. I, for one, welcome our AI overlords. Mark Manson; 2016. Available at: https:// markmanson.net/artificial-intelligence. Accessed April 14, 2021.

89. Perrault R, Shoham Y, Brynjolfsson E, et al. The AI Index 2019 annual report. Stanford, CA: AI Index Steering Committee, Human-Centered AI Institute, Stanford University; 2019. Available at: https://hai. stanford.edu/research/ai-index-2019.

90. 2021-AI-Index-Report_Master.pdf. Available at: https://aiindex.stanford.edu/wp-content/uploads/ 2021/03/2021-AI-Index-Report_Master.pdf. Accessed on June 29, 2021.

91. Ruspoli T. Being in the world - on the subject of the #Heideggerian Dasein. Alive mind Cinema; 15 Apr 2018. Available at: https://www.youtube.com/ watch?v=dlFsZ9uTrpE. Accessed June 25, 2021.

92. Taylor T. When machines that think, learn, and create Arrived 1957. Available at: https://www.bbntimes. com/global-economy/1957-when-machines-that-

think-learn-and-create-arrived. Accessed June 29, 2021.

93. Vincent J. Forty percent of 'AI startups' in Europe don't actually use AI, claims report 2019. Available at: https://www.theverge.com/2019/3/5/18251326/ai-startups-europe-fake-40-percent-mmc-report. Accessed April 17, 2021.

94. Lipton ZC, Steinhardt J. Troubling trends in machine learning scholarship. arXiv [stat.ML]. 2018. Available at: http://arxiv.org/abs/1807.03341. Accessed on May 27, 2021.

95. Roberts M, Driggs D, Thorpe M, et al. Common pitfalls and recommendations for using machine learning to detect and prognosticate for COVID-19 using chest radiographs and CT scans. Nat Machine Intelligence 2021;3:199–217.

96. Contributor IW-B. What machine learning can and cannot do. In: WSJ online [internet]. 27 Jul 2018. Available at: https://www.wsj.com/articles/what-machine-learning-can-and-cannot-do-1532714166?tesla=y. Accessed April 18, 2021.

97. AI set to exceed human brain power. CNN. Available at: http://edition.cnn.com/2006/TECH/science/07/24/ai.bostrom/. Accessed April 29, 2021.

98. Brown TB, Mann B, Ryder N, et al. Language models are few-Shot Learners. arXiv [cs.CL]. 2020. Available at: http://arxiv.org/abs/2005.14165. Accessed on May 28, 2021.

99. Floridi L. Establishing the rules for building trustworthy AI. Nat Machine Intelligence 2019;1: 261–2.

100. Gunning D, Aha D. DARPA's explainable artificial intelligence (XAI) program. AI Mag 2019;40: 44–58.

101. Barredo Arrieta A, Díaz-Rodríguez N, Del Ser J, et al. Explainable Artificial Intelligence (XAI): concepts, taxonomies, opportunities and challenges toward responsible AI. Inf Fusion 2020;58:82–115.

102. Gunning D. Explainable artificial intelligence (xai). Defense advanced research projects agency (DARPA), nd Web. 2017;2. Available at: http://www.cc.gatech.edu/~alanwags/DLAI2016/(Gunning)%20IJCAI-16%20DLAI%20WS.pdf. Accessed on June 18, 2021.

103. Sarker K, Zhou L, Eberhart A, Hitzler P. Neuro-symbolic artificial intelligence: current trends. arXiv e-prints. 2021; arXiv:2105.05330.

Anatomy and Physiology of Artificial Intelligence in PET Imaging

Tyler J. Bradshaw, PhD*, Alan B. McMillan, PhD

KEYWORDS

- Artificial intelligence • Machine learning • Nuclear medicine • PET • Neural network

KEY POINTS

- Modern artificial intelligence algorithms are built on the foundation of a traditional artificial neural network.
- The key components of a simple convolutional neural network are the convolution layer, pooling operation, fully connected layer, and output layer.
- The U-Net is a widely used network for image segmentation and image synthesis.

INTRODUCTION

Artificial intelligence (AI) has seen an explosion in interest within nuclear medicine.[1] This interest has been driven by the rapid progress and eye-catching achievements of machine learning (ML) algorithms over the past decade. AI, and in particular computer vision, is now receiving attention from many outside of computer science, hoping to apply the promising technologies within their own field of study. Nuclear medicine, like many other medical specialties, is poised to benefit from AI in several ways.[2–4] However, newcomers to ML may be overwhelmed by the nearly limitless acronyms, network architectures, and publications claiming "state-of-the-art performance," all of which is challenging for beginners to navigate.

This article provides an illustrated guide to foundational concepts in AI. Given the breadth of AI, this article focuses on topics and networks that are most relevant to PET imaging. There are many classes of AI algorithms, many of which are beyond the scope of this article. For example, there are supervised learning algorithms that are trained using datasets with paired inputs and labels, and unsupervised learning algorithms that learn relationships using unlabeled data (eg, clustering). Algorithms can also be classified based on application, such as computer vision algorithms that are applied to images, and natural language processing algorithms that are applied to text. Algorithms are further classified according to the structure and function of the network, such as artificial neural networks, decision forests, support vector machines, transformers, and so forth. Algorithms are designed with certain structures (anatomy) and functions (physiology) so that they are capable of handling specific tasks (eg, image classification). This article focuses on supervised learning algorithms that process images, with a specific focus on convolutional neural networks (CNN), because these are currently the most relevant algorithms to PET imaging. The target audience is nontechnical, future consumers of AI algorithms in nuclear medicine who wish to better understand this emerging technology. We aim to convey a high level conceptual understanding of AI, whereas readers interested in a deeper treatment of its mathematical underpinnings are referred to other publications.[5–7]

The article is organized as follows. First, we provide an overview of the pipeline for AI algorithm development. We then give a step-by-step survey of the components and operations of AI

Department of Radiology, University of Wisconsin, 3252 Clinical Science Center, 600 Highland Avenue, Madison, WI 53792, USA
* Corresponding author.
E-mail address: tbradshaw@wisc.edu
Twitter: @tybradshaw11 (T.J.B.); @alan_b_mcmillan (A.B.M.)

PET Clin 16 (2021) 471–482
https://doi.org/10.1016/j.cpet.2021.06.003

algorithms, particularly the basic CNN, which is the principal ingredient of most modern computer vision algorithms. We then describe the process of model training. Finally, we explain the components of the widely used U-Net architecture, which is arguably the most widely used CNN in the medical imaging community.[8]

STEPS OF ALGORITHM DEVELOPMENT

There is a common pipeline used when developing ML algorithms. Understanding the development life cycle of an ML algorithm is important for placing promising studies or newly Food and Drug Administration–cleared AI software in proper context. The steps of the pipeline begin once an investigator has a clearly defined task that they would like to perform (which can itself be a challenge). The task is a prediction task: given some input data, the model predicts the expected output. To build the prediction model, investigators then collect data, label data, build the network, train the model, evaluate the model, and deploy the model. This pipeline is shown in **Fig. 1**.

Each step of the pipeline is deserving of its own in-depth treatment. Indeed, many review and educational articles have been dedicated to the individual steps.[9–11] When developers take shortcuts or fail to follow best practices anywhere along the pipeline, they risk seeing their algorithms fail during evaluation or postdeployment.[12] Most of the important terms and concepts of ML algorithm development are beyond the scope of this article; however, many of them are listed in **Fig. 1** and readers are encouraged to explore them further. Also, a glossary of terms used in this article is found in **Table 1**.

Data collection and labeling are arguably the most critical but time-consuming steps of building an ML model. If the dataset does not reflect the clinical task (eg, using radiotherapy contours for PET lesion detection algorithm) or the clinical patient population (eg, lacking obese patients), then the algorithm will likely reflect those limitations. High-quality, large, and diverse datasets are needed for ML algorithm development.

A key concept for users to understand is generalizability, together with its counterpart overfitting. The primary goal and also the primary challenge of ML algorithm development is to create an algorithm that performs well when applied to unseen data (ie, data not available to the model during training). ML algorithms can easily memorize training samples: they can detect noise patterns or features that are highly specific to the training dataset and then rely on those features to make predictions. However, those features are not useful, and in fact are misleading, when used to make predictions for a new dataset. Therefore, significant effort is spent during algorithm development to preventing overfitting. Data also need to be collected and labeled from diverse sources, matching the diversity of the expected population, to avoid overfitting to a specific subpopulation. Then, once the model is trained, its performance must be evaluated with new data that are external to the development dataset.[13]

BUILDING BLOCKS OF MACHINE LEARNING NETWORKS

The primary assumption underpinning many ML algorithms is that simple mathematical operations, when intelligently stacked together, can be used to represent highly complex relationships between input data and training labels. Motivated by the "simple" functions of individual biologic neurons in the brain, many modern ML networks are in fact a long series of simple operations. The operations rely on numerical weights or parameters that are learned during training. These building blocks often include weighted sums, or binary yes/no decisions, or convolutions, as illustrated in **Fig. 2**. Most modern ML networks are primarily composed of these simple operations, such as artificial neural networks (weighted sums), random

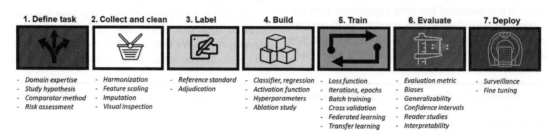

1. Define task	2. Collect and clean	3. Label	4. Build	5. Train	6. Evaluate	7. Deploy

- Domain expertise
- Study hypothesis
- Comparator method
- Risk assessment

- Harmonization
- Feature scaling
- Imputation
- Visual inspection

- Reference standard
- Adjudication

- Classifier, regression
- Activation function
- Hyperparameters
- Ablation study

- Loss function
- Iterations, epochs
- Batch training
- Cross validation
- Federated learning
- Transfer learning

- Evaluation metric
- Biases
- Generalizability
- Confidence intervals
- Reader studies
- Interpretability

- Surveillance
- Fine tuning

Fig. 1. The steps of machine learning algorithm development, together with key concepts for each step. Many of the key concepts are beyond the scope of this article and readers are encouraged to explore these concepts further through other sources.

Table 1
Glossary of terms

Term	Definition
1×1 convolution	A convenient tool for changing the number of channels in a layer
Activation function	A function that transforms the output of a layer; often used to add nonlinearity to a network
Activation (feature) map	The result of network operations performed on input data; often represents salient features of the input data
Backpropagation	A method used by an optimizer to compute the network's gradients
Batch (minibatch)	Datasets are partitioned into batches for training; one batch is used during each iteration
Batch normalization	An operation that normalizes the values of an activation map
Channel	The number of activation maps or input depth; for images, the size of the third dimension (eg, red-green-blue = 3 channels)
Concatenation	Often used to stack two sets of activation maps together
Convolution layer	A network layer in which a bank of filters is convolved with an input matrix, producing an activation map for each filter
Cross-validation	A data partitioning technique where the dataset is repeatedly sampled into different training and testing sets
Decision tree	A series of binary yes/no operations performed on input data; trees are often combined together to create decision forests
Encoder-decoder	A type of network that consists of a series of downsampling operations followed by a series of upsampling operations
Epoch	Passing over the entire dataset (all batches) during training
Filter	A set of weights that is convolved with an input image as part of a convolution layer; updated during training
Fully connected (dense) layer	A single layer of a traditional neural network; each node connects to each element of the input
Generative adversarial network	A framework for training models by having two models compete and learn from each other
Hyperparameters	Model parameters not explicitly learned during training; often design choices (eg, number of layers, channels, epochs)
Iteration	An individual update step during training, often using a single batch of data
Linear layer	An activation function that only scales the input; used for continuously valued outputs
Loss function	A measurement of how far off the model's predictions are from the labels; used to guide model training
Max pooling	A downsampling operation that passes on the highest value in each patch after an image has been partitioned into patches
Neuron/node	A single operation within an artificial neural network
Optimizer	The method used to update the model's weights based on the loss function
Overfitting	The network memorizing training examples; often results in poor generalization performance
Rectified linear unit	An activation function that sets all negative valued inputs to zero and passes through all positive values
Sigmoid	An activation function that yields a value between 0 and 1; used for binary classification
Softmax	An activation function that provides the probabilities for each possible class the sample might belong to; for multiclass classification

(continued on next page)

Table 1 *(continued)*	
Term	**Definition**
Stochastic gradient descent	A commonly used optimizer
Supervised learning	Methods by which an algorithm learns to map input data to a desired output by training with a dataset of paired input-label examples
Tensor	A data object; often a multidimensional data array
U-Net	An encoder-decoder network that is commonly used for segmentation and image synthesis
Upsampling (upconvolution, transpose convolution)	An operation that increases the dimensions of the input data
Unsupervised learning	Methods by which an algorithm learns patterns in an unlabeled dataset (eg, clustering)
Weights (parameters)	Coefficients that are used in network operations and are updated/learned during training

forests (binary decisions), and CNNs (convolutions). The building blocks are typically combined with additional operations (eg, nonlinear functions) and organized into complex pathways to better represent the complex relationships they are tasked to learn.

THE CONVOLUTIONAL NEURAL NETWORK

This section walks the reader step-by-step through all the major components of a CNN.

Diagrams

CNNs are often represented using diagrams like the one shown in **Fig. 3**. There are different conventions for representing networks in literature, which is a source of confusion. In general, diagrams either illustrate the series of operations that are performed on the input data (eg, showing a series of convolution operations as in He and colleagues[14]) or diagrams illustrate the data that result from the network operations (eg, showing how the dimensions of the data change following network operations as in Simonyan and Zisserman[15]). The latter style is used in **Fig. 3**. Often the weights of a network, such as the bank of convolutional filters, are not represented in the diagrams but are implied.

Convolution Layers

The network depicted in **Fig. 3** is a simple three-layer CNN. The three components of this network that are considered "layers" are the convolution layer, the fully connected (FC) layer, and the output layer. This small network serves as a toy example that allows us to understand the foundational components of a CNN. In

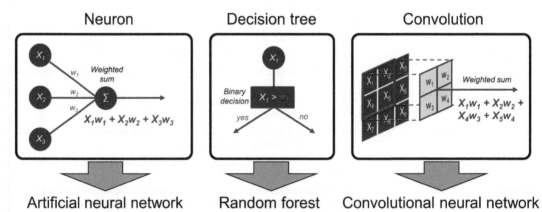

Fig. 2. Simple functions are used as the main building blocks of most AI networks. Learnable weights (w_i) are used to perform basic operations on input data (X_i). When stacked together in large numbers, these building blocks can create complex and powerful networks.

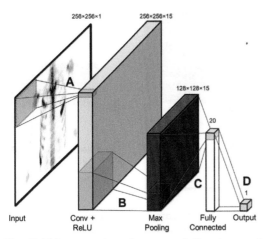

Fig. 3. This example of a convolutional neural network is dissected throughout the article. The key steps are labeled. (A) The convolution operation (see Fig. 4). (B) Max pooling (see Fig. 5). (C) Fully connected layer (see Fig. 6). (D) The output (see Fig. 7). The numbers above each layer indicate the dimensions of the activation maps or number of nodes: $N_x \times N_y \times N_{channels}$. ReLU, rectified linear unit.

Fig. 3A–D, each operation performed by the network is represented. Each operation is discussed next and illustrated in more detail in Figs. 4–7.

The first convolution operation is shown in Fig. 3A. This is a two-dimensional (2D) convolution and is depicted in greater detail in Fig. 4. The first convolution layer takes two arrays as input: the input image and a bank of learnable 2D filters or kernels. The convolution layer produces a third array as output: the activation map. Each filter (the number of filters is a parameter selected by the developer) is convolved with the input image and consequently creates its own independent and unique activation map as output: J filters produce J activation maps. The filters are conceptually understood to represent "feature detectors." They begin as random numbers and then during training they evolve into useful filters, such as edge detectors. The activation maps (also called feature maps or internal representations) reflect the part of the input image that is "activated" by the filter. For example, an edge-detecting filter produces an activation map with high values in the pixels that correspond to edges in the input image. This is depicted in Fig. 4. Activation maps in the early layers of the network are thought to reflect simple features (eg, edges), whereas activation maps deep within the network are thought to reflect high-level, abstract features (eg, ribcage). By convention, the number of activation

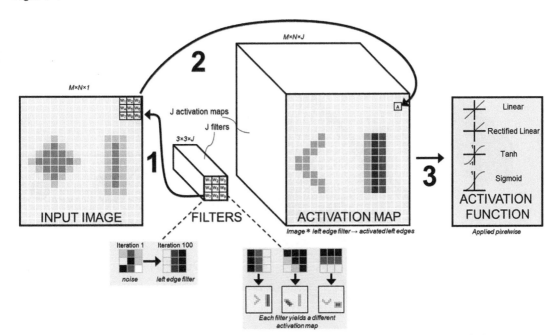

Fig. 4. A convolutional layer consists of three operations. (1) A bank of filters is convolved with the image in a sliding window fashion. The filters start as random numbers and evolve over the course of training to become feature detectors, such as edge detectors. Each of the J filters is convolved with the input image. (2) The convolution operation produces an activation map. The activation map reflects the locations of the input image that contain whichever feature the filter has learned to detect (eg, the left edge is activated by left edge filters). Each filter produces a different activation map. (3) An activation function is applied pixel-wise to the activation maps so that the network is capable of learning nonlinear relationships between the input image and the training label.

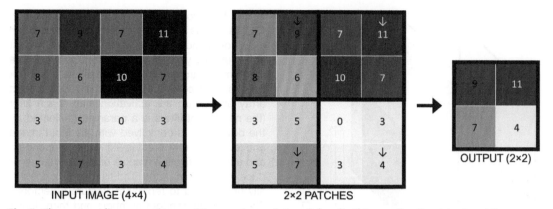

INPUT IMAGE (4×4)   2×2 PATCHES   OUTPUT (2×2)

Fig. 5. The max pooling operation partitions an image into patches (in this case 2 × 2 patches) and then passes along the highest value in the patch to the next layer. This has the effect of downsampling the image/activation map.

maps produced in a given layer is also called the number of channels in that layer (100 activation maps = 100 channels).

Activation Functions

Following each convolution layer, the resulting activation map is passed through an activation function. The activation function is a mathematical function applied to each element of the activation map (ie, pixel-wise). The purpose of the activation function is to introduce nonlinearity into the network, otherwise the sequence of convolutions (which are linear operations) would be limited to only learning linear relationships between the input data and target labels. There are a variety of functions that can serve as activation functions, the most common being the rectified linear unit and

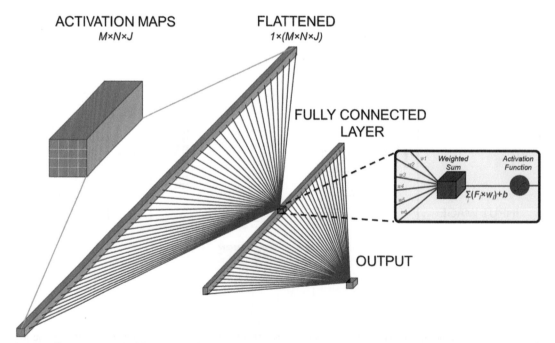

Fig. 6. Fully connected (FC) layers are often used before the output layer of a CNN. The activation maps are first flattened (ie, converted to a one-dimensional vector) and then fed to an FC layer. Each element of the flattened activation maps, F_i, is connected to each node of the FC layer, with each connection assigned a learnable weight, w_i (for convenience, this figure only shows F_i connected to a single FC node). The output of a node is the weighted sum of all elements feeding into the node, plus a learned bias weight, followed by an activation function.

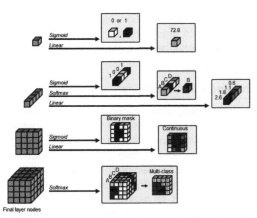

Fig. 7. The output node and its activation function dictate the output of the network. The output layer can have a single node, a vector of nodes, a 2D array of nodes, or (for multiclass segmentation using softmax) a three-dimensional array of nodes.

the sigmoid, as shown in **Fig. 4**. The rectified linear unit is a simple function whose output is 0 if the input (ie, pixel in the activation map) is less than 0, otherwise its output is identical to the input. The rectified linear unit effectively sets all negative values in the activation maps to zero, which is surprisingly simple yet effective.

Convolution operations are often repeated multiple times in a row. The activation maps resulting from the first convolution layer act as the input for a second convolution layer. These activation maps are convolved with a new, independent bank of learned filters, yielding another set of activation maps in the second layer. Some CNNs have dozens of convolution layers.

Pooling Layers

Pooling layers (see **Fig. 3**B), are a key component of most CNNs. Pooling layers are downsampling operations, which are necessary because of the GPU's limited memory. A succession of convolution layers producing multichannel activation maps can quickly surpass the GPU's memory capacity when applied to high-resolution images. For a given memory budget, the empirical rule-of-thumb is that one can get greater performance when activation maps are downsampled. This saves memory, which effectively allows one to build a deeper network with more layers and/or channels. Large networks typically have several pooling layers.

The most common type of pooling is max pooling, which is depicted in **Fig. 5**. In 2 × 2 max pooling, the activation map is first partitioned into 2 × 2 patches. The highest pixel value in each patch is passed to the next layer, whereas the other three

pixel values are thrown away. This has the effect of reducing the dimensions of the activation maps by half (512 × 512 → 256 × 256) and memory by a factor of four. Conceptually, by passing the maximum pixel value in a patch to the next layer, the network is indicating to the next layer that there is a high activation (ie, there is an important feature) within the patch.

Fully Connected Layers

FC layers are often used before the final output of the network (see **Fig. 3**C). An FC layer, or dense layer, is equivalent to a traditional artificial neural network comprised of neurons or nodes. The FC layer is depicted in detail in **Fig. 6**. Often the purpose of placing an FC layer at the end of a CNN is to learn complex relationships between the last set of activation maps and the final output of the network. The developer selects the number of nodes in the FC layer, and each element of the input to the layer, which we call F_i, is conceptually "connected" to each node in the FC layer. These connections are often illustrated in diagrams by lines connecting two nodes. Each connection is assigned a learnable weight, w_i. The output of each node in the FC layer is a weighted sum, meaning the total sum of all input values multiplied by their respective weights: $\Sigma(F_i \times w_i)$. In practice, this is simply a matrix multiplication of the input vector and the weight vector. Often a learned bias value, b, is added to the output of the node and then it is passed through an activation function, as shown in **Fig. 6**. Note that in the figure, the input to the FC layer is not the activation map itself, but rather a flattened version of the activation map, in which the three-dimensional array gets collapsed to a 1 × N vector. This is a necessary step before feeding the activation map to the FC layer.

Final Layer

The final layer of a network together with its corresponding activation function dictate the output of the model. For our toy network, the final layer (see **Fig. 3**D) consists of a single node. The last layer can be a single node, a vector of nodes, or even a 2D or three-dimensional array of nodes, depending on the desired output of the model. The different possible forms that the last layer might take and options for activation functions are depicted in **Fig. 7**. The most common activation functions for the last layer are sigmoid, linear, and softmax. Sigmoid activation functions are ideal for binary tasks (eg, disease present or disease absent).[7] The output of a sigmoid is a continuous value between 0 and 1 (see **Fig. 4**), but in practice its output gets rounded to either 0 or 1. Sigmoids are used for binary classification or two-class image segmentation (for which the last layer would have dimensions $N_x \times N_y$). Linear activation functions are for continuously valued outputs, such as predicting a risk score or for image synthesis. Softmax activation functions are used in multiclass classification problems. Softmax returns a probability score for each of the possible output classes, and the class with the highest score is then used as the model output. Layers using softmax must therefore have an extra dimension whose size is the number of possible classes (see **Fig. 7**). For example, if classifying an image into one of four disease groups, softmax would output four values, one for each disease group, representing the probability of the image belonging to each group. So the final layer should be of dimensions 1×4.

NETWORK TRAINING

A detailed treatment of network training is beyond the scope of this article, but the following is a brief overview of the key components.

Optimization

Training is an optimization process. This means that with each iteration of training, the weights of the network (which start off as random numbers) are tweaked in a way that makes the output of the network better (ie, the network's output gets closer in value to the labels of the training data). For the network shown in **Fig. 3**, the weights that get updated during training are the convolutional filters and the FC layer weights (both of which are not depicted in the figure). Weights can number in the tens of millions for large networks.

An optimization problem requires a loss function. A loss function quantifies the difference between the model's output and the training labels. The overall goal of training is to minimize the network's loss function. For example, a potential loss function for problems with continuously valued outputs might be mean squared error: (predicted – true)^2. For classification problems, classification accuracy could be used as a loss function, but researchers have found that a measure called cross-entropy produces better results for classification and is therefore more widely used.[7]

The training algorithm, or the optimizer, is the method that determines the magnitude and direction that each weight should be changed during training so that the loss function gets smaller. For example, stochastic gradient descent is a commonly used optimizer for CNNs.[16] Most optimizers, including stochastic gradient descent,

use the backpropagation algorithm to compute the network's gradients (the gradients tell how a directional change in a weight will impact the loss function).

Training Considerations

During training, precautions are taken to prevent the network from overfitting the training dataset. To avoid overfitting, developmental datasets are often partitioned into two or three distinct sets: the training set for training the model, the test set for estimating the performance of the model on unseen data, and (if needed) a validation set for model selection. The validation set lets developers try out different models without the risk of accidently selecting a model that is by chance overfitting the test set. An even better method than one-time data splitting is the use of cross-validation, in which the dataset is repeatedly split into training and testing sets and a new model is trained with each split. With cross-validation, the whole dataset is used for training and for testing across the different splits.

Because of memory constraints, developers often train the model on batches of examples from the training dataset, updating the model with each batch of data. When enough batches have passed through the model to encompass the full size of the entire training dataset, this is called an epoch. Model training typically proceeds through many epochs and stops when the error in the validation set begins to rise (even if the error in the training set continues to improve).

THE U-NET

Most CNNs used in academic or commercial applications are more complicated than the toy network shown in **Fig. 3**. In this section, we describe in detail the well-known and widely used U-Net architecture. The U-Net architecture was proposed by Ronneberger and colleagues in 2015 and is depicted in **Fig. 8**.[8] The U-Net forms a U-shape, with the left-hand descending side called the encoder, and the right-hand ascending side called the decoder. The U-Net was developed to solve a problem that was challenging at the time: how to produce high-resolution segmentation maps using CNNs. The "funnel" shape of CNNs, in which high-resolution images get repeatedly downsampled to low-resolution activation maps, causes the high-resolution information (eg, sharp edges) to get lost along the way. The U-Net solves this problem in two ways: upsampling and concatenation operations. **Fig. 8** shows that the upsampling operations begin halfway through the network. An upsampling operation

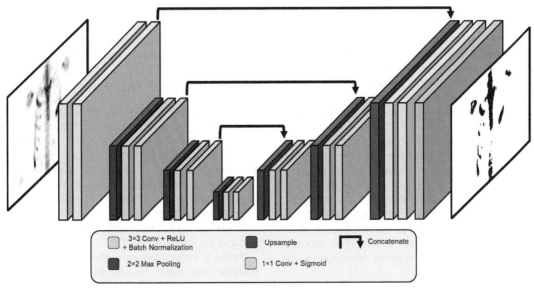

3×3 Conv + ReLU + Batch Normalization

2×2 Max Pooling

Upsample

1×1 Conv + Sigmoid

Concatenate

Fig. 8. The U-Net is an encoder-decoder network, with the encoder (left side) consisting of downsampling operations via max pooling and the decoder (right side) consisting of upsampling operations. This U-Net is producing a binary segmentation map from a nuclear medicine image.

doubles the X-Y dimensions of an activation map, and if repeated enough, eventually allows for the network's output (eg, a segmentation map) to match the dimensions of the input image. It also allows for features from the lowest-resolution level of the network, which represent the most abstract and contextually aware features, to be passed to the high-resolution output map. Upsampling can be performed using nearest neighbor upsampling, in which one pixel value is replicated four times into a 2 × 2 patch, or through upconvolution (also called transpose convolution or deconvolution), in which one pixel gets multiplied by four learned weights to produce a 2 × 2 patch. The number of channels often remains the same after upsampling. Note that in **Fig. 8** the channel depth (ie, number of activation maps) is not accurately depicted: all layers appear to have the same number of channels. In fact, the U-Net increases in channel number with each stage of the encoder, and then decreases in channel number with each stage of the decoder. **Fig. 8** ignores this for convenience only.

The second novel component of the U-Net is the concatenation operations. These operations allow the network to combine the abstract features learned at the lowest resolution layer with the high-resolution features of the input images. It works in the following manner: the activation maps on the encoder side of the network, which are produced by convolutional layers acting on the input image and its descendants, are combined with the activation maps on the decoder side of the network, which are produced by upsampling the lowest-resolution features. Because the X and Y dimensions of some activation maps match on the encoder and decoder sides of the network, the activation maps are combined by simply stacking them together channel-wise. If the activation maps in the encoder side are of dimensions $N_x \times N_y \times N_A$, and the activation maps on the decoder side are $N_x \times N_{y-} \times N_B$, the concatenated maps will be of dimension $N_x \times N_y \times N_{A + B}$.

Finally, there are a few other components of the U-Net in **Fig. 8** that are not included in our original toy example: batch normalization (BN) and 1 × 1 convolutions. BN is a surprisingly powerful operation that is frequently used after every convolutional layer.[17] For each iteration of training (ie, for each batch of training samples), BN causes the output values of a given layer to have a fixed mean and variance. This means that the activation maps are scaled such that the average value of all the elements in the activation maps is equal to some number (this number is a learned weight and changes with each batch) and the variance of the activation maps is equal to some number (also a learned weight). This prevents the values in the activation maps from drifting to large difficult-to-handle numbers during training. Empirically, BN results in faster convergence and helps regularize a network. The 1 × 1 convolution, which is applied in the last layer of the U-Net in **Fig. 8**, is a means of converting a stack of activation maps into a single 2D output image: $N_x \times N_y \times N_z \rightarrow N_{x-} \times N_y$. Conceptually, every individual X-Y index in the activation maps before the last layer will have multiple values in the z-dimension, N_z, one for each activation map. A 1×1 convolution performs a weighted sum of those N_z values to produce a single *X-Y* output. The weights of this weighted sum are learned during training. Consequently, the 1×1 convolution is used as a convenient tool for changing the number of channels of a layer.

The U-Net is used for more than just segmentation. By simply changing the last layer activation function from sigmoid (binary output) to linear (continuously valued output), and using an appropriate loss function and training set, the U-Net can perform image synthesis. BN often needs to be removed for image synthesis applications, however, because BN can make it difficult to produce consistent quantitative outputs because of the constantly shifting values of the activation maps. The U-Net has been used in several image synthesis applications, such as computed tomography synthesis for attenuation correction.[2]

OTHER NETWORKS AND MODELS

CNNs, including the U-Net, have gained wide popularity in nuclear medicine, but they are not always the best option for every application. Furthermore, not all CNNs are designed to perform the same function. Developers must select a model type and architecture (anatomy) matched with the proper functionality (physiology) that is appropriate for their prediction task. For example, a model designed for classification is often not suitable for image synthesis.

Table 2 shows several different classes of AI models and their typical uses. It also lists

Table 2
Different classes of AI models and their typical uses

Model Classes	Input	Output	Typical Uses	Example Architectures
Convolutional neural network				
Deep CNN	Image	Class, score[a]	Image classification, risk score prediction	AlexNet, ResNet
Encoder-decoder CNN	Image	Image, mask	Image segmentation, image synthesis	U-Net, SegNet, FCN
Detection CNN	Image	Pixel indices	Object detection/ localization	R-CNN, YOLO
Generative adversarial network	Image	Image, mask	Image-to-image translation	CycleGAN, pix2pix
Artificial neural network				
Feed forward artificial neural network	Features	Class, score	Radiomics, risk score prediction	Perceptron, multilayer perceptron
Recurrent artificial neural network	Features	Class, score, text	Language modeling, time series	LSTM
Transformer	Features	Class, score, text	Language modeling	BERT, GPT-3
Decision forest				
Random forests	Features	Class, score	Radiomics, risk score prediction, classification	CART, bagged trees
Gradient-boosted decision forest	Features	Class, score	Radiomics, risk score prediction, classification	XGBoost
Clustering	Features	Class	Unsupervised classification	k-means, k-NN,
Support vector machines	Features	Class	Classification	RBF SVM

[a] Score can mean any continuous variable, such as age, size, or risk.

examples of published architectures for each class. The structure and function of each type of model dictates applications for which it is suitable. For example, a radiomics model should be designed to take a list of numerical values (radiomics features) as input and produce a numerical output (eg, risk score). Hence, radiomics models often use artificial neural networks or decision forests with the appropriate structure (eg, number of input/output nodes) and function (eg, activation functions).[18]

Novel classes of model are continuing to be developed. For example, a generative adversarial network is a unique type of model that is gaining popularity in medical imaging. Generative adversarial networks can often perform the same tasks as CNNs but may require fewer labeled data samples.[19] Generative adversarial networks pit two networks against one another (often two CNNs). One network is tasked with producing realistic and accurate outputs (eg, segmentation masks) and the other network is tasked with predicting whether a sample was generated by the first network or came from a set of true labels. Each network gets penalized when the other network succeeds, which causes both networks to compete and improve. Novel unsupervised and semisupervised model types are also showing promise. Readers are encouraged to explore benchmark datasets and data science competitions to become familiar with the ever-growing variety of AI architectures.[20]

SUMMARY

As the foothold of AI within PET imaging continues to grow, more and more people in nuclear medicine will be exposed to concepts and principles of AI. Here, we have described the core structure and function of CNNs, starting basic and then building up to the more complicated U-Net. It is hoped that this establishes a foundation of knowledge that readers can build on and familiarizes readers with the building blocks that are used in most ML applications. With a greater familiarity of AI principles, readers are better positioned to develop, evaluate, and use AI tools in future clinical practice.

DISCLOSURE

T.J. Bradshaw and A.B. McMillan receive research support from GE Healthcare. Research reported in this publication was supported by the National Institute of Biomedical Imaging and Bioengineering of the National Institutes of Health under award number R01EB026708.

REFERENCES

1. Visvikis D, Cheze Le Rest C, Jaouen V, et al. Artificial intelligence, machine (deep) learning and radio(geno)mics: definitions and nuclear medicine imaging applications. Eur J Nucl Med Mol Imaging 2019;46(13):2630–7.
2. Liu F, Jang H, Kijowski R, et al. A deep learning approach for 18F-FDG PET attenuation correction. EJNMMI Phys 2018; 5(1):24
3. Weisman AJ, Kim J, Lee I, et al. Automated quantification of baseline imaging PET metrics on FDG PET/CT images of pediatric Hodgkin lymphoma patients. EJNMMI Phys 2020;7(1):76.
4. Capobianco N, Meignan M, Cottereau A, et al. Deep learning FDG uptake classification enables total metabolic tumor volume estimation in diffuse large B-cell lymphoma. J Nucl Med 2021;62(1):30–6.
5. Torres-Velazquez M, Chen W-J, Li X, et al. Application and construction of deep learning networks in medical imaging. IEEE Trans Radiat Plasma Med Sci 2021;5(2):137–59.
6. Rawat W, Wang Z. Deep convolutional neural networks for image classification: a comprehensive review. Neural Comput 2017;29(9):2352–449.
7. Chollet F. Deep learning with Python. Shelter Island, NY, USA: Manning Publications Co; 2017.
8. Ronneberger O, Fischer P, Brox T, et al. U-Net: Convolutional networks for biomedical image segmentation. Cham (Switzerland): Springer International Publishing; 2015.
9. Harvey H, Glocker B. A standardised approach for preparing imaging data for machine learning tasks in radiology. In: Ranschaert ER, Morozov S, Algra PR, editors. Artificial intelligence in medical imaging: opportunities, applications and risks. Cham (Switzerland): Springer International Publishing; 2019. p. 61–72.
10. Willemink MJ, Koszek WA, Hardell C, et al. Preparing medical imaging data for machine learning. Radiology 2020;295(1):4–15.
11. Kohli M, Prevedello LM, Filice RW, et al. Implementing machine learning in radiology practice and research. AJR Am J Roentgenol 2017;208(4):754–60.
12. Sambasivan N, Kapania S, Highfill H, et al. Everyone wants to do the model work, not the data work": data Cascades in High-Stakes AI. In SIGCHI CHI. Yokohama: Japan; 2021. https://doi.org/10.1145/3411764.3445518.
13. Kleppe A, Skrede OJ, De Raedt S, et al. Designing deep learning studies in cancer diagnostics. Nat Rev Cancer 2021;21(3):199–211.
14. He K, Zhang X, Ren S, et al. Deep residual learning for image recognition. In 2016 IEEE Conference on Computer Vision and Pattern Recognition (CVPR). 27-30 June 2016:Las Vegas, NV, USA.

15. Simonyan K, Zisserman A. Very deep convolutional networks for large-scale image recognition. 2015. arXiv:1409.1556 [cs.CV].

16. Ketkar N. Stochastic gradient descent, in deep learning with Python: a hands-on introduction. Berkeley, CA: Apress; 2017. p. 113–32.

17. Ioffe S, Szegedy C. Batch normalization: accelerating deep network training by reducing internal covariate shift. 2015. arXiv:1502.03167.

18. Zwanenburg A. Radiomics in nuclear medicine: robustness, reproducibility, standardization, and how to avoid data analysis traps and replication crisis. Eur J Nucl Med Mol Imaging 2019;46(13):2638–55.

19. Yi X, Walia E, Babyn P. Generative adversarial network in medical imaging: a review. Med Image Anal 2019;58:101552.

20. Available at: https://paperswithcode.com/. Accessed May 17, 2021.

Artificial Intelligence in PET: An Industry Perspective

Arkadiusz Sitek, PhD[a],*, Sangtae Ahn, PhD[b], Evren Asma, PhD[c], Adam Chandler, PhD[d], Alvin Ihsani, PhD[e], Sven Prevrhal, PhD[f], Arman Rahmim, PhD, DABSNM[g,h], Babak Saboury, MD, MPH, DABR, DABNM[i,j,k], Kris Thielemans, PhD[l,m]

KEYWORDS

- Industry • AI • List-mode • Ecosystem • Workflow • PET

KEY POINTS

- Industry faces unique challenges to bring artificial intelligence (AI) to positron emission tomography (PET) clinical workflows.
- There are new AI ecosystems created to facilitate the use of AI in clinics.
- New computing ecosystems can include reconstructions of vendor neutral format raw PET list-mode data.
- Custom workflows including image reconstructions and list-mode data processing can be used in new AI ecosystems.

GLOSSARY

Artificial intelligence, convolutional neural networks, Positron Emission Tomography, Radiology, AI ecosystem, AI workflows, federated learning, industry perspective, data acquisition, list-mode data, standardization, cost, data access, robustness, underspecification of AI model, clinical value, regulations, AI failures, adversarial attacks, uncertainty estimation, explainability, decision making, decision support, human-machine decision making, liability, custom data processing, adoption of AI, trust in AI recommendations, PET list-mode standardization, standardized image reconstruction.

INTRODUCTION

The recent popularity of *artificial intelligence* (AI) heralded as a game-changing technology has generated high hopes for breakthrough advancements and changes across the entire health care industry. The specific area of clinical positron emission tomography (PET) imaging is no exception. In this work, we provide an industry perspective on specific opportunities and challenges for PET arising by the emergence of AI and deep learning (DL) methods.

DL[1] is a machine learning technique which uses deep neural networks to create a variety of models which can process raw data. In recent years, DL

[a] Sano Centre for Computational Medicine, Nawojki 11 Street, Kraków 30-072, Poland; [b] GE Research, 1 Research Circle KWC-1310C, Niskayuna, NY 12309, USA; [c] Canon Medical Research, 706 N Deerpath Drive, Vernon Hills, IL 60061, USA; [d] Global Scientific Collaborations Group, United Imaging Healthcare, America, 9230 Kirby Drive, Houston, TX 77054, USA; [e] NVIDIA, 2 Technology Park Drive, Westford, MA 01886, USA; [f] Philips Research Europe, Röntgenstr. 22, Hamburg 22335, Germany; [g] Department of Radiology, University of British Columbia, BC Cancer, BC Cancer Research Institute, 675 West 10th Avenue, Office 6-112, Vancouver, British Columbia V5Z 1L3, Canada; [h] Department of Physics, University of British Columbia, BC Cancer, BC Cancer Research Institute, 675 West 10th Avenue, Office 6-112, Vancouver, British Columbia V5Z 1L3, Canada; [i] Department of Radiology and Imaging Sciences, Clinical Center, National Institutes of Health, 9000 Rockville Pike, Bethesda, MD 20892, USA; [j] Department of Computer Science and Electrical Engineering, University of Maryland Baltimore County, Baltimore, MD, USA; [k] Department of Radiology, Hospital of the University of Pennsylvania, 3400 Spruce Street, Philadelphia, PA 19104, USA; [l] Institute of Nuclear Medicine, University College London, UCL Hospital Tower 5, 235 Euston Road, London NW1 2BU, UK; [m] Algorithms and Software Consulting Ltd, 10 Laneway, London SW15 5HX, UK
* Corresponding author.
E-mail address: a.sitek@sanoscience.org

PET Clin 16 (2021) 483–492
https://doi.org/10.1016/j.cpet.2021.06.006
1556-8598/21/© 2021 Elsevier Inc. All rights reserved.

has demonstrated significantly promising results for several PET applications, including segmentation, reconstruction, outcome modeling, decision support, and so forth.[2–8]

In this work, a *manufacturer* is defined as an industry member manufacturing PET scanners, and a *vendor* as an industry member providing AI and other processing software solutions. These two groups are not exclusive. In the present work, we sometimes interchangeably use the terms *deep learning* and *artificial intelligence*, although AI (and its subset machine learning) are wider fields. The recent spike of interest in AI is due to increased popularity of DL, especially the use of convolutional neural networks (CNNs), which is why we use this convention in this article.

The article is organized as follows. Section Challenges for commercialization identifies selected challenges in the adoption of AI from the industry point of view. They are general and not PET specific. The goal of this section is not to discuss potential solutions to those challenges but rather paint a perspective on specific challenges from the industry point of view. In section Looking into the future of AI in PET, specific applications of AI in PET are discussed in more detail. In particular, a concept of reconstruction of the list-mode (LM) data on demand is combined with AI algorithms and presented.

CHALLENGES FOR COMMERCIALIZATION

One of the main concerns for industry is to release reliable, extensively tested and validated products that impact disease and patient management. For the purpose of this article, we define a reliable product as working as intended and within a set of predefined specifications. Equally important, the product should demonstrate clinical utility. In this section, we discuss some of the major concerns and obstacles the industry has to overcome.

Development and Clinical Evidence

Access to data

Obtaining large amounts of data to develop AI products is challenging, and often ownership of the data is not with the industry. The need for obtaining sufficient amounts of data for training, which encompass all expected variations in the data, that is, population-based variations (both locally and geographically), body locations, disease state variations (including normal/nondisease cases), and so forth, adds further challenges. *Federated learning* (FL) is an approach that may at least partially alleviate the issue. In FL, AI models are trained based on data that never leave the medical institutions[9] and therefore data security and privacy are much less of a concern. The paradigm of FL is being widely explored (eg, the work on FL from the London Medical Imaging & AI Center for Value-Based Healthcare[10,11]).

Ground truth

In some applications of AI such as supervised learning, obtaining ground truth will present a great challenge. Ground truth can be obtained from an independent measurement (eg, biopsy, postmortem analysis), clinical outcomes (death, morbidity), or previous diagnoses (eg, radiology reports), or new reads or annotations can be used. Ideally, the data sets should be large, but new reads and annotations make data preparation a lengthy and expensive process.

Robustness

Of particular, commercial interest is a reliable, regulatory cleared product that performs according to specifications regardless of geographic location, patient mix, and local preferences and guidelines. Unfortunately, AI algorithms can generalize poorly and are dependent on the data sets used to train and test the algorithms. An AI algorithm may produce unreliable results if characteristics of the input deviate from the training data. This has critical consequences. It is acceptable to publish an AI algorithm tested on homogeneous data (eg, from a single or small number of institutions using well-defined study inclusion criteria) as long as those limitations are transparently disclosed in the publication. However, a commercially available product ought to be applied to real life data that may be more diverse and complex than single-center study data, which may render certain limitations of an algorithm as nonacceptable. In general radiology, there are many large publicly available data sets which can be used to test generalization of developed AI algorithms. Unfortunately, there are few such sets available that include PET data, making the development of AI algorithms for PET more difficult.

Underspecification

Another obstacle to generalization of AI is a recently documented problem of *underspecification*.[12] This term denotes the problem that if we train the same model a number of times with slightly different initial weights on the same large data set and achieve similar performance on the test set, there is no guarantee that those models will perform the same in the real world. This is a very difficult problem to tackle and extremely important from the industry point of view as the real-world performance is what matters. When many models are trained on the same set of data with random initial weights and applied to a certain unseen real-world scenario, some models may work and some other models may not. At the phase of model development, it is difficult to tell which of those models will work and which ones will not. Testing models with diverse real-world data will alleviate the problem although not entirely. Therefore, we emphasize the importance of postmarket surveillance after algorithm deployment which becomes even more important than classical (not DL) offerings.

Clinical value

When commercializing AI algorithms, there is a need to demonstrate that the product provides clinical value and evidence that supports the intended use. To generate such data that can be used as evidence for potential regulatory claims that translate into customer value, often multicenter, multireader studies are required. Here, we emphasize that often one develops an excellent technological solution to a clinical problem, but when introduced to clinical workflows, it is not widely used in routine clinical practice by clinicians. Appropriately designed external evaluation studies at clinical sites by clinicians could mitigate the problem.

Regulatory Pathways

AI's towering dependence on data exposes MedTechś regulatory and privacy challenges more than ever before: compounded by the sharp teeth that GDPR has afforded the EU, with global effects, academia and industry are only now learning to safely share massive amounts of data.

Regulatory bodies, too, increasingly demand being shown the data used to train the AI parts of software submitted for their approval. However, basing approval on the data creates the conundrum as once approved that retraining with new data would invalidate it and burden industry and administration with incessant reapproval cycles. Luckily, everybody agrees a solution is direly needed. In the United States, the FDA is working on an action plan, and the EU has just released a white paper with very similar thoughts.[13-15] Obviously, an eventual worldwide joint framework will be key for industry and data-owning individuals alike.

Return on Investment

The health care industry requires a reasonable return of investment to create or sustain a viable business. For applications of AI in PET products, investment in development should be properly justified by balancing the growth potential of the AI technology with the considerable risks. AI may require a nontraditional business model in which subscription approaches, architectures open to third parties such as marketplaces, and new ecosystems are used. It is an industry challenge to figure out why and how clients would pay for AI innovations.

Understanding AI

Explainability

Explainability is an important factor associated with the adoption of AI from the commercial point of view. In short, in DL methods, the decisions made by AI are often opaque, black box decisions. For more details on this problem, please refer to the study by Arrieta and colleagues.[16] For AI algorithms to succeed in the commercial world, the users of the algorithms have to gain trust in them. For example, a clear explanation on how the AI algorithm arrived at a certain classification can increase trust in the subsequent clinical decisions which AI recommends.

Education and trust

It is critically important to educate users about AI's capabilities and, even more importantly, its limitations. Most current applications of neural networks are some form of image denoising where very noisy images, presumably from short- or low-dose scans, are converted into images that appear less noisy. However, this does not mean that nothing is lost because of shorter or lower dose scans. Users need to understand that the quantitative lesion/region of Interest performances of their images are still governed by the statistics of the acquisition. AI can mimic longer or higher dose scans by making backgrounds smoother but cannot create the information that is lost due to shorter or lower dose scans. Nonetheless, we note that AI can improve image quality such as lesion detectability or signal-to-noise ratio by using better priors, system models, data correction, or noise models learned from data.

Another related topic is how clinicians determine the reliability of lesion standardized uptake values. They may look at how noisy a large, approximately constant region such as the liver is and decide that smoother regions indicate more reliable lesion quantitation. For typical reconstruction algorithms such as Ordered-subset expectation maximization (OSEM), this approach works reasonably well because if the noise correlation lengths are short, the single-image-noise in the liver is related to the standard deviation of a single liver voxel, which is in turn related to the standard deviations of individual lesion voxels which finally determine the standard deviation of the lesion SUV. In contrast, when the background is smoothed using

AI-based methods, this connection is lost. The single-image-noise in the liver may be greatly reduced without any significant changes to the lesion ensemble noise properties. Therefore, a clinician looking at an image denoised with neural networks should be cautious about interpreting the variability (or uncertainty) of the lesion SUV. It should also be noted that denoising could introduce an additional bias in the lesion SUV.

Combining human and AI insights
In the foreseeable future, human decision-makers will be augmented/assisted and not replaced by automated algorithms. Unavoidably there will be situations where a human opinion is different from that of an algorithm. This creates opportunities and challenges because the combination of AI and humans may create a better and more accurate decision.[17,18] However, it creates a problem on how to meaningfully combine human and AI insights. The final decision in the foreseeable future will be made by humans, and some solutions are needed to deal with disagreements. One such approach could be that AI provides explanations or examples from the past of similar images with known outcomes, which may persuade the physician. Another resolution of such conflicts could be that we teach the AI algorithm to consider the physician's arguments for the different opinion (similarly as the difference in opinions is resolved between two physicians) and then to recompute the estimates. It is however unclear how this can be accomplished in the current workflows and requires future research. These are important ethical issues of paramount importance to industry which need to be resolved with cooperation with stakeholders including clinical and ethical experts, patient advocacy groups, governmental bodies, and of course, the industry.[19] Finally, we anticipate that, when AI makes a clinical decision without human intervention some day perhaps in the not-too-distant future, we will face a complex problem of who is liable for a wrong decision made by AI, similar to self-driving car liability.

Failures

Critical failures
If algorithms do not perform according to specifications, it constitutes a major problem for vendors. For example, DL-based image reconstruction can be unstable resulting in severe artifacts.[20] This risk is often a consequence of the poor generalization of the AI algorithms and the fact that results presented by an AI algorithm are often not explainable. If a spectacular error is made by AI, it is very damaging to the perception of a product even if it works within specified characteristics.

When publishing an article, the same penalty is applied if the algorithm had an error or a spectacular error. However, when we deploy an AI product, a spectacular failure could be much more detrimental to the trust in the algorithm. These types of errors, although very damaging, are very hard to mitigate with the current state of knowledge about neural networks. On a positive note, as much as critical failures of AI are damaging to its reputation, they are at least easily identifiable as errors. There are some safety features that can be used ("graceful failure"). For example, if we use AI to compute quantitative values and if the computed values are outside of the physiologic range, one may display a message that AI failed to compute the value rather than providing it to the user. For classification problems, these types of mitigations are much more difficult to implement. This is certainly important from an industry point of view and an important direction of future research.

Uncertainty estimation
Clear communication to the interpreting physician of uncertainty in the AI result is crucial in building trust in the AI system because, as previously discussed, no AI system will be perfect or able to handle the huge range of real-world inputs. It is not practical, or even possible, for AI developers to aim for a perfect result every time, so communication of uncertainty is of paramount importance.[21,22] Large uncertainty alerts about low confidence in provided inference. This is particularly true for nuclear imaging techniques which produce data with high noise compared with other modalities, and this noise may translate to uncertainty in reconstructed images and AI decisions. Suppose we develop an AI algorithm which automatically detects the volume of interest (VOI) of abnormal uptake of FDG, ideally the algorithm would also provide an estimation of uncertainty on the VOI size and SUV. This uncertainty can be expressed by providing a range of values that with a high likelihood contains the true value (confidence intervals). This can also be done using Bayesian approaches where each value of the volume or SUV is assigned probability of being true.[23] Estimation of such uncertainty can be accomplished with neural networks using approximations to Bayesian approaches[24,25] or some other approximate methods.[26,27]

Malicious AI, adversarial attacks
Another potential concern is that AI and DL methods either by accident or maliciously may introduce perturbations in the images. Some of these perturbations can be imperceptible to

humans but may have a drastic effect on AI outcomes. For example, in an image manufactured by malicious AI, the analyzing AI may detect a tumor with 100% certainty which remains completely invisible to a human observer. For more on adversarial attacks refer to the study by Ma and colleagues.[28] When used for PET image reconstruction, AI may also introduce perturbations with image textures different from those obtained by standard iterative methods, which may be misinterpreted as abnormalities.

To Err is Human. How Does This Apply to AI?

Another issue that industry faces is to roll out products that will over time earn the trust of radiologists and nuclear medicine physicians and convince them to use algorithmic advice. We already drew the reader's attention to challenges associated with explainability. *Algorithm aversion* is another, potentially more serious, obstacle which may prevent seamless acceptance of AI solutions. Human decision-makers are averse to algorithmic predictions after seeing them perform; even with evidence of noninferiority of the AI algorithm, humans still tend to follow advice given by humans because people more quickly lose confidence in algorithms than in human forecasters after observing them repeating a mistake.[29] Algorithmic aversion may be a major obstacle to adoption of AI. AI algorithms used in augmenting human decision-making will likely have to be held to very high standards by enforcing interuser and extrauser reproducibility. If we can, we should also provide quantitative values with confidence measures (see also section Regulatory Pathways). Confidence is also important for yes/no or other classification decision tasks, and some type of confidence measures should always be provided.

LOOKING INTO THE FUTURE OF AI IN PET

Various academic medical centers worldwide are currently investing to incorporate AI in both research and clinical research settings as a prelude to AI-supported clinical workflows. For those applications, AI is largely used to scale and automate data analysis for large cohorts in multiyear studies whereby thousands of images are analyzed retrospectively. In clinical research, AI is typically used for clinical decision support as a "second opinion" to that of the clinician, to increase the saliency of structures and functions of interest in images while increasing efficiency of acquisition, and/or to identify possible regions or planes of interest in images so the clinician may improve diagnosis, increase efficiency, and minimize fatigue.[30-32]

The important question for the industry is how we bring AI into the clinical workflow in an efficient and scalable way. In section AI During PET Data Acquisition, we consider using AI during PET data acquisition. In section Vendor-Neutral Data-Processing Platforms, we explore new AI ecosystems already proposed elsewhere[33-35] and discuss how to leverage the uniqueness of PET raw data (eg, LM) in such ecosystems.

AI During PET Data Acquisition

AI offers a whole new array of promising approaches that have the potential to optimize the utility of PET imaging by adjusting controllable parameters based on the specific patient anatomy, patient physiology, and scanner type. The basic idea of how to achieve this is summarized in **Fig. 1**. We present the ability of AI algorithms to combine various types of information to provide just-in-time inferences which help to create high-fidelity PET data at the PET scanner while data are being acquired.

In this section, we provide example scenarios of how such AI inferences can be applied. In *scenario 1*, while the data are being acquired during a single-bed position, AI analyses the *data acquired* (**Fig. 1**) and uses criteria of *acceptable data quality* to determine if a sufficient number of counts were acquired up to this moment. An example of what problem this may partially solve is patient motion. If AI detects substantial patient motion, it triggers additional time for data acquisition also informing the operator. In *scenario 2*, suppose we scan a patient to determine whether the SUV in a given VOI changed versus the SUV measured in a previous PET scan. We provide the AI the *previous PET/CT scan*, *data acquired*, and maximum threshold for uncertainty of a decision (**Fig. 1**). We want to know if the SUV increased/decreased by 20%

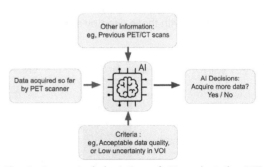

Fig. 1. Conceptual depiction of AI used at the PET scanner during data acquisition. *Gray arrows* indicate input to AI (data acquired so far, other data acquired in the past, and criteria for decision-making) and *red arrow* indicates output from AI.

with 95% certainty. AI analyzes the data and computes the maximum possible certainty that can be reached and the additional acquisition time to reach it.

The PET scanner is also a location where manufacturer-specific AI can be deployed. Once the raw data are created and the image is reconstructed, an AI algorithm can generate insights which can be sent to Picture archiving and communication system (PACS) or other destinations along with the data. Such solutions may be very effective as the manufacturer controls the type of data the AI algorithm is exposed to. The downside is of course that it is limited to individual manufacturers.

Vendor-Neutral Data-Processing Platforms

An effective approach to deployment of AI in radiology and other clinical environments is unclear. It is likely however that in the near future, we will have hundreds of AI algorithms approved for use in clinics and operating on different parts of clinical workflow and data. If we do not have a common platform to deploy them and rather depend on each AI vendor to use their own methods, the deployment and growth of AI in PET could stall as the complexity quickly becomes unmanageable.

To address this, new vendor-neutral data-processing platforms (VNDPs) are proposed.[33–35] In radiology, the VNDPs are interfaced with PACS. AI and other algorithms can process the data pulled from PACS and other hospital IT systems. After processing, the output can be sent back to the PACS, be saved on different archives, or displayed as shown in **Fig. 2**. We will not discuss these workflows in detail here and refer the reader to references available on this topic (vid.[33–35]). Software units that operate in VNDPs can be stacked together if their output/input type fits. Once stacked, blocks can be replaced by different blocks or stack of blocks. Such an architecture has a similarity with those used by smartphones[34]

because software units are "sitting" on the platform and are activated if the "right" data arrives and they can be swapped/updated on user requests. Using this analogy, we will refer to the software units as "apps" (**Fig. 2**).

To provide an example of data processing in a VNDP platform, let us consider **Fig. 2** and processing by apps 4, 5, and 6. The input consists of PET/CT images. App 4 segments the liver using CT, app 5 detects liver lesions using PET and CT, and app 6 performs diagnosis and computes SUV using PET and CT if lesions were detected. Note that outputs from apps 4 and 5 are used by app 6.

Extended VNDP platform—processing standardized LM

Archiving PET data in a raw LM format has many advantages as it gives the ability to retrospectively reconstruct images on demand. There are many examples of where such flexibility is beneficial. For example, when training AI algorithms, it allows the developer to create a larger variety of images in terms of resolution and noise from just a single raw datafile. It also allows the developer to vary the total number of counts simulating different doses. The LM format may contain information about deposited energy and time-of-flight per event information, exact crystal pairs in which the gamma photons were detected, which may lead to development of improved reconstruction algorithms or correction algorithms compared with histogram (sinogram) data. As timing information is available for each event, it allows for various patient motion corrections.

The availability of LM data in new ecosystems would open opportunities to processing PET data, training new AI algorithms, and deriving AI inferences. The data reconstruction in such an ecosystem would just be another processing app which can be inserted in the processing pipeline (recon apps in **Fig. 3**). An example of such processing could be, for example, raw LM data

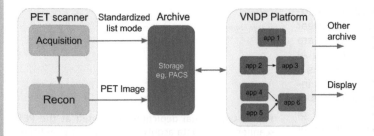

Fig. 2. Simplified PET data flows in new AI ecosystems. Data stored in, for example, PACS is pulled to the VNDP platform where they are processed by software units ('apps'). Apps can be used as a single processor (app 1) or stacked (eg, app 2 and 3 or apps 4, 5, and 6). VNDP platforms allow for creation of custom workflows with custom apps. Output from VNDP platform can be sent back to original storage, other archive, or displayed. Interactions with hospital information systems and other sources of information are omitted for clarity. Applications of AI before data reach storage are not shown.

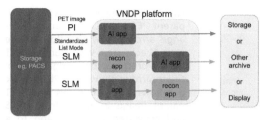

Fig. 3. PET data flow in VNDP. *Orange arrows* show dataflow in the new AI ecosystem with standard PET images processed by a single AI app. *Green arrows* show new PET-specific dataflows proposed in this work. SLM can be reconstructed by recon app and processed by AI app. In the third example, SLM is pre-processed (eg, randoms correction) and then reconstructed by the recon app. Interactions with hospital information systems and other sources of information are omitted for clarity.

correction for randoms or scatter which could be performed before image reconstruction. Ideally, in such an ecosystem, one would like to standardize the format of LM data to make it easier for vendors to develop apps which would work directly on LM data irrespective of the type of scanner the data were generated on. We refer to such a format as standardized LM (SLM) format. To perform state-of-the-art reconstruction, reconstruction applications need information including geometry, detector calibration, sensitivity, and so forth, which would have to be included in the SLM. We note that such a format does not exist at the time of writing this article as each scanner vendor uses a proprietary format. We note that standards for raw data are long established in Single Photon Computed Tomography (SPECT),[36,37] and more recently in MRI.[38] The SLM format for PET needs to be designed and approved by all stakeholders. A first step toward this goal would be that manufacturers disclose nonsensitive parts of their file formats, as some have already agreed to in the context of open-source projects.[39–41]

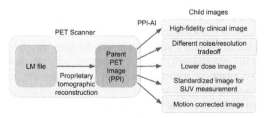

Fig. 4. LM data are reconstructed using vendor-specific proprietary software at the scanner. Each manufacturer creates manufacturer-specific AI models (PPI-AI) to transform the parent PET image to child images needed for various clinical and research tasks.

Extended VNDP platform—processing parent PET image

Although SLM in the VNDP platform provides enormous flexibility in constructing custom processing pipelines, handling LM files presents challenges. They are very large files (3–20 GB), and storage and network demands are considerable. Each vendor has a proprietary highly optimized software program which reconstructs images directly from the LM or sinograms created from the LM. Reconstruction software may have specific computing hardware requirements that may not be readily available in the VNDP platform.

AI offers an alternative approach toward creating a practical platform for generalization of the reconstruction process across different scanners and manufacturers without explicitly using LM files. The suggested approach gives up some generalizability compared with the SLM approach described in section 3.2.1, but it is more practical and well suited for use within a VNDP platform. We refer to this concept as the *parent PET image* (PPI) and summarize it in **Fig. 4**.

The main idea is that instead of handling SLM in the new ecosystem as shown in **Fig. 3**, we reconstruct on the scanner a parent image (or images) and use it instead of SLM in the VNDP platform. In the VNDP platform, PPI is then used to generate on demand various child images (**Fig. 4**). The generation of child images from the PPI is performed using deep CNNs referred to in this article as PPI-AI. The PPI-AI are types of apps in the ecosystem (**Fig. 2**) that convert PPIs to child images.

The PPI can be, for example, the high-fidelity image. PPI can actually also be a set of images, such as high-fidelity images with and without attenuation correction, resolution modeling, and so forth. If time-of-flight is available, it could also contain back-projections at different angles, as used by the DIRECT method.[42] There are many possibilities on how to define PPI, and research is needed to determine which of those choices would be optimal. The PPI is reconstructed on the scanner, and it is stored in PACS possibly along with some child images. The PPI can be pulled to the VNDP platform and almost instantaneously converted to any child image as the inference using the PPI-AI CNN model is fast. Once converted to a child image, it can be further processed by AI apps or other apps as a regular PET image (**Fig. 5**).

Looking at **Fig. 4**, the PPI can be converted to a high-fidelity image, the best utility image that a vendor can generate from the LM file. When training AI apps to be used in new ecosystems (**Fig. 2**), we would like to use images of various quality with various artifacts for the app to be more robust and general. A PPI-AI model can be

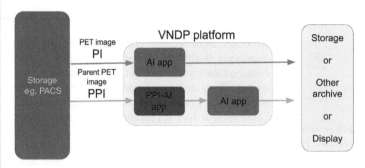

Fig. 5. PET data flow in VNDP with parent PET image (PPI) concept. *Orange arrows* show dataflow in the new AI ecosystem with standard PET images processed by a single AI app. *Green arrows* show new PET-specific dataflows proposed in this work. PET parent image is pulled from PACS and converted by PPI-AI app to a PET image which is processed by a single AI app. Interactions with hospital information systems and other sources of information are omitted for clarity.

trained to generate poorer quality images from the PPI. Examples of such are shown as different noise/resolution tradeoff and lower dose child images in **Fig. 4**.

There are ongoing efforts to harmonize and standardize results obtained on different scanners.[43,44] This can also be done using the PPI by creating harmonized child images. For this, we would require collaboration between vendors to create a single PPI-AI CNN model which could generate harmonized images from PPIs of different vendors. We can take this concept further and imagine a situation where the user points a cursor on a lesion when viewing a high-fidelity image, the standardized image is created in the background transparently to the user, and the viewing system displays standardized SUV values.

The fifth child image example provided in **Fig. 4** is physiologic motion (eg, respiratory) correction using PPI-AI. If no motion correction is applied, regions of the PPI with motion will appear blurry. PPI-AI models can be trained to recover resolution from blurred PPIs. Alternatively, a PPI could contain several images, for example, in different motion states, or one in end-expiration and one without motion correction, from which a fully motion-corrected image can be produced.

The training of PPI-AI models is conceptually straightforward. Suppose we want to create a PPI-AI model that generates from the PPI a half-dose image, first, we identify a training set which contains, for example, 1000 PET scans from some patient population. Then, we reconstruct those 1000 images from LM data using only half of the counts available in the LM. Then, we create PPIs by reconstructing images using all counts and high-fidelity reconstructions. We train neural networks (PPI-AI) with PPIs as the input and half-dose images as the target. This completes the creation of the PPI-AI model. Similarly, any other PPI-AI model can be trained. In the aforementioned steps, we assumed that

high-fidelity reconstruction image is the PPI, but this may not necessarily be the optimal choice as already discussed.

A disadvantage of using the PPI compared with SLM is that the PPI contains less information than the LM file. Timing information is not available, and although the PPI can in general be a dynamic (or ECG-gated) sequence, it cannot be time reframed to a different sequence. We also do not have access to deposited energy, time of flight, and so forth. However, we remember that some of the information is transferred to PPI-AI models during training. Intuitively, during PPI-AI inference, when child images are generated from the PPI, not only the information in the PPI is used but also the information "stored" in PPI-AI models.

Another disadvantage of PPI is that if a manufacturer improves the tomographic reconstruction algorithm and wants to update it on the scanner, all PPI-AI models have to be retrained, which could be an automated process, but it is computationally intensive. If novel reconstruction is to be applied retrospectively to data acquired in the past, the PPIs have to be updated as well.

SUMMARY

In section Challenges for commercialization, we presented important challenges for creating and adopting AI solutions in clinics from the point of view of the industry. In section Looking into the future of AI in PET, we concentrated on PET explored unique to PET applications of AI during data acquisition. We examined a flexible and scalable ecosystem for deployment of AI and described a synergy of such systems with an idea of SLM data and the other solution presented here based on the PPI concept.

There are emerging new workflows and data ecosystems in radiology. In addition to facilitating AI deployment, they provide a tremendous opportunity for the PET community to transform the current paradigm of PET data processing.

CLINICS CARE POINTS

- Reconstruct PET data on demand (eg, just before or during reading) from raw data such as standardized list-mode data or parent PET images.

- Use raw data as a part of the "patient medical record."

- Include "DICOM push" for ease of raw data transfer/storage/management.

- Archive raw data which is essential for future improved reconstruction with motion correction, harmonization, or comparison with prior images.

- Process raw data in new AI ecosystems.

DISCLOSURE

S.A., E.A., A.C., A.I., and S.P. are employees of GE, Canon, United Imaging, NVIDIA, and Philips, respectively. K.T. is the owner of Algorithms and Software Consulting Ltd.

ACKNOWLEDGMENTS

Authors would like to thank Sven Zuehlsdorff, PhD, Siemens Medical Solutions USA, Inc., Hoffman Estates, IL, USA, sven.zuehlsdorff@siemens-healthineers.com for his input. The opinions expressed by authors in this article may not necessarily represent the official opinions of their employers. This publication is partly supported by the European Union's Horizon 2020 research and innovation programme under grant agreement Sano No 857533 and the International Research Agendas programme of the Foundation for Polish Science, co-financed by the European Union under the European Regional Development Fund.

REFERENCES

1. LeCun Y, Bengio Y, Hinton G. Deep learning. nature. 2015;521(7553):436–44.
2. Sharif MS, Abbod M, Amira A, et al. Artificial neural network-based system for PET volume segmentation. J Biomed Imaging 2010;4:2010.
3. Zhao X, Li L, Lu W, et al. Tumor co-segmentation in PET/CT using multi-modality fully convolutional neural network. Phys Med Biol 2018;64:015011.
4. Ypsilantis P-P, Siddique M, Sohn H-M, et al. Predicting response to neoadjuvant chemotherapy with PET imaging using convolutional neural networks. PLoS One 2015;10:e0137036.
5. Gong K, Kim K, Cui J, et al. The evolution of image reconstruction in PET: from filtered back-projection to artificial intelligence. PET Clinics. Current issue. doi:10.1016/j.cpet.2021.06.004.
6. Sanaat A, Zaidi H. Depth of interaction estimation in a preclinical PET scanner equipped with monolithic crystals coupled to SiPMs using a deep neural network. Appl Sci 2020;10(14):4753.
7. Berg E, Cherry SR. Using convolutional neural networks to estimate time-of-flight from PET detector waveforms. Phys Med Biol 2018;63(2):02LT01.
8. Gong K, Berg E, Cherry SR, et al. Machine learning in PET: from photon detection to quantitative image reconstruction. Proc IEEE 2019;108(1):51–68.
9. Sheller MJ, Edwards B, Reina GA, et al. Federated learning in medicine: facilitating multi-institutional collaborations without sharing patient data. Sci Rep 2020;10(1):1–2.
10. Sheller MJ, Reina GA, Edwards B, Martin J, Bakas S. Multi-institutional deep learning modeling without sharing patient data: A feasibility study on brain tumor segmentation. International MICCAI Brainlesion Workshop September 16-20, 2018 (pp. 92-104). 21st International Conference, Granada, Spain Springer, Cham.
11. Crimi A, Bakas S, Kuijf H, Menze B, Reyes M, editors. Brainlesion: Glioma, Multiple Sclerosis, Stroke and Traumatic Brain Injuries: Third International Workshop, BrainLes 2017, Held in Conjunction with MICCAI 2017, Quebec City, QC, Canada, September 14, 2017, Revised Selected Papers. Springer; 2018 Feb 16.
12. D'Amour A, Heller K, Moldovan D, et al. Underspecification presents challenges for credibility in modern machine learning. arXiv preprint arXiv:2011.03395. 2020 Nov 6.
13. European Commission. White Paper on Artificial Intelligence: A European Approach to Excellence and Trust. Report. 2020. Available at: https://ec.europa.eu/info/sites/default/files/commission-white-paper-artificial-intelligence-feb2020_en.pdf.
14. Artificial intelligence/machine learning (AI/ML)-Based. Software as a medical Device (SaMD) action plan. Available at: https://www.fda.gov/media/145022. Accessed July 22, 2021.
15. Proposed regulatory framework for Modifications to artificial intelligence/machine learning-based software as a medical Device. Available at: https://www.fda.gov/media/122535. Accessed July 22, 2021.
16. Arrieta AB, Díaz-Rodríguez N, Del Ser J, et al. Explainable Artificial Intelligence (XAI): Concepts, taxonomies, opportunities and challenges toward responsible AI. Inf Fusion 2020;58:82–115.
17. Wu N, Phang J, Park J, et al. Deep neural networks improve radiologists' performance in breast cancer screening. IEEE Trans Med Imaging 2019;39(4):1184–94.

18. Sitek A, Wolfe JM. Assessing cancer risk from mammograms: deep learning is superior to conventional risk models. Radiology 2019;292(1):67–8.

19. Fenech M, Strukelj N, Buston O. Ethical, social, and political challenges of artificial intelligence in health. London: Wellcome Trust Future Advocacy; 2018.

20. Antun V, Renna F, Poon C, et al. On instabilities of deep learning in image reconstruction and the potential costs of AI. PNAS 2020;117(48):30088.

21. Begoli E, Bhattacharya T, Kusnezov D. The need for uncertainty quantification in machine-assisted medical decision making. Nat Machine Intelligence 2019;1(1):20–3.

22. Kompa B, Snoek J, Beam AL. Second opinion needed: communicating uncertainty in medical machine learning. NPJ Digital Med 2021;4(1):1–6.

23. Sitek A. Data analysis in emission tomography using emission-count posteriors. Phys Med Biol 2012; 57(21):6779.

24. Neal RM. Bayesian learning for neural networks. New York: Springer Science & Business Media; 2012.

25. Wilson AG. The case for Bayesian deep learning. arXiv preprint arXiv:2001.10995. 2020 Jan 29.

26. Lakshminarayanan B, Pritzel A, Blundell C. Simple and scalable predictive uncertainty estimation using deep ensembles. arXiv preprint arXiv:1612.01474. 2016.

27. Abdar M, Pourpanah F, Hussain S, Rezazadegan D, Liu L, Ghavamzadeh M, Fieguth P, Khosravi A, Acharya UR, Makarenkov V, Nahavandi S. A review of uncertainty quantification in deep learning: Techniques, applications and challenges. arXiv preprint arXiv:2011.06225. 2020 Nov 12.

28. Ma X, Niu Y, Gu L, et al. Understanding adversarial attacks on deep learning based medical image analysis systems. Pattern Recognition 2021;110: 107332.

29. Dietvorst BJ, Simmons JP, Massey C. Algorithm aversion: people erroneously avoid algorithms after seeing them err. J Exp Psychol Gen 2015;144(1): 114.

30. Demirer M, Candemir S, Bigelow MT, et al. A user interface for optimizing radiologist engagement in image data curation for artificial intelligence. Radiol Artif Intelligence 2019;1(6):e180095.

31. White RD, Erdal BS, Demirer M, et al. Artificial Intelligence to Assist in Exclusion of Coronary Atherosclerosis during CCTA Evaluation of Chest-Pain in the Emergency Department: Preparing an Application for Real-World Use. arXiv preprint arXiv:2008.04802. 2020 Aug 10.

32. Hashemian B, Manchanda A, Li M, et al. Review (2020). Clinical deployment and validation of a radiology artificial intelligence system for COVID-19.

33. Leiner T, Bennink E, Mol CP, et al. Bringing AI to the clinic: blueprint for a vendor-neutral AI deployment infrastructure. Insights Imaging 2021;12(1):1.

34. Enzmann DR, Arnold CW, Zaragoza E, et al. Radiology's information architecture could Migrate to one emulating that of smartphones. J Am Coll Radiol 2020;17(10):1299–306.

35. Allen B, Dreyer K. The artificial intelligence ecosystem for the radiological sciences: ideas to clinical practice. J Am Coll Radiol 2018;15(10): 1455–7.

36. National Electrical Manufacturers Association. NEMA PS3/ISO 12052, Digital Imaging and Communications in Medicine (DICOM) Standard. Available at: http://dicom.nema.org/medical/dicom/current/output/html/part01.html.

37. Todd-Pokropek A, Cradduck TD, Deconinck F. A file format for the exchange of nuclear medicine image data: a specification of Interfile version 3.3. Nucl Med Commun 1992;13(9):673–99.

38. Inati SJ, Naegele JD, Zwart NR, et al. ISMRM Raw data format: a proposed standard for MRI raw datasets. Magn Reson Med 2017;77(1):411–21.

39. Wadhwa P, Thielemans K, Efthimiou N, et al. PET image reconstruction using physical and mathematical modelling for time of flight PET-MR scanners in the STIR library. Methods 2021;185:110–9.

40. Ovtchinnikov E, Brown R, Kolbitsch C, et al. SIRF: synergistic image reconstruction framework. Computer Phys Commun 2020;249:107087.

41. Markiewicz PJ, Ehrhardt MJ, Erlandsson K, et al. NiftyPET: a high-throughput software platform for high quantitative accuracy and precision PET imaging and analysis. Neuroinformatics 2018;16(1):95–115.

42. Matej S, Surti S, Jayanthi S, et al. Efficient 3-D TOF PET reconstruction using view-grouped histo-images: DIRECT—Direct image reconstruction for TOF. IEEE Trans Med Imaging 2009;28(5):739–51.

43. Sullivan DC, Obuchowski NA, Kessler LG, et al. Metrology standards for quantitative imaging biomarkers. Radiology 2015;277(3):813–25.

44. Boellaard R, Delgado-Bolton R, Oyen WJ, et al. Fdg PET/CT: EANM procedure guidelines for tumour imaging: version 2.0. Eur J Nucl Med Mol Imaging 2015;42(2):328–54.

Objective Task-Based Evaluation of Artificial Intelligence-Based Medical Imaging Methods:
Framework, Strategies, and Role of the Physician

Abhinav K. Jha, PhD[a],*, Kyle J. Myers, PhD[b], Nancy A. Obuchowski, PhD[c], Ziping Liu, BS[d], Md Ashequr Rahman, BS[d], Babak Saboury, MD, MPH, DABR, DABNM[e], Arman Rahmim, PhD, DABSNM[f], Barry A. Siegel, MD[g]

KEYWORDS

- Artificial intelligence (AI) • Task-based evaluation • Medical imaging
- Positron emission tomography (PET) • Role of physician • Machine learning

KEY POINTS

- There is an important need for strategies for rigorous objective evaluation of artificial intelligence-based methods for medical imaging on clinical task.
- We lay out a framework for objective task-based evaluations of artificial intelligence-based methods.
- Techniques to conduct objective task-based evaluations, specifically in the context of PET, are presented.
- The role of physicians in conducting these evaluations is presented.
- Examples of applying the framework to evaluate hypothetical artificial intelligence-based methods for PET data acquisition and analysis are presented.
- Future areas of research on task-based evaluation are outlined.

INTRODUCTION

Artificial intelligence (AI)-based methods for medical imaging, and more specifically PET, hold exciting promise in multiple stages of the imaging–technology–development lifecycle ranging from data acquisition to image reconstruction, image processing, clinical assessment, and toward

[a] Department of Biomedical Engineering, Mallinckrodt Institute of Radioly, Alvin J. Siteman Cancer Center, Washington University in St. Louis, 510 S Kingshighway Boulevard, St Louis, MO 63110, USA; [b] Division of Imaging, Diagnostics, and Software Reliability, Office of Science and Engineering Laboratories, Center for Devices and Radiological Health, Food and Drug Administration (FDA), Silver Spring, MD, USA; [c] Quantitative Health Sciences, Cleveland Clinic, Cleveland, OH, USA; [d] Department of Biomedical Engineering, Washington University in St. Louis, 1 Brookings Drive, St Louis, MO 63130, USA; [e] Department of Radiology and Imaging Sciences, Clinical Center, National Institutes of Health, 9000 Rockville Pike, Bethesda, MD 20892, USA; [f] Department of Radiology, Department of Physics, University of British Columbia, BC Cancer, BC Cancer Research Institute, 675 West 10th Avenue, Office 6-112, Vancouver, British Columbia V5Z 1L3, Canada; [g] Division of Nuclear Medicine, Mallinckrodt Institute of Radiology, Alvin J. Siteman Cancer Center, Washington University School of Medicine, 510 S Kingshighway Boulevard #956, St Louis, MO 63110, USA
* Corresponding author.
E-mail address: a.jha@wustl.edu

PET Clin 16 (2021) 493–511
https://doi.org/10.1016/j.cpet.2021.06.013

clinical decision support.[1–3] Thus, there is substantial interest in the clinical translation of these methods. Although AI encompasses a broad range of methods, in this article, AI specifically refers to methods that are based on artificial neural networks, such as deep-learning approaches. These methods have been showing the most promise in medical imaging over the past few years.

For the translation of any technology, the need for rigorous evaluation is well recognized.[4] The need for such evaluation is even more critical for AI methods. These methods are not generally programmed with user-defined rules and instead learn rules by analysis of training data. For example, a neural network-based method for tumor segmentation is not provided any guidance or rules on the defining traits of a lesion boundary (eg, difference in tumor and background intensities). Instead, the method is trained on example images (referred to as training images) where a delineation of the tumor boundaries is given, and the method learns the rules to segment these tumors. These rules are implicit and not necessarily interpretable (although there are several efforts toward interpretability), thereby often making the output of these methods unpredictable and not explainable. This can have major implications. One implication is the possible inability to detect a failure of the method. Evaluations are required to identify such failures, assess the reliability of the methods, and thus provide guidance on clinical applicability. Next, because the rules learned by the AI methods are derived from a certain training dataset, their performance with new unseen datasets, such as from a different patient population or acquired with a different imaging protocol, may be subpar (issue of generalizability).[5,6] Evaluation would assess this generalizability. A related issue is that AI-based methods may learn spurious correlations from training data that may be unrelated to disease state.[7–9] A recent study, rather alarmingly, showed that even highly publicized AI-based systems for the detection of the coronavirus disease 2019 from chest radiographs relied on confounding factors rather than medical pathology.[9] Evaluations can help to identify such issues. Further, AI methods are being explored in new areas such as fully automating medical imaging applications that currently require some level of manual intervention[10] and in making critical therapeutic decisions.[11] The high costs associated with inaccuracy in these decisions make rigorous evaluation even more critical. Consequently, there have been multiple calls for rigorous evaluation of AI methods.[12–15]

Concept of Clinical Task in Medical Imaging

In medical imaging, images are acquired for specific clinical tasks such as detection, quantification, or a combination. For example, an oncological PET image in a patient showing symptoms of lung cancer may be acquired for the task of tumor detection, tumor–tracer–uptake quantification, or both. Thus, it is widely recognized that evaluation of medical-imaging methods should be performed on the clinical task that is required from the images. However, current evaluations of AI methods are typically task agnostic. For example, AI-based reconstruction and postprocessing methods are typically being evaluated using figures of merit (FoMs) such as the root mean square error that measure fidelity between the estimated image and a certain reference standard (see Liu and colleagues' article, "Artificial Intelligence-based Image Enhancement in PET Imaging: Noise Reduction and Resolution Enhancement," in this issue for a listing of some of these FoMs). However, studies are showing that these FoMs may provide misleading interpretations.[16–20] For example, the evaluation of an AI-based reconstruction approach for whole body PET using these FoMs suggested that the method was yielding similar performance as a conventional approach. However, evaluation on the task of lesion detection revealed that the method was yielding false negatives owing to blurring or missing lesions, and false positives owing to pseudo low uptake patterns.[16] Another study quantitatively compared task-based evaluation with evaluation using fidelity-based FoMs for an AI-based denoising method for low-dose cardiac single photon emission computed tomography (SPECT).[17] In that study, the fidelity-based FoMs suggested that the AI-based denoising led to improved performance. However, on the task of detecting cardiac perfusion defects, the clinical task for which these images are acquired, the performance with AI-based denoising method was almost equivalent, if not worse, compared with not conducting the denoising. Similar findings have been observed in subsequent studies.[18–20] Similarly, AI-based methods for PET segmentation are commonly evaluated using FoMs such as Dice scores, which quantify some measure of distance between the estimated segmentation and a reference standard (e.g., manual segmentation). However, again, these FoMs are not designed to correlate directly with the task required from the image, such as an estimation of quantitative features[21] or PET-based radiotherapy planning.[22] In summary, the current task-agnostic approaches to evaluating AI methods have limitations. Thus, there is an important and timely need for strategies to conduct task-based evaluation of these methods.

The literature on the objective assessment of image quality (OAIQ) has proposed multiple techniques to achieve the goal of objective task-based evaluation.[23–26] Further, OAIQ techniques have been applied widely to evaluate imaging methods,[27] including in PET.[28–30] However, designing OAIQ studies to evaluate AI methods requires special considerations given the unique working principles of these methods in terms of learning rules from training data. Our goal in this work is to propose an OAIQ-based framework that is fine tuned for evaluating AI methods. Although the framework is general, it is presented in the context of PET. A list of important factors to consider when designing an OAIQ study to evaluate AI methods are summarized in **Table 2**.

A few remarks: the framework presented here is readily extendible to SPECT and a number of other imaging modalities. In fact, recent studies have investigated evaluating AI-based SPECT methods using this framework.[17,31] Further, we focus on evaluation of AI methods that are intermediate to performing the eventual clinical task. These methods include those for optimizing imaging system instrumentation and acquisition protocols, image reconstruction, any kind of image processing, and image analysis. Finally, although we propose this framework in the context of evaluating neural network-based approaches, the framework could also be applied to evaluate other categories of AI methods.

FRAMEWORK FOR OBJECTIVE TASK-BASED ASSESSMENT

A rigorous and structured evaluation of imaging methods using the OAIQ framework requires 4 essential steps[27]:

1. Specification of the task
2. Defining the patient population and the imaging process
3. Method to extract task-specific information
4. Figure of merit

We discuss each of these components in the context of evaluation of AI-based methods for PET scans. A well-designed evaluation study should yield a claim that quantitatively defines the performance of the method.[32,33] Following this 4-component framework would yield such a claim, as we will see in the evaluation of hypothetical AI-based methods later in this article.

Objective Assessment of Image Quality (OAIQ) Terminology

We first introduce some OAIQ terminology with reference to clinical imaging. As per this terminology, the biological property of the patient that is measured during the imaging process is referred to as the object. In PET, this would be the distribution of the tracer within the patient. The object consists of signal and background. The signal typically refers to the abnormality in the patient, and the background refers to regions in the patient in the absence of the signal. For example, consider a patient showing symptoms of cancer who has been injected with, say, the 18F-fluoro-deoxy-glucose (FDG) tracer. The concentration of this tracer in the cancer cells and in the normal tissues would be referred to as the signal and background, respectively. The measured data are referred to as the image. In PET, this can be the sinogram, but often also refers to the reconstructed image.

We next introduce the imaging equation, which will assist with illustrating the framework. Consider a PET system described by an operator H that is imaging radiotracer distribution, denoted by a vector f, within a patient. This tracer distribution is a continuous function. The imaging process leads to measured projection data g, a finite-dimensional vector. Further, during imaging, noise, denoted by the vector n, is introduced. The imaging equation is then given by[27]

$$g = Hf + n \qquad (1)$$

Often, the projection data are reconstructed, yielding a reconstructed image denoted by $\hat{f}$. In these cases, to describe the transformation from the object f to the image $\hat{f}$, the reconstruction operator also needs to be incorporated into the imaging equation.

With this background, we provide the 4-component evaluation framework next.

Specification of the Task

PET images are acquired for multiple clinical tasks. Typically, these tasks can be divided into 3 broad categories (**Fig. 1**). They are briefly described with corresponding examples.

Classification task

A task that results in a decision-maker or observer deciding in favor of a particular hypothesis from a finite hypothesis space is termed a classification task. If the space contains only 2 hypotheses (yes/no decision), then the task is termed as binary classification. Examples include lung-tumor detection using FDG-PET, cardiac defect detection using myocardial perfusion PET, and differential diagnosis of Alzheimer's disease from frontotemporal dementia using FDG-PET in patients with dementia. This binary-classification

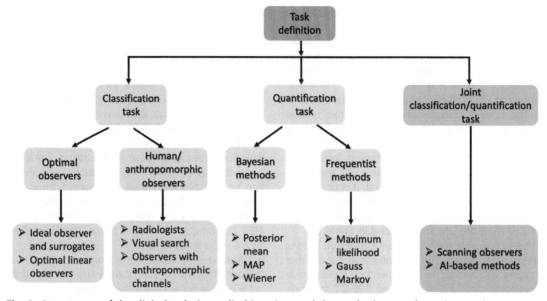

Fig. 1. A taxonomy of the clinical tasks in medical imaging, and the methods to perform these tasks.

task is also termed as a signal-detection task where the presence of a signal (increased uptake in lung nodule, decreased blood flow in myocardium, decreased uptake in brain regions) typically corresponds with an abnormality.

Depending on the information available about the to-be-detected signal and the background, the detection task can be classified into different categories. The signal can be known exactly (SKE) or statistically (SKS), and likewise, the background can be known exactly (BKE) or statistically (BKS). Note that an SKE or BKE task does not imply that the signal or background is flat. Instead, the implication is that the tracer uptake at each point within the signal or background, whether homogeneous or heterogeneous, is known. In contrast, for an SKS or BKS task, only a statistical description of this tracer uptake would be available. In clinical settings, both the signal and the background are known only statistically. However, tasks that are SKE or BKE can help to get insights on imaging system performance.[34] Another point to emphasize here is that even in a task that is both SKE and BKE, the image will only be known statistically, because imaging systems introduce noise (see Eq. 1).

In some cases, the task can be posed as one where the signal properties are variable, but in each image presented to the observer, the observer knows the signal properties, although they do not know whether the signal is present. This is referred to as a signal known exactly but variable (SKEV) task. For example, in each image presented to the observer, the lesion location is

different, but known to the observer. The observer only has to decide if the lesion is present at that location.

When evaluating imaging methods, realistic modeling of variability in the patient population is important. Thus, tasks that model this variability, which include SKS/BKS and SKEV/BKS tasks should preferably be considered. The data collected for these tasks should be representative of patient population, as we further describe in the section on Defining the Patient Population and the Imaging Process. However, in certain settings, an SKE/BKS task may be considered to evaluate the performance of the method for specific signal sizes or amplitudes, or study the sensitivity of the method to these signal properties.

Estimation/quantification task

The goal in estimation/quantification tasks is to measure some numerical or statistical feature of the object that has been imaged. In PET and SPECT, this includes quantifying features such as tracer uptake within a certain region of interest,[35–38] and volumetric parameters such as metabolic tumor volume (MTV) and total lesion glycolysis.[10] Additionally, in tracer kinetic modeling, parameters that describe the physiologic characteristics of a region of interest, such as blood flow and receptor binding potential, are estimated.[39] Further, quantitative PET (and SPECT) are being actively explored for targeted radionuclide therapy dosimetry.[40] In summary, a broad range of quantification tasks are performed using radionuclide imaging.

When evaluating AI methods, the task should be posed as one where the features of both the signal (eg, tumor) and the background are varying, preferably realistically as in clinical settings. This is equivalent to an SKS/BKS setting in the context of estimation tasks.

Joint classification and quantification task

Often, the clinical task in PET involves both classification and quantification of some features of an abnormality.[41] For example, to quantify the MTV of the primary lung tumor in a patient with lung cancer from an FDG-PET image, the primary tumor has to be first detected. These are referred to as joint classification and quantification tasks. Again, when evaluating AI methods, the detection and quantification components of the task should account for patient variability.

Define the Patient Population and the Imaging Process

Rigorous image quality assessment should model the physical and statistical properties of the objects (ie, the patients) being imaged through the imaging system. Thus, the patient population selected for evaluation should be representative of populations seen in clinical practice. Factors that would impact method performance, which could include sex, age, ethnicity, and disease prevalence, should be accounted for in the study. Further, depending on the method, the image acquisition protocol, including the system(s) over which the patient images were acquired, whether the study was single center or multicenter, and other acquisition settings, should be modeled. Accounting for these factors would also help to evaluate the generalizability of the AI method to different populations and/or different image acquisition protocols. For example, a multicenter evaluation will provide more confidence about generalizability compared to a single-center evaluation.

An OAIQ study typically requires some level of statistical description of the image data to extract task-specific information. We see from Eq. 1 that defining the patient population and the imaging process can yield such a description. This description can be obtained through analytical approaches, clinical studies, and realistic simulations. Of these 3 approaches, clinical studies typically provide the most confidence for clinical translation. However, conducting these studies presents several challenges (high costs, patient risks, time consuming) and thus may not be feasible for each AI method. Further, clinical studies may not have ground truth available for conducting the evaluation. Clinically realistic simulations, as conducted in virtual clinical trials (VCTs),[42,43] provide a mechanism to address these issues and identify promising methods for further clinical evaluation. In the next subsection, we describe the tools to conduct clinically realistic simulations.

Tools to conduct clinically realistic simulations

In clinically realistic simulations, image data corresponding to a clinically realistic digital model of the patient population are generated using software that models the imaging scanners. These simulations provide multiple advantages such as known ground truth, the ability to simulate patient variability and imaging physics, generation of numerous images relatively quickly and inexpensively, minimal risks (e.g. no radiation dose), and no patient discomfort. These images can then be used to conduct an OAIQ study. In the rest of this subsection, we list tools available to simulate patient populations, simulate PET systems and factors to consider while reconstructing the images.

Description of the patient population

To ensure clinical relevance in simulation-based evaluations, accurate modeling of in vivo anatomic and physiologic properties of the patient and variability in patient population is essential. Anthropomorphic digital phantoms can be used to achieve this goal. Kainz and colleagues[44] provide a library of available anthropomorphic phantoms. A widely used anthropomorphic phantom is the extended cardiac and torso phantom,[45] which can generate digital phantom populations with variable anatomies, including scaling the size of the body or specific organs, modeling normal and diseased patients, and modeling cardiac and respiratory motions. Additionally, hybrid phantoms can be used where simulated signals are added to real clinical images[46,47] to ensure background realism. Another option is stochastic approaches that estimate parameters that describe the object distribution directly from patient images.[48] Generative adversarial network–based approaches have also been explored to simulate phantom populations.[49]

Next, realistic modeling of lesions (the signal) is important. Assuming simplistic models such as spherically shaped lesions can provide misleading interpretations. To develop realistic models, we can obtain a distribution of the parameters of lesions, such as size, shape, and signal-to-background uptake ratio, from clinical images. These distributions could be sampled to generate lesions. Leung and colleagues[46] used such an approach to simulate the primary tumor in patients with lung cancer. Additionally, it is preferable to account for heterogeneity within the lesion, such as intratumor heterogeneity in oncological PET. We can define this heterogeneity directly from the manually delineated tumor on PET images.[50] However, this practice may limit the number of simulated lesion types. An alternative is sampling heterogeneity descriptors from a distribution.[47]

In simulation studies, the phantom must be generated at a higher resolution than the reconstructed image. This simulates the continuous radiotracer distribution, is clinically realistic, and has been shown to yield realistic reconstructed images.[51] Also, imaging systems are typically unable to measure certain components of the object function. For example, a low-resolution imaging system, as PET and SPECT systems often are, will not pass the high frequency components in spatial domain. Similarly, a system that records the measurements as detector pixel values will inherently transform a continuous object to a discrete vector (see Eq. 1), leading to loss of high-frequency components.[12,26,52] These components of the object that the imaging system is unable to measure are referred to as null functions.[12,26] Almost all biomedical imaging systems have a null space. Simulating the phantom at a higher resolution enables investigating the impact of null space of the imaging system on task performance.

Modeling PET instrumentation

The next step is to generate PET measurements (in projection data or list-mode format) for the digital phantom population. Realistic simulations should accurately model clinical PET scanner configurations, including transaxial and axial fields of view, detector crystal pitch, and other acquisition parameters. Additionally, modeling photon propagation and detector physics including attenuation, scatter, random coincidences, noise, and resolution degradation owing to positron range, photon noncollinearity, and inter-crystal penetration increases the realism of simulations.

Multiple PET simulation tools have been developed for modeling PET systems and can be divided into 2 major categories, namely, those that perform photon tracking vs. those that rely on analytical modeling (**Table 1**). The photon-tracking-based simulation tools, such as GATE,[53,54] SimSET,[39] and PeneloPET,[55] accurately model imaging physics, but are computationally expensive. The model-based simulation software may have limited accuracy in modeling the physics and may only model the major image-degrading processes. However, these methods are typically computationally faster, which is important since task-based evaluation may require simulations of hundreds, or even thousands of images. Considering these tradeoffs can help decide the appropriate simulation software for the study.[46,47,56,57]

Modeling image reconstruction and postprocessing protocols

Multiple AI methods, such as those for postprocessing and segmentation, are designed to operate on reconstructed images. To evaluate these methods, reconstructed images must be simulated. To obtain these images from simulated sinograms, clinical protocols should be followed. For example, when reconstructing using ordered subsets expectation maximization–based methods, the number of iterations and subsets should be similar to those in clinical protocols. Further, depending on the clinical protocol, the reconstruction process may have to compensate for image-degrading processes.

Process to Extract Task-specific Information

The third step in the OAIQ evaluation framework is defining the process to extract task-specific

Table 1
Comparison of PET simulation software tools

Software	GATE	SimSET	PeneloPET	PETSTEP	SMART PET	ASIM
Category	Photon-tracking based	Photon-tracking based	Photon-tracking based	Model-based	Model-based	Model-based
Computational expense	High	Medium	Medium	Low	Low	Low
PSF modeling	Yes	Yes	Yes	Analytically modeled	Analytically modeled	Analytically modeled
Attenuation modeling	Yes	Yes	Yes	Analytically modeled	Analytically modeled	Analytically modeled
Scatter modeling	Yes	Yes	Yes	Limited accuracy	Limited accuracy	Limited accuracy
Random modeling	Yes	Yes	Yes	Limited accuracy	Limited accuracy	Limited accuracy

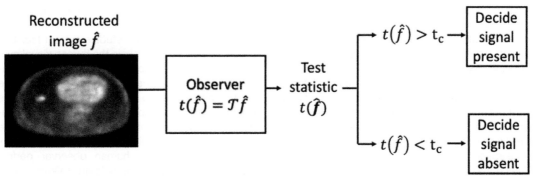

Fig. 2. A schematic demonstrating the process that an observer follows to decide on the presence of a signal when interpreting a reconstructed image. In the figure, t_c denotes the decision threshold.

information from the acquired image. The entity that extracts this information is termed as an observer. In general, any observer can be described by an operator τ that operates on some projection data g or the reconstructed image $\hat{f}$ to estimate a statistic. For a detection task, this statistic can be compared with a threshold to decide about the presence of the signal (**Fig. 2**). For a quantification task, this statistic could be the feature that was intended to be estimated (**Fig. 3**). The process to extract this information for various tasks is summarized next.

Classification task

For a classification task, the term "observer" conjures the image of a trained radiologist. The radiologist belongs to the class of human observers. However, human-observer studies can be expensive, time consuming, and tedious. Further, often OAIQ studies need to be performed over hundreds or even thousands of images and several different

configurations, exacerbating these issues. As an alternative, numerical observers, referred to as model observers,[58,59] have been proposed. These observers are mathematical algorithms that extract a test statistic from the projection data or the reconstructed image. This test statistic can then be compared with a certain threshold for decision making on the detection task.

Of these model observers, the observer that uses all statistical information available regarding the task to maximize task performance is referred to as the ideal observer (IO). The IO provides the best possible performance for the detection task. Computation of the IO for SKS/BKS tasks can be challenging, but strategies have been developed to address this issue. Park and colleagues[60] and Zhou and colleagues[61] proposed strategies to compute the IO test statistic for parametric object models. Clarkson and colleagues proposed and applied Fisher information-based surrogates to

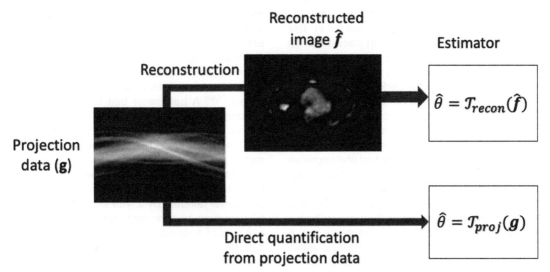

Fig. 3. Schematic demonstrating the process to estimate a parameter of interest from projections and reconstructed images.

the IO.[62,63] However, the IO can still be challenging to compute in clinically realistic settings.

An alternative to IO is using optimal *linear* observers. These have been developed for SKS/BKS and SKEV/BKS tasks.[64–66] For example, Li and colleagues proposed and theoretically demonstrated the optimality of a multitemplate linear discriminant observer for SKS tasks.[66] However, computing these observers can still be computationally challenging owing to the large dimension of the image data g. The use of channels provides a mechanism to address this issue.[67–69] Briefly, an operator, columns of which correspond to a channels, are applied to the image data g, yielding a lower dimensional vector. To approximate the performance of the IO, a class of channels referred to as efficient channels should be used.[27]

Some commonly used linear observers in OAIQ studies are the Hotelling observer and non–prewhitening matched filter, but these should be used with caution when applied to SKS/BKS tasks as they make certain assumptions that may not hold for these tasks.[70]

When the goal of the AI method is optimizing a system hardware design or an acquisition protocol, performing the detection task directly on projection data has several advantages. This process enables the OAIQ study to purely evaluate system performance and be agnostic to the choice of the reconstruction method. Additionally, the noise statistics are typically easier to describe with projection data, facilitating observer development. For system optimization, use of an optimal observer, such as the IO, is recommended.[27]

Many AI methods are developed for applications where the detection task is performed on a reconstructed image that is displayed for visual interpretation. These include applications such as reconstruction and image processing. In this case, psychophysical studies with trained human observers, such as radiologists, are the gold standard. Standardized methods are available to conduct studies to evaluate performance on detection tasks.[71] These include the 2-alternative forced choice test and the rating scale–based experiments. Owing to the inherent variability in readers' diagnostic accuracy, on account of differences in training, experience, and perceptual and cognitive abilities, studies to evaluate performance on detection tasks usually involve several trained readers to capture the spectrum of performances. For this purpose, a rich literature on multireader multicase study design and analysis methods exists.[72,73] A key criterion while designing these studies within an OAIQ framework is to evaluate performance on diagnostic tasks, and not on factors such as goodness of images, ease of interpretation, or fidelity-based similarity to some benchmark.

When human observer studies are not feasible, model observers that mimic the human visual system, also referred to as anthropomorphic observers, are an alternative. Classic studies in the field of vision science show that humans process data through the use of frequency-selective channels. By incorporating such channels in the observer model, studies have shown that model observers can mimic human observer performance.[34,67,74] These channels are referred to as anthropomorphic channels. Multiple anthropomorphic observers have been proposed in literature,[59] including for SKS/BKS tasks.[75,76] Recently, deep learning–based observers have shown promise in predicting human performance in SKS/BKS tasks.[77] When using an AI-based observer to evaluate an AI-based imaging method, it should be ensured that the method and the observer are both independently designed and validated.

Estimation/quantification task

In an OAIQ study, the goal of the estimation task is to use image data to estimate parameters that define the object.[26] In contrast, in fields such as texture analysis and computer-aided diagnosis, the typical practice is estimating parameters that define the image. For example, when estimating the parameters of MTV or intratumor heterogeneity, an OAIQ study will define these parameters as the properties of the tumor and then estimate them from the image by incorporating the transformation of the imaging system and the noise (see Eq. 1). In contrast, in most texture-analysis studies, the tumor-image heterogeneity (which may also arise due to noise and image-degrading processes),[78] and not tumor heterogeneity is estimated.

Another important concept is that of estimability. The null space of the imaging system impacts the estimation of parameters of the object.[79,80] A parameter that can be estimated accurately from the measured image data for all true values of the parameter in the presence of these null functions is referred to as an estimable parameter.

Consider an object described by some parameters, of which we are interested in estimating the parameter denoted by θ. The estimation task can be posed as an operator that maps from g to an estimate of θ, denoted by $\hat{\theta}$. These tasks are typically performed by first reconstructing the PET image over a voxelized grid, and then estimating the parameter of interest from that reconstructed image (see **Fig. 3**). A less common but highly effective approach is to directly estimate the unknown parameters from the projection data.[38,79,81] Similar to detection tasks, when the goal is system optimization, quantifying the parameters directly from projection data provides several advantages. However, when evaluating AI methods for reconstruction or post-reconstruction operations, the quantification task should be performed on reconstructed images.

Multiple quantification methods have been developed[27,82] that can be broadly categorized into 2 categories, frequentist and Bayesian methods.

Frequentist methods In frequentist methods, the parameter θ for a given patient is assumed fixed. A widely used method in this category is maximum likelihood estimation.[27] This estimator has multiple desirable properties. In particular, the estimator achieves the lowest bound of variance for any unbiased estimator (Cramer–Rao lower bound), if this bound can be achieved. An estimator that achieves this bound is referred to as efficient, so the maximum likelihood estimator is efficient if an efficient estimator exists.

Bayesian methods In Bayesian methods, for a given patient, θ is assumed to be a random variable and a prior PDF on θ is assumed. The development of these methods starts with defining a cost function. When the cost function is the ensemble mean square error (EMSE) between true and estimated value of the parameter of interest, the posterior mean of θ minimizes that cost function.[27] The posterior mean also minimizes binary cross-entropy loss,[83] and, in fact, any symmetric convex upward cost function between the measured and the true values.[27] Similarly, the maximum-a-posteriori estimator minimizes a cost function that is constant everywhere other than when the difference between the measured and true values is small, where it is zero.

The estimators mentioned above are typically nonlinear in data. Linear estimators have also been proposed. These estimators map the data to the estimate using a linear transformation. Among all linear estimators, Weiner estimator achieves the lowest EMSE and has been used for optimizing imaging systems.[84] A scanning linear estimator has been proposed[85] that has exhibited reliable performance in tasks such as estimating signal location.

Joint classification and quantification task
Research on developing observers for the joint classification and estimation task is relatively in its infancy. Some proposed observers include the channelized joint observer[86–88] and the channelized scanning linear observer.[89] AI-based approaches are also showing promise in this area.[90]

Figures of Merits to Measure Task Performance

FoMs provide a quantitative measure of the performance of the imaging method on a certain task. Here we summarize the FoMs for the tasks discussed in this article.

Classification task
Consider a binary classification task where the object being imaged (the patient) belongs to 1 of 2 classes: signal present versus signal absent. In this task, the true-positive fraction (TPF) and false-positive fraction (FPF) are defined as the proportion of correctly defined signal-present decisions and incorrectly defined signal-absent decisions (**Fig. 4**A). Commonly, the TPF is referred to as sensitivity and 1– FPF is referred to as specificity. However, the sensitivity and specificity are computed based on a specified decision threshold, and thus can vary based on the strictness of this threshold. A complete characterization of observer performance can be obtained by plotting the TPF and FPF at different threshold values. This yields a receiver operating characteristic (ROC) curve

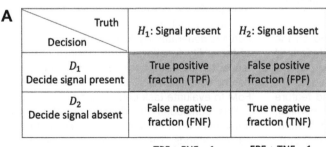

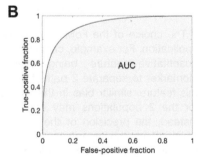

Fig. 4. Schematics illustrating the concepts of (*A*) true positive fraction and false positive fraction and (*B*) ROC curve and AUC.

(**Fig. 4**B). This curve provides a comprehensive description of the detection task performance.[91] Further, the area under the ROC curve (AUC) provides a summary FoM to evaluate detection task performance. The observer yielding a higher AUC is more accurate on the corresponding detection task. For tasks that involve classifying the object into more than 2 classes, multiclass ROC analysis techniques have been proposed.[92–96]

Quantification task

In quantification tasks, criteria to evaluate performance can include accuracy, precision, and overall reliability. We describe these criteria here, along with the corresponding FoMs to evaluate performance on these criteria.

a. The accuracy of a measurement is the closeness between the true and average measured values and is commonly quantified by measurement bias. However, the bias is often a function of the true value. A bias profile, which shows the bias as a function of the true value, provides a more complete measure of performance on accuracy.[97,98] To account for variability in the parameter of interest across populations, ensemble bias, which is the bias averaged over the distribution of the true values, provides a summary FoM for accuracy.
b. The precision of an estimate is the repeatability of the estimate over multiple noise realizations of the projection data. This precision is quantified by the variance, the standard deviation, or the coefficient of variation. This can then be averaged over the distribution of true values to obtain an ensemble variance. The precision profile, which is the precision over the range of true values, again provides a more complete measure of performance.[97,98]
c. Finally, a summary FoM that quantifies the overall reliability while accounting for the variability in the parameter to be estimated, is the EMSE. The EMSE is the mean square error averaged over the distribution of the true values and the image acquisitions. The EMSE incorporates the effects of both bias and variance.

The choice of the FoM should depend on the application. For example, consider a PET-derived quantitative feature being evaluated as a biomarker to separate 2 patient populations. For this feature, similar bias in the estimated feature for the 2 populations may not be concerning. Instead, the precision of the estimated feature, which affects the separability between the 2 populations, would be more relevant. As another example, suppose we are interested in the change in a quantitative PET-derived feature over time;

assuming constant bias over time, the precision of the measurements determines when a true change over time can be discerned from just measurement noise.[98,99]

Clinical Evaluation without Gold Standard

The FoMs described above for quantification tasks are applicable when the true values of the parameter of interest are known. This is the case in simulation or physical-phantom studies. However, such ground truth is typically unavailable during clinical evaluation of different quantitative imaging methods. To address this issue, no-gold-standard evaluation techniques have been developed.[100-103] In these techniques, the key idea is that even though the ground truth corresponding to a measured value is unknown, because the measured value results from a specific image-formation and quantification process, a relationship between the true and measured values is expected. If the relationship is linear, it can be modeled using slope, bias, and standard deviation of a normally distributed noise term. If we can assume that the ground truth is sampled from a bounded distribution, then maximum-likelihood-based procedures can be developed to statistically estimate these terms for the different methods without knowledge of the true value. For a linear relationship between the true and measured quantitative values, the ratio of the noise standard deviation and slope terms can be used as an FoM to evaluate the different methods on the basis of precision of the measured values. These no-gold-standard evaluation techniques have shown the ability to rank quantitative imaging methods in multiple imaging modalities.[102,104-106] Further, these have also been developed in the context of PET.[103,107,108]

Joint classification and quantification task

The estimation ROC curve provides a comprehensive description of performance on joint detection and estimation tasks.[41] To define the estimation ROC curve, we first define a utility function that represents the closeness between the estimated and true signal parameters. The estimation ROC curve is generated by plotting the expected value of the utility function in true positive cases with respect to the false positive fraction. The area under the estimation ROC curve provides a summary FoM to evaluate task performance.

This concludes the description of the OAIQ framework from evaluating AI-based medical imaging methods. The framework is summarized in **Fig. 5**. A set of key factors to consider when designing OAIQ studies for AI methods are summarized in **Table 2**.

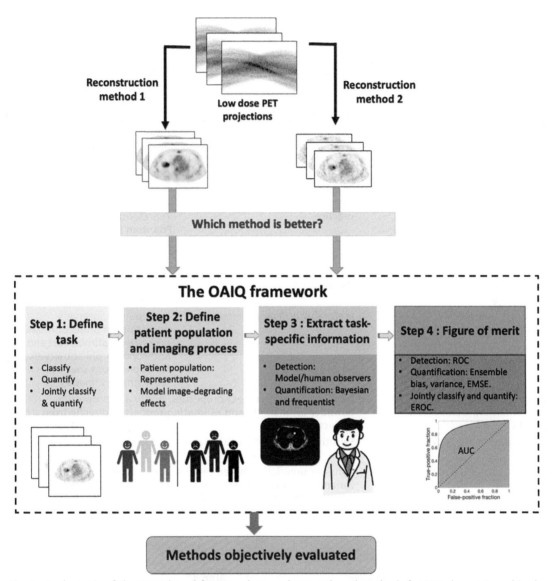

Fig. 5. A schematic of the OAIQ-based framework to evaluate AI-based methods for PET, demonstrated in the context of evaluating 2 low-dose reconstruction methods.

TASK-BASED EVALUATION OF ARTIFICIAL INTELLIGENCE METHODS: ROLE OF PHYSICIANS

Physicians, including radiologists, nuclear medicine physicians, and disease specialists, have a crucial role in OAIQ-based evaluation studies of AI methods. Their inputs are vital to designing clinically relevant study designs, and their participation substantially improves the rigor of the evaluation study. They have a role in each of the 4 steps of the OAIQ-based framework, as summarized in **Fig. 6** and described here.

a. *Step 1: Defining the task*: Physicians can help to define the clinically most relevant task for the

evaluation of the AI method. For example, consider an AI-based oncological PET reconstruction method. The physicians can specify, from a clinical perspective, whether the method should be evaluated on just the tumor-detection task or whether the task should include quantification of some parameter such as tracer uptake or MTV. Alternatively, the physician may specify that the goal of quantification is to use the parameter as a prognostic marker, in which case, the task becomes one of classification.

b. *Step 2: Choosing patient population*: Physicians can help define patient populations that are representative and diverse as in clinical practice. Additionally, in simulation studies,

Table 2
Certain key factors to consider when designing task-based evaluation studies for AI methods

OAIQ Study Step	Factors to Consider during Study Design	
	Task-Based Clinical Evaluation	Additional Considerations for Evaluation with Simulation Studies
Definition of task	Consider clinically relevant tasks	Consider tasks that model defect and background variability in patient populations: SKS or SKEV tasks
Choosing patient populations	Should be representative of that observed in clinical practice	Anthropomorphic phantoms that are realistic and representative Phantom resolution should be higher than reconstructed image resolution
Defining the imaging process	Image acquisition protocol should be clearly reported	Model clinical scanners realistically Follow clinical protocols
Extract task-specific information: Detection tasks	Preferably human observers	Use optimal observers operating on projection data for system optimization and anthropomorphic observers for applications that use reconstructed images
Extract task-specific information: Quantification tasks	Goal is estimating object properties, not image properties. Consider estimability and estimating properties directly from projection data.	
Figure of merit: Detection tasks	Sensitivity, specificity, ROC analysis, and AUC values	
Figure of merit: Quantification tasks	Consider population-based metrics, such as ensemble bias and variance (or bias and variance profiles), and EMSE, to quantify accuracy, precision and overall reliability of quantification.	

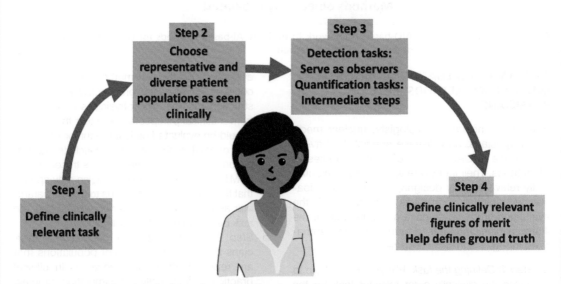

Fig. 6. A schematic showing the key role of physicians in task-based evaluation of AI methods.

physicians can help define the physical and statistical properties of the simulated population. In simulation-based evaluations, validating that the simulated and real images have similar distributions is important for clinically relevant evaluations. Observer studies with physicians can help to quantitatively evaluate this similarity.[46]

c. *Step 3: Extract task-specific information*: For a detection task conducted on reconstructed images, it is preferable if physicians can serve as observers. This point is true regardless of whether the images are simulated or real. Similarly, for quantitative tasks, physicians can assist in the intermediate steps. For example, for a PET reconstruction method being evaluated on the task of quantifying regional uptake, the physicians can delineate the boundaries of the different regions.

d. *Step 4: Figures of merit (FoMs)*: Physicians can help to define the most clinically relevant FoMs. For example, an ROC analysis is a comprehensive description of performance on detection tasks. However, in clinical practice, the AI method will operate at 1 point on the ROC curve with a certain sensitivity and specificity. Depending on the clinical application, sensitivity or specificity may be more important. Inputs from physicians can help to choose these specificity and sensitivity values for the clinical application. Further, when conducting clinical evaluation, the ground truth is typically not known. Sometimes multiple reference standards are needed in the same study. For example, for studies of breast cancer detection, biopsy might be used for subjects with suspicious lesions but 1-year follow-up would be the reference standard for those subjects without detected suspicious lesions. In other applications where no reference standards are available, a panel of 3 to 5 expert radiologists might serve as truthers, where each truther independently interprets the sample of images and makes the relevant measurements, blinded to the results of the AI algorithm and the other truthers. Then the results of the truthers can be averaged, using a priori defined rules, to create the reference standard. Reference standards from panelists may have uncertainties associated with them. Approaches have been proposed to obtain this uncertainty.[109] In fact, the approach proposed by Miller and colleagues [109] was used in the evaluation of the first FDA-approved computer-aided diagnosis algorithm for lung nodule detection. Physicians have an important role in defining these reference standards.

Imaging scientists developing AI-based methods for medical imaging should closely collaborate with physicians to ensure a clinically relevant and rigorous evaluation of these methods.

EXAMPLE EVALUATION STUDIES

In this section, we present examples of using the described OAIQ-based framework to evaluate hypothetical AI-based methods for 2 applications in PET, namely, data acquisition and image segmentation. Both of these examples are based on using realistic simulation studies. Readers are referred to recent studies using the OAIQ framework to objectively evaluate AI-based methods for 2 other important nuclear-medicine imaging applications, namely, reconstruction[55] and denoising.[31]

Evaluation of a Hypothetical Artificial Intelligence–Based Approach for Data Acquisition

AI-based methods for improving PET system instrumentation are showing much promise. For example, a convolutional neural network–based approach to estimate time-of-flight from PET detector waveforms yielded improved performance compared with existing methods.[110] Further, incorporating time-of-flight information has been shown to help improve performance on lesion-detection tasks.[111] In this section, we demonstrate the application of OAIQ to evaluate a hypothetical AI-based method for improving timing resolution in a time-of-flight PET system.

Definition of the task
The task is posed as detecting cardiac perfusion defects using myocardial perfusion PET, where the defect as well as the anatomy and physiologic uptake varies across the patient population. This leads to an SKS/BKS task.

Defining the patient population and imaging process
Realistic simulations using the tools outlined earlier provide a feasible mechanism to conduct this study.

Observer
Because the goal is system optimization, an optimal observer, such as the IO or optimal linear observers, should be used.

Figure of merit
ROC analysis and AUC would quantify performance on the defect-detection task.

Claim from the evaluation study

On the task of defect detection in myocardial perfusion PET for a SKS/BKS task, an AI-based approach to data acquisition yielded an increase in AUC from X (obtained without the AI approach) to Y, with a change of ΔZ (95% confidence intervals), as evaluated using a realistic simulation study with a channelized linear discriminant.[66]

Evaluation of a Hypothetical Artificial Intelligence–Based Tumor Segmentation Method

AI-based segmentation methods are showing significant promise in oncological PET, where they are being explored for tasks such as radiotherapy planning, and estimating quantitative features, such as MTV, total lesion glycolysis, and features that describe intratumor heterogeneity and shape. We consider the evaluation of a hypothetical AI-based oncological PET segmentation method on the task of quantifying MTV from FDG-PET images.

Defining the task

Measuring MTV of the primary tumors from FDG-PET images in patients with lung cancer.

Defining patient population and imaging process

Because segmentations are performed on reconstructed images, for clinical realism, it is important that the reconstruction protocol be similar to those in clinical settings. Further, it is important that aspects such as intratumor heterogeneity and tumor shape are realistically simulated.

Observer

To estimate the MTV for an OAIQ study, we recognize that tumors are continuous regions, whereas PET images are voxelized. Voxels in reconstructed images may contain a mixture of tumor and normal tissue. Thus, to estimate the MTV, we should preferably measure the volume that tumor occupies in each voxel.[83] MTV can then be computed as the sum of tumor fraction volumes within each voxel, multiplied by the volume of the voxel. However, if the segmentation method classifies each voxel as either tumor or background, then the MTV can be defined as the product of the number of tumor voxels and the volume of each voxel.

Figure of merit

MTV is being explored as a biomarker for separating patient populations into categories, for example, identifying patients likely to respond to therapy versus those who do not. Thus, if the bias is observed to be the same across the 2 populations, then standard deviation of the estimated MTV values may be a relevant FoM.

Claim from the evaluation study

An AI-based tumor segmentation method yielded MTV values that had an average normalized standard deviation of X (95% confidence intervals) in patients with stage III non-small cell lung cancer, as evaluated using a realistic simulation study.

DISCUSSIONS AND SUMMARY

The OAIQ framework provides a comprehensive and rigorous framework to objectively evaluate imaging systems and methods on performance in clinical tasks. Given the unique training-based nature of neural network-based AI methods, in this work we have outlined a fine-tuned OAIQ framework to evaluate these methods on performance in clinical tasks. In the process, we have highlighted factors that should be considered while designing the OAIQ study. Further, tools have been summarized to implement the concepts of this framework. Certain key factors to consider when designing OAIQ studies for AI-based methods are summarized in **Table 2**.

The OAIQ-based evaluation strategy quantifies method performance over populations, rather than a single individual. This, in addition to being clinically realistic and comprehensive, also allows the evaluation to study aspects such as generalizability of the approach to different patient populations and acquisition protocols. For example, if there is a method that claims to be generalizable across different age groups, step 2 of the OAIQ framework would require the method to include these different age groups in their patient population description, and use these to define the distribution of the patient images while extracting the task-specific information. The OAIQ framework can also evaluate methods for specific subsets of the population if the method is only suitable for that subset. Thus, the framework can help to generate appropriate claims on generalizability of the method. More generally, an OAIQ-based evaluation provides inputs to specify a descriptive and statistically rigorous claim for a method.

A focus in this article has been providing tools to conduct OAIQ-based evaluation *in silico* using a VCT framework, where the patient population, imaging system, and human observer are replaced by anthropomorphic phantoms, simulated systems, and model observers, respectively. One reason for the limited usage of task-based evaluation of imaging methods has been the perception that they always require expensive and time-consuming clinical studies with human observers. A reason that task-agnostic FoMs such as root mean square error and Dice scores are widely used in medical imaging is that they can be evaluated without requiring such studies. However, we note that OAIQ using a VCT framework can be performed relatively inexpensively and entirely *in silico* without having to address the logistical challenges associated with clinical studies. These studies can help to identify promising candidate methods for further clinical evaluation. We hope that the framework and methods provided in this article will stimulate wider task-based evaluation of AI methods using VCTs.

There are multiple areas of future research to improve OAIQ-based evaluation techniques. An important area is developing OAIQ-based methods for quantification tasks. Multiple important topics require investigation in this area. To begin with, current quantification methods operate on reconstructed images. However, it is recognized that such methods suffer from reconstruction-related information loss and have limited efficacy in modeling noise. Additionally, methods to quantify regional radiotracer uptake directly from projection data[79,81] have shown improved performance compared with reconstruction-based quantification. This factor motivates efforts to estimate other object parameters directly from projection data. Also, in estimation tasks, there is an important need to develop clinically relevant FoMs. Although FoMs such as bias, variance, and EMSE quantify the error between true and measured values, FoMs that quantify the impact of this error in making clinical decisions are needed. For example, if the objective using a quantitative method is separating patient populations into 2 categories, then that becomes a 2-class classification task, and FoMs that quantify performance on this task, such as an ROC analysis, may be more appropriate. Another example is FoMs for prediction, for example, evaluating and optimizing AI methods to maximize the hazard ratio in a Cox regression analysis to best stratify patients in terms of their outcome. Another area of research is developing observers for joint classification and quantification tasks. Clinically realistic quantification tasks typically have a detection step, so developing observers for these tasks would make the evaluation study even more clinically relevant.

Clinical task-based evaluation of AI-based methods is another exciting research frontier. Current evaluations of AI methods with clinical data are typically restricted to some measure of "goodness" of the image, as subjectively defined through closeness to some reference standard, noise properties, or ease of interpretability of the image. An OAIQ-based evaluation paradigm should instead focus on the evaluation of the clinical task. This area requires close collaborations between physicians and AI developers, as we outline in a previous section. Further Rubin[112] provides descriptive guidelines for the specific ways through which radiologists can get involved in evaluation of AI tools and other aspects of AI method development. The Society of Nuclear Medicine and Molecular Imaging AI taskforce is also composing a set of best practices for evaluation of AI methods.[33]

A key issue confronting the AI community is the inability of AI methods to generalize well to new unseen data. Models trained with 1 group of patients (say with a certain ethnicity) may underperform, or may even provide misleading results with other groups. The lack of interpretability in AI compounds this issue. Thus, when conducting OAIQ studies to evaluate AI methods, it is important that the patient populations chosen are representative and diverse as in clinical practice. This principle should also be followed when conducting OAIQ studies using VCTs. Here, an area that requires attention is developing techniques to ensure that the distributions of the digital phantom populations match those seen in clinical practice. In other words, it is not just important that the patient anatomies and physiologies are realistic for each patient, but that the distribution of these properties should also be realistic and representative. Developing methods that can generate such phantom populations and techniques that can evaluate clinical realism are important areas of future research.

SUMMARY

The elucidated objective assessment of image quality (OAIQ)-based framework presents a rigorous and comprehensive paradigm to evaluate the emerging AI-based imaging methods on clinically relevant tasks. Such evaluation will increase the confidence in the clinical usefulness of these methods and thus strengthen the potential for clinical translation. Our vision is that OAIQ-based virtual clinical trial (VCT) studies will identify promising AI-based methods for further clinical evaluation and then OAIQ-based clinical studies will help to evaluate these methods on clinical tasks. This process will provide trust in the clinical application of these methods, ultimately leading to improvements in quality of health care. Software to conduct task-based image quality evaluation studies is available at multiple locations such as the University of Arizona Image quality toolbox and the Metz ROC software at the University of Chicago.

ACKNOWLEDGMENTS

The authors thank Richard Wahl, MD, Craig Abbey, PhD, Prabhat K.C., PhD, Paul Kinahan, PhD, Charles Ross Schmidtlein, PhD and Ronald Boellaard, PhD for helpful discussions and the anonymous reviewers for their review.

DISCLOSURE

Nancy Obuchowski is a statistician for the Quantitative Imaging Biomarkers Alliance (QIBA). Other authors have no relevant financial disclosures.

REFERENCES

1. Arabi H, AkhavanAllaf A, Sanaat A, et al. The promise of artificial intelligence and deep learning in PET and SPECT imaging. Phys Med 2021;83: 122–37.
2. Ding Y, Sohn JH, Kawczynski MG, et al. A deep learning model to predict a diagnosis of Alzheimer disease by using (18)F-FDG PET of the brain. Radiology 2019;290(2):456–64.
3. Reader AJ, Corda G, Mehranian A, et al. Deep learning for PET image reconstruction. IEEE Trans Radiat Plasma Med Sci 2021;5(1):1–25.
4. Food and Drug Administration. Proposed regulatory framework for modifications to artificial intelligence/Machine learning (AI/ML)-based software as a medical Device (SaMD). Department of Health and Human Services (United States); 2019.
5. Zech JR, Badgeley MA, Liu M, et al. Variable generalization performance of a deep learning model to detect pneumonia in chest radiographs: a cross-sectional study. Plos Med 2018;15(11): e1002683.
6. Pan I, Agarwal S, Merck D. Generalizable inter-institutional classification of abnormal chest radiographs using efficient convolutional neural networks. J Digit Imaging 2019;32(5):888–96.
7. Narla A, Kuprel B, Sarin K, et al. Automated classification of skin lesions: from pixels to practice. J Invest Dermatol 2018;138(10):2108–10.
8. Winkler JK, Fink C, Toberer F, et al. Association between surgical skin markings in dermoscopic images and diagnostic performance of a deep learning convolutional neural network for melanoma Recognition. JAMA Dermatol 2019;155(10): 1135–41.
9. DeGrave AJ, Janizek JD, Lee S-I. AI for radiographic COVID-19 detection selects shortcuts over signal. Nat Mach Intell 2021. https://doi.org/ 10.1101/2020.09.13.20193565.
10. Weisman AJ, Kim J, Lee I, et al. Automated quantification of baseline imaging PET metrics on FDG PET/CT images of pediatric Hodgkin lymphoma patients. EJNMMI Phys 2020;7(1):76.
11. Wei L, El Naqa I. Artificial intelligence for response evaluation with PET/CT. Semin Nucl Med 2021; 51(2):157–69.
12. Barrett HH. Is there a role for image science in the brave new world of artificial intelligence? J Med Imag 2019;7(1):1–6.
13. Wu E, Wu K, Daneshjou R, et al. How medical AI devices are evaluated: limitations and recommendations from an analysis of FDA approvals. Nat Med 2021;27(4):582–4.
14. Gaube S, Suresh H, Raue M, et al. Do as AI say: susceptibility in deployment of clinical decision-aids. Npj Digit Med 2021;4(1):31.
15. van Leeuwen KG, Schalekamp S, Rutten MJCM, et al. Artificial intelligence in radiology: 100 commercially available products and their scientific evidence. Eur Rad 2021;31(6):3797–804.
16. Yang J, Sohn JH, Behr SC, et al. CT-less Direct correction of attenuation and scatter in the image space using deep learning for whole-body FDG PET: potential benefits and pitfalls. Radiol AI 2020;3(2):e200137.
17. Yu Z, Rahman M, Schindler T, et al. AI-based methods for nuclear-medicine imaging: need for objective task-specific evaluation. J Nucl Med 2020;61(supplement 1):575.
18. Prabhat KC, Zeng R, Farhangi MM, et al. Deep neural networks-based denoising models for CT imaging and their efficacy. Proc. SPIE Med Imag 2021;11595, 115950H.
19. Kelkar VA, Zhang X, Granstedt J, et al. Task-based evaluation of deep image super-resolution in medical imaging. Proc. SPIE Med Imag 2021; 11599: 115990X.
20. Li K, Zhou W, Li H, et al. Task-based performance evaluation of deep neural network-based image denoising. Proc. SPIE Med Imag 2021; 11599: 115990L.
21. Zhu Y, Yousefirizi F, Liu Z, et al. Comparing clinical evaluation of PET segmentation methods with reference-based metrics and no-gold-standard evaluation technique. J Nucl Med 2021; 62(supplement 1):1430.
22. Barrett HH, Wilson DW, Kupinski MA, et al. Therapy operating characteristic (TOC) curves and their application to the evaluation of segmentation algorithms. Proc SPIE Med Imag 2010;7627: 76270Z.
23. Barrett HH. Objective assessment of image quality: effects of quantum noise and object variability. J Opt Soc Am A 1990;7:1266–78.
24. Barrett HH, Abbey CK, Clarkson E. Objective assessment of image quality. III. ROC metrics, ideal observers, and likelihood-generating functions. J Opt Soc Am A Opt Image Sci Vis 1998; 15:1520–35.
25. Barrett HH, Denny JL, Wagner RF, et al. Objective assessment of image quality. II. Fisher information,

Fourier crosstalk, and figures of merit for task performance. J Opt Soc Am A Opt Image Sci Vis 1995;12:834–52.

26. Barrett HH, Myers KJ, Hoeschen C, et al. Task-based measures of image quality and their relation to radiation dose and patient risk. Phys Med Biol 2015;60(2):R1–75.

27. Barrett HH, Myers KJ. Foundations of image science, vol. 1. John Wiley & Sons; 2003.

28. Gifford HC, Kinahan PE, Kinahan PE, et al. Evaluation of Multiclass model observers in PET LROC studies. IEEE Trans Nucl Sci 2007;54:116–23.

29. Rahmim A, Tang J. Noise propagation in resolution modeled PET imaging and its impact on detectability. Phys Med Biol 2013;58(19):6945–68.

30. Kadrmas DJ, Casey ME, Conti M, et al. Impact of time-of-flight on PET tumor detection. J Nucl Med 2009;50(8):1315–23.

31. Yu Z, Rahman MA, Laforest R, et al. A physics and learning-based transmission-less attenuation compensation method for SPECT. Proc. SPIE Med Imag 2021; 11595: 1159512.

32. Obuchowski NA, Buckler A, Kinahan P, et al. Statistical issues in testing conformance with the quantitative imaging biomarker alliance (QIBA) profile claims. Acad Radiol 2016;23(4):496–506.

33. Jha AK, et al. Nuclear medicine in artificial intelligence: best practices for evaluation. In: SNMMI AI Taskforce; in preparation.

34. Frey EC, Gilland KL, Tsui BM. Application of task-based measures of image quality to optimization and evaluation of three-dimensional reconstruction-based compensation methods in myocardial perfusion SPECT. IEEE Trans Med Imaging 2002; 21:1040–50.

35. Meikle SR, Badawi RD. Quantitative techniques in PET. In: Bailey DL, Townsend DW, Valk PE, et al, editors. Positron emission tomography: basic sciences. London: Springer London; 2005. p. 93–126.

36. Mhlanga JC, Chirindel A, Lodge MA, et al. Quantitative PET/CT in clinical practice: assessing the agreement of PET tumor indices using different clinical reading platforms. Nucl Med Commun 2018;39(2):154–60.

37. Wahl RL, Jacene H, Kasamon Y, et al. From RECIST to PERCIST: evolving Considerations for PET response criteria in solid tumors. J Nucl Med 2009;50(Suppl 1):122s–50s.

38. Li Z, Benabdallah N, Abou D, et al. A projection-domain quantification method for absolute quantification with low-count SPECT for alpha-particle radiopharmaceutical therapy. J Nucl Med 2021; 62(supplement 1):1539.

39. Bentourkia M, Zaidi H. Tracer kinetic modeling in PET. PET Clin 2007;2(2):267–77.

40. Li T, Ao ECI, Lambert B, et al. Quantitative imaging for targeted radionuclide therapy Dosimetry - technical review. Theranostics 2017;7(18):4551–65.

41. Clarkson E. Estimation receiver operating characteristic curve and ideal observers for combined detection/estimation tasks. J Opt Soc Am A Opt Image Sci Vis 2007;24(12):B91–8.

42. Abadi E, Segars WP, Tsui BMW, et al. Virtual clinical trials in medical imaging: a review. J Med Imaging (Bellingham) 2020;7(4):042805.

43. Badano A, Graff CG, Badal A, et al. Evaluation of digital breast tomosynthesis as replacement of full-field digital mammography using an in silico imaging trial. JAMA Netw Open 2018;1(7):e185474.

44. Kainz W, Neufeld E, Bolch WE, et al. Advances in computational human phantoms and their applications in biomedical engineering - a topical review. IEEE Trans Radiat Plasma Med Sci 2019;3(1):1–23.

45. Segars WP, Sturgeon G, Mendonca S, et al. 4D XCAT phantom for multimodality imaging research. Med Phys 2010;37(9):4902–15.

46. Leung KH, Marashdeh W, Wray R, et al. A physics-guided modular deep-learning based automated framework for tumor segmentation in PET. Phys Med Biol 2020;65(24):245032.

47. Liu Z, Laforest R, Mhlanga J, et al. Observer study-based evaluation of a stochastic and physics-based method to generate oncological PET images. Proc SPIE Med Imag 2021; 11599: 1159905.

48. Kupinski MA, Clarkson E, Hoppin JW, et al. Experimental determination of object statistics from noisy images. J Opt Soc Am A Opt Image Sci Vis 2003; 20(3):421–9.

49. Zhou W, Bhadra S, Brooks F, et al. Learning stochastic object model from noisy imaging measurements using AmbientGANs Proc. SPIE Med Imag 2021; 10952: 109520M.

50. Hatt M, Cheze le Rest C, Descourt P, et al. Accurate automatic delineation of heterogeneous functional volumes in positron emission tomography for oncology applications. Int J Radiat Oncol Biol Phys 2010;77(1):301–8.

51. Stute S, Carlier T, Cristina K, et al. Monte Carlo simulations of clinical PET and SPECT scans: impact of the input data on the simulated images. Phys Med Biol 2011;56(19):6441–57.

52. Jha AK, Barrett HH, Frey EC, et al. Singular value decomposition for photon-processing nuclear imaging systems and applications for reconstruction and computing null functions. Phys Med Biol 2015;60(18):7359–85.

53. Jan S, Santin G, Strul D, et al. GATE: a simulation toolkit for PET and SPECT. Phys Med Biol 2004; 49(19):4543–61.

54. Barret O, Carpenter TA, Clark JC, et al. Monte Carlo simulation and scatter correction of the GE

advance PET scanner with SimSET and Geant4. Phys Med Biol 2005;50(20):4823–40.

55. España S, Herraiz JL, Vicente E, et al. PeneloPET, a Monte Carlo PET simulation tool based on PENELOPE: features and validation. Phys Med Biol 2009;54(6):1723–42.

56. Elston B, Comtat C, Harrison RL, et al. ASIM: an analytic PET simulator. Monte Carlo calculations in nuclear medicine: applications in diagnostic imaging. 2017:201-220.

57. Pfaehler E, De Jong JR, Dierckx RAJO, et al. SMART (SiMulAtion and ReconsTruction) PET: an efficient PET simulation-reconstruction tool. EJNMMI Phys 2018;5(1):16.

58. Barrett HH, Yao J, Rolland JP, et al. Model observers for assessment of image quality. Proc Natl Acad Sci U S A 1993;90(21):9758–65.

59. He X, Park S. Model observers in medical imaging research. Theranostics 2013;3(10):774–86.

60. Park S, Kupinski MA, Clarkson E, et al. Ideal-Observer Performance under Signal and Background Uncertainty. Biennial International Conference on Information Processing in Medical Imaging 2003. Springer, Berlin, Heidelberg .pp. 342-353.

61. Zhou W, Li H, Anastasio MA. Approximating the ideal observer and Hotelling observer for binary signal detection tasks by use of supervised learning methods. IEEE Trans Med Imaging 2019; 38(10):2456–68.

62. Clarkson E, Shen F. Fisher information and surrogate figures of merit for the task-based assessment of image quality. J Opt Soc Am A Opt Image Sci Vis 2010;27(10):2313–26.

63. Jha AK, Clarkson E, Kupinski MA. An ideal-observer framework to investigate signal detectability in diffuse optical imaging. Biomed Opt Express 2013; 4(10):2107–23.

64. Eckstein MP, Abbey CK. Model observers for signal-known-statistically tasks (SKS). Proc. SPIE Med Imag 2001;4324: 91-102.

65. Eckstein MP, Pham B, Abbey CK. Effect of image compression for model and human observers in signal-known-statistically tasks. Proc. SPIE Med Imag 2002; 4686: 13-24.

66. Li X, Jha AK, Ghaly M, et al. Use of sub-ensembles and multi-template observers to evaluate detection task performance for data that are not multivariate normal. IEEE Trans Med Imaging 2017;36(4): 917–29.

67. Myers KJ, Barrett HH. Addition of a channel mechanism to the ideal-observer model. J Opt Soc Am A 1987;4(12):2447–57.

68. Gallas BD, Barrett HH. Validating the use of channels to estimate the ideal linear observer. JOSA A 20.9 2003;1725–38.

69. Barrett HH, Abbey CK, Gallas BD, et al. Stabilized estimates of Hotelling-observer detection performance in patient-structured noise. Proc. SPIE Med Imag 1998;3340:27–43.

70. Elshahaby FE, Ghaly M, Jha AK, et al. Factors affecting the normality of channel outputs of channelized model observers: an investigation using realistic myocardial perfusion SPECT images. J Med Imaging (Bellingham) 2016;3(1):015503.

71. Gifford HC, King MA, de Vries DJ, et al. Channelized hotelling and human observer correlation for lesion detection in hepatic SPECT imaging. J Nucl Med 2000;41(3):514–21.

72. Obuchowski NA, Beiden SV, Berbaum KS, et al. Multireader, multicase receiver operating characteristic analysis: an empirical comparison of five methods. Acad Radiol 2004;11(9):980–95.

73. Zhou X-H, McClish DK, Obuchowski NA. Statistical methods in diagnostic medicine, vol. 569. John Wiley & Sons; 2009.

74. Abbey CK, Barrett HH. Human- and model-observer performance in ramp-spectrum noise: effects of regularization and object variability. J Opt Soc Am A Opt Image Sci Vis 2001;18(3): 473–88.

75. Sen A, Kalantari F, Gifford HC. Task equivalence for model and human-observer comparisons in SPECT localization studies. IEEE Trans Nucl Sci 2016; 63(3):1426–34.

76. Gifford HC, Liang Z, Das M. Visual-search observers for assessing tomographic x-ray image quality. Med Phys 2016;43(3):1563–75.

77. Li Y, Chen J, Brown J, et al. DeepAMO: a multi-slice, multi-view anthropomorphic model observer for visual detection tasks performed on volume images. J Med Imaging 2021;8(4):041204.

78. Nyflot MJ, Yang F, Byrd D, et al. Quantitative radiomics: impact of stochastic effects on textural feature analysis implies the need for standards, J. Med. Imag. 2(4) 041002.

79. Jha AK, Frey EC. Estimating ROI activity concentration with photon-processing and photon-counting SPECT imaging systems. Proc SPIE Med Imag 2015;9412:94120r.

80. Clarkson E, Kupinski M. Quantifying the loss of information from binning list-mode data. J Opt Soc Am A Opt Image Sci Vis 2020;37(3):450–7.

81. Carson RE. A maximum likelihood method for region-of-interest evaluation in emission tomography. J Computer Assisted Tomography 1986;10(4):654–63.

82. Trees HLV. Detection, estimation, and modulation theory: radar-sonar signal processing and Gaussian signals in noise. Krieger Publishing Co., Inc.; 1992.

83. Liu Z, Mhlanga JC, Laforest R, et al. A Bayesian approach to tissue-fraction estimation for oncological PET segmentation. Phys Med Biol 2021;66(12). https://doi.org/10.1088/1361-6560/ac01f4.

84. Lin A, Kupinski MA, Peterson TE, et al. Task-based design of a synthetic-collimator SPECT system

used for small animal imaging. Med Phys 2018; 45(7):2952–63.

85. Whitaker MK, Clarkson E, Barrett HH. Estimating random signal parameters from noisy images with nuisance parameters: linear and scanning-linear methods. Opt Express 2008;16:8150–73.

86. Zhang L, Cavaro-Menard C, Le Callet P, et al. A perceptually relevant channelized joint observer (PCJO) for the detection-localization of parametric signals. IEEE Trans Med Imaging 2012;31(10): 1875–88.

87. Zhang L, Goossens B, Cavaro-Ménard C, et al. Channelized model observer for the detection and estimation of signals with unknown amplitude, orientation, and size. J Opt Soc Am A Opt Image Sci Vis 2013;30(11):2422–32.

88. Goossens B, Luong H, Platiša L, et al. Objectively measuring signal detectability, contrast, blur and noise in medical images using channelized joint observers. Proc. SPIE Med Imag 2013; 8673:86730J.

89. Tseng H-W, Fan J, Kupinski MA. Combination of detection and estimation tasks using channelized scanning linear observer for CT imaging systems. Proc. SPIE Med Imag 2015;9416: 94160H.

90. Li K, Zhou W, Li H, et al. Supervised learning-based ideal observer approximation for joint detection and estimation tasks Proc. SPIE Med Imag, 11599. SPIE; 2021. p. 115990F.

91. Metz CE. Receiver operating characteristic analysis: a tool for the quantitative evaluation of observer performance and imaging systems. J Am Coll Radiol 2006;3(6):413–22.

92. He X, Gallas BD, Frey EC. Three-class ROC analysis–toward a general decision theoretic solution. IEEE Trans Med Imaging 2010;29(1):206–15.

93. Mossman D. Three-way ROCs. Med Decis Making 1999;19(1):78–89.

94. Kijewski MF, Swensson RG, Judy PF. Analysis of rating data from multiple-alternative tasks. J Math Psychol 1989;33(4):428–51.

95. Obuchowski NA. Estimating and comparing diagnostic tests' accuracy when the gold standard is not binary. Acad Radiol 2005;12(9):1198–204.

96. Obuchowski NA, Goske MJ, Applegate KE. Assessing physicians' accuracy in diagnosing paediatric patients with acute abdominal pain: measuring accuracy for multiple diseases. Stat Med 2001;20(21):3261–78.

97. Kessler LG, Barnhart HX, Buckler AJ, et al. The emerging science of quantitative imaging biomarkers terminology and definitions for scientific studies and regulatory submissions. Stat Methods Med Res 2015;24(1):9–26.

98. Raunig DL, McShane LM, Pennello G, et al. Quantitative imaging biomarkers: a review of statistical methods for technical performance assessment. Stat Methods Med Res 2015;24(1):27–67.

99. Obuchowski NA, Reeves AP, Huang EP, et al. Quantitative imaging biomarkers: a review of statistical methods for computer algorithm comparisons. Stat Methods Med Res 2015;24(1):68–106.

100. Hoppin JW, Kupinski MA, Kastis GA, et al. Objective comparison of quantitative imaging modalities without the use of a gold standard. IEEE Trans Med Imaging 2002;21(5):441–9.

101. Kupinski MA, Hoppin JW, Clarkson E, et al. Estimation in medical imaging without a gold standard. Acad Radiol 2002;9(3):290–7.

102. Jha AK, Caffo B, Frey EC. A no-gold-standard technique for objective assessment of quantitative nuclear-medicine imaging methods. Phys Med Biol 2016;61(7):2780–800.

103. Liu J, Liu Z, Moon HS, et al. A no-gold-standard technique for objective evaluation of quantitative nuclear-medicine imaging methods in the presence of correlated noise. J Nucl Med 2020; 61(supplement 1):523.

104. Jha AK, Kupinski MA, Rodriguez JJ, et al. Task-based evaluation of segmentation algorithms for diffusion-weighted MRI without using a gold standard. Phys Med Biol 2013;57(13):4425. https://doi.org/10.1088/0031-9155/57/13/4425.

105. Jha AK, Kupinski MA, Rodriguez JJ, et al. Corrigendum: task-based evaluation of segmentation algorithms for diffusion-weighted MRI without using a gold standard. Phys Med Biol 2013;58(1):183.

106. Lebenberg J, Buvat I, Lalande A, et al. Nonsupervised ranking of different segmentation approaches: application to the estimation of the left ventricular ejection fraction from cardiac cine MRI sequences. IEEE Trans Med Imaging 2012;31(8):1651–60. https://doi.org/10.1109/TMI.2012.2201737.

107. Jha AK, Mena E, Caffo B, et al. Practical no-gold-standard evaluation framework for quantitative imaging methods: application to lesion segmentation in positron emission tomography. J Med Imaging (Bellingham) 2017;4(1):011011.

108. Zhu Y, Liu Z, Bilgel M, et al. No-gold-standard evaluation of partial volume compensation methods for brain PET. J Nucl Med 2021;62(supplement 1):1409.

109. Miller DP, O'shaughnessy KF, Wood SA, et al. Gold standards and expert panels: a pulmonary nodule case study with challenges and solutions. Proc SPIE Med Imag 2004;5372: 173-184.

110. Berg E, Cherry SR. Using convolutional neural networks to estimate time-of-flight from PET detector waveforms. Phys Med Biol 2018;63(2):02LT01.

111. El Fakhri G, Surti S, Trott CM, et al. Improvement in lesion detection with whole-body oncologic time-of-flight PET. J Nucl Med 2011;52(3):347–53. https://doi.org/10.2967/jnumed.110.080382.

112. Rubin DL. Artificial intelligence in imaging: the radiologist's role. J Am Coll Radiol 2019;16(9 Pt B): 1309–17.

Artificial Intelligence and the Future of Diagnostic and Therapeutic Radiopharmaceutical Development:
In Silico Smart Molecular Design

Bahar Ataeinia, MD, MPH, Pedram Heidari, MD*

KEYWORDS

- Artificial intelligence • Computer-aided drug design • In silico • Positron emission tomography
- Radiopharmaceuticals

KEY POINTS

- Artificial intelligence is a novel way to develop new radiopharmaceuticals.
- Artificial intelligence methods enable designing lead radiotracers with favorable pharmacokinetics and pharmacodynamics.
- Using artificial intelligence methods decreases the time and costs of radiopharmaceutical development.
- Artificial intelligence does not obviate the need for in vivo testing of the lead compounds, given that the accuracy of the methods is greatly affected by the assumptions put in the models.
- Radiopharmaceuticals developed by artificial intelligence have a wide range of applications including central nervous system, cancer, infection, and inflammation imaging.

INTRODUCTION

Radiopharmaceuticals play a pivotal role in the rapidly emerging field of personalized medicine.[1] In disease states, altered expression or aggregation of specific molecules allow for noninvasive diagnosis and/or targeted radiotherapy using radiopharmaceuticals.[2–4] Thus, the development of new radiopharmaceuticals is key to improved diagnosis and therapy in a broader range of diseases. However, the design, validation, and translation of these compounds are time consuming and require considerable effort and financial investment.[5,6]

A translatable radiopharmaceutical has structural and functional characteristics that result in high affinity for its target, low nonspecific binding, and favorable pharmacokinetics. Whether the structure of a compound is novel or similar to an existing compound, substantial effort is required to ensure optimal radiopharmaceutical performance. Despite all the care in designing a compound, there is high likelihood that it fails to adequately engage its target in vivo, owing to unpredicted parameters that were not considered during the development phase.[7]

The term "in silico medicine" refers to using computer modeling and simulation for conducting biomedical research. In silico approaches can predict outcomes for crucial variables that are quite taxing by conventional in vitro and in vivo radiopharmaceutical development methods.[7,8]

Funded by: NIH. Grant number(s): K08CA249047.
Department of Radiology, Massachusetts General Hospital, 55 Fruit St, Wht 427, Boston, MA 02114, USA
* Corresponding author.
E-mail address: pheidari@mgh.harvard.edu

PET Clin 16 (2021) 513–523
https://doi.org/10.1016/j.cpet.2021.06.008
1556-8598/21/© 2021 Elsevier Inc. All rights reserved.

Computational models can predict target-binding properties of a compound, and critical pharmacokinetic characteristics such as absorption, distribution, metabolism, excretion, and toxicity (ADMET).[9] Therefore, incorporation of in silico methods could facilitate faster and more cost-effective design and testing of new radiopharmaceuticals, by informing in vitro and in vivo studies, which decreases the need for animal models to evaluate the lead compounds.[10–14]

Artificial intelligence (AI) methods have been used to improve drug discovery since the 1990s.[15] With ever growing rapid expansion of our knowledge about the structure and function of biological targets, AI can expedite radiopharmaceutical design research, resulting in more rapid incorporation of these compounds in routine medical practice (**Fig. 1**).[16–18] It is important to note that computational modeling is not a replacement for in-laboratory experiments, but rather a complementary tool that facilitates radiopharmaceutical development; currently, no modeling can emulate the complexity of human body.[12,19]

Herein, we summarize the current computer-aided drug design methods, their potential application, and challenges in radiopharmaceutical development research, and provide real-world examples of radiopharmaceutical design using the input from computer-aided drug design methods.

APPROACH

In general, in silico approaches focus on structure and behavior of compounds for modeling (**Fig. 2**). Structural models predict binding affinity of a radiopharmaceutical for its target, while behavioral approaches focus on its pharmacokinetics. Both approaches are complementary and essential because a translatable radiopharmaceutical should have high specificity and affinity for the target, optimal biodistribution, stability, practical effective half-life and a desirable clearance kinetic based on its intended diagnostic or therapeutic applications.[20]

Structure-based computational modeling approaches are classified into 2 main categories, structure-based drug design (SBDD) and ligand-based drug design (LBDD). SBDD is used to predict radiopharmaceutical–target interaction when the structure of the target is known. For instance, chemical structure of some of the most studied targets such as prostate-specific membrane antigen and chemokine receptor-4 is known and can be used for modeling in SBDD.[21,22] If the structure of the target is not available, LBDD models can be used, which analyze the structure of known ligands for the target (**Fig. 3**).[12,23,24] Here we discuss structural and behavioral approaches in more detail.

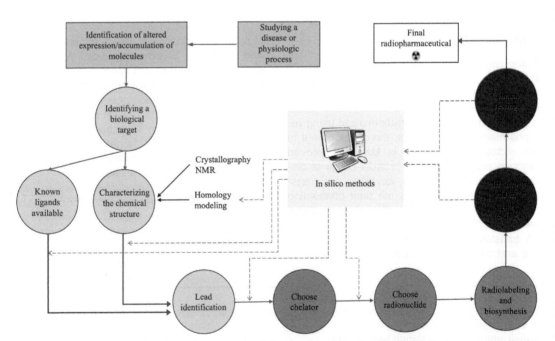

Fig. 1. Incorporation of in silico drug design methods in routine approach toward developing novel radiopharmaceuticals for unmet clinical needs. NMR, nuclear magnetic resonance.

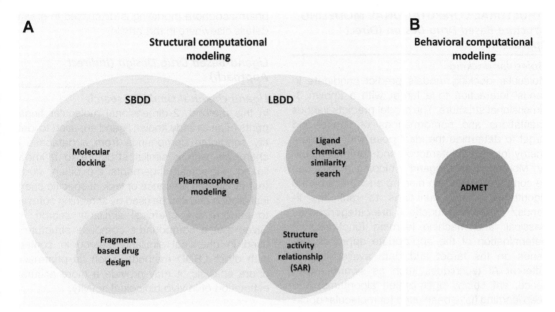

Fig. 2. Categories of computer-aided drug design methods. (*A*) Structural computational modeling. (*B*) Behavioral computational modeling. LBDD, ligand-based drug design; SBDD, structure-based drug design.

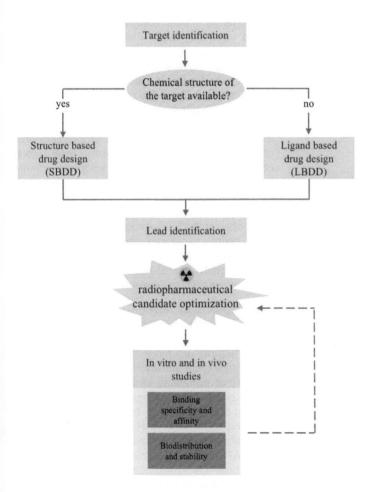

Fig. 3. Basic workflow of structural computational modeling techniques in radiopharmaceutical design and optimization.

STRUCTURAL COMPUTATIONAL MODELING
Structure-Based Drug Design (Direct Approach)

Molecular docking
Molecular docking models predict candidate ligands' interaction to a target with a known 3-dimensional structure. The model predicts various orientations and conformations of ligand and target to determine the ideal pose with minimum energy for best fit interaction and complex stability. Moreover, each ligand's binding affinity can be computed based on binding energetics by the algorithm's scoring functions to rank the ligands.[25,26] Scoring functions are categorized as classical, and machine learning functions.[27,28] Determination of the appropriate approach depends on the target and data availability.[25,29] Different AI techniques such as swarm intelligence, ant colony optimization algorithms, and deep learning have been used for molecular docking.[30–32] Selecting the most appropriate software and scoring function is a critical step and can significantly affect outcomes.[33] Docking models cannot be used reliably if the chemical structure of the ligand or the specific binding site are unknown, unless protein homology modeling and binding site identification is performed before docking.[34–36] Molecular docking models are commonly used in radiopharmaceutical development studies to predict the effect of labeling with different radionuclides and chelators on ligand's binding affinity to the target.[37–41]

Fragment-based drug design
Fragment-based drug design is an alternative for the modeling of compounds with a high molecular weight and low solubility. In fragment-based drug design, low-molecular-weight fragments that interact with biological targets are first identified and appropriate fragments are then expanded by adding chemical groups or merging with other fragments to design the final compound.[42,43]

Pharmacophore modeling
Pharmacophore analysis is applicable in both SBDD and LBDD, although it is used more commonly with LBDD. This method mainly focuses on the molecular features important for the target–ligand interaction. Such features include hydrophobic groups, aromatic rings, polar groups, and hydrogen bond vectors.[23,44] Structure-based pharmacophore modeling is an SBDD pharmacophore analysis that is used if the 3-dimensional structure of the target is known. The model can include structural properties of both target and ligand or the target exclusively.[45,46] LBDD

pharmacophore modeling is discussed in greater details elsewhere in this article.

Ligand-Based Drug Design (Indirect Approach)

Ligand chemical similarity search
In this method, 2-dimensional molecular fingerprints of an already known ligand are used to identify candidate compounds from a database of chemicals with a similar structure to a known ligand. Molecular fingerprints are binary codes that record the presence or lack of specific chemical groups and can be used by screening software to perform the chemical similarity search.[23,47] Given that a compound's complete structure is used in chemical similarity search in contrast with other LBDD methods, such as pharmacophore analysis, it may provide a more accurate estimation of in vivo biological activity.

Pharmacophore analysis
As mentioned elsewhere in this article, pharmacophore analysis incorporates crucial features for ligand–target interaction into the model. Initially, a wide range of biologically active ligands is studied to train the model. The main 2 goals are to distinguish overlapping structures for optimal ligand–target interaction and create conformational space for the studied ligands to determine structural flexibility in the model. However, there are several challenges in designing a pharmacophore model, including the modeling of ligand flexibility, molecular alignment, and proper selection of training set compounds, which is even more challenging in designing radiopharmaceuticals.[23,44] Even when a radionuclide is added to the backbone structure and not the active binding site, it can alter the radiopharmaceutical's biological behavior.[48–53] Pharmacophore analyses are used mainly to screen potential ligands or to design a new radiopharmaceutical.[44] Pharmacophore models can also be used in SBDD approaches as discussed elsewhere in this article.

Structure–activity relationships analysis
Structure–activity relationship (SAR) is based on the assumption that molecules with similar chemical structures are more likely to demonstrate a similar biological activity.[54,55] Using a regression model that correlates structural properties of a known group of similar ligands to their biological activity, such as binding to the desired target or inhibiting an enzyme, SAR can predict a pharmaceutical's biological behavior.[56] Quantitative SAR is an SAR that quantifies bioactivity level of a pharmaceutical. Using artificial neural networks and deep learning algorithms, quantitative SAR has

been used for drug design.[15,57] The crucial step in SAR is carefully choosing molecular properties used in the regression model to avoid overfitting. An overfitted model has optimal performance on the training dataset, but fails when used on new data.[15] Note should be made that structural similarity does not necessarily imply similar activity, indicating the need for cautious use of this assumption given the complexity of in vivo biochemical interactions.[58] SAR models can predict whether adding chelators, radionuclides, or chemical groups to a bioactive compound will alter the binding properties and potency of the proposed radiopharmaceutical or cause undesired interactions leading to toxicity or off-target binding.[59]

BEHAVIORAL COMPUTATIONAL MODELING

ADMET modeling is used to predict the ligand's in vivo behavior based on the pharmacokinetics of similar ligands and modeling the interaction of the candidate compound with enzymes involved in toxicity, insolubility, and undesired metabolism.[60] Inputs from SBDD models and SAR, as well as other in silico approaches, are used to predict ADMET characteristics.[61] A fundamental step to ensure optimal accuracy of ADMET models is using a chemically diverse dataset of ligands to train the model.[62]

In addition to proper target specificity and affinity, a translatable radiopharmaceutical should have appropriate pharmacokinetics and stability for optimal performance in vivo. Even slight alterations in radiopharmaceutical structure, such as changes in chelator and linker, can still dramatically affect biodistribution and stability. Hence, using computational ADMET modeling before in vivo experiments can help to predict serum stability and target organ uptake.[63] Absorption is often not an issue for radiopharmaceuticals because they are generally administered intravenously. In certain situations such as targeting a receptor in the central nervous system or an intracellular target, ADMET algorithms can be additionally beneficial to model the passage of a radiopharmaceutical through these natural barriers.[7,13,14,64] ADMET models can also help to predict the effect of individual components of the radiopharmaceutical on the overall pharmacokinetics. In this regard, using computer-aided drug design models, one can alter the design of a radiopharmaceutical to improve the pharmacokinetics without adversely affecting the binding affinity to the target.[65] This strategy has been implemented successfully for radiolabeled analogs of somatostatin, integrins, bombesin, cholecystokinin, and vasoactive intestinal peptide analogues. Lastly, ADMET can help in ensuring that the radiopharmaceutical has minimal toxicity, especially if the ligand is not a naturally occurring molecule or an established pharmaceutical.[66]

APPLICATIONS

To date, molecular docking, SAR, and ADMET models are the most commonly used approaches in radiopharmaceutical development. These methods can predict a bioactive compound's interaction with its target after radiolabeling and whether altering radionuclides and chelators affects radiopharmaceutical's performance (see **Fig. 1**). In this section, we review some of the applications of these methods in radiopharmaceutical design in caner, neurologic disorders, and other disease processes.

Cancer

Radiopharmaceuticals are used extensively for imaging various nodes in cancer pathways. One common approach is radiolabeling chemotherapy agents to study their pharmacokinetics and their ability to engage the target in the tumor. Molecular docking models have been used to ensure that the addition of a chelator or a radionuclide does not adversely affect the binding affinity to the target. For instance, a recent study investigated ^{99m}technetium (^{99m}Tc)-labeled ifosfamide, an alkylating chemotherapy agent, for solid tumor imaging. Molecular docking showed that ^{99m}Tc labeling did not affect the radiotracer's affinity for the binding site.[38] A similar approach was used with iodine-labeled cladribine, a chlorinated purine analogue, showing that its binding affinity to DNA polymerase was not changed.[67] Another example of using molecular docking is to evaluate effect of changing chelators on binding properties of a commonly used radiopharmaceutical. For instance, Cai and colleagues[68] showed that the in vivo binding affinity of a somatostatin receptor subtype 2 agonist was not affected by using a new generation of chelators for ^{64}copper (^{64}Cu) (**Fig. 4**).

Some studies used a combination of approaches to develop radiopharmaceuticals targeting receptors or enzymes, overexpressed by cancer cells or other cells in tumor microenvironment. An example is development of PET tracers for imaging focal adhesion kinase, a tyrosine kinase overexpressed in a number of cancers. Inputs from molecular docking and molecular dynamics were used to ensure binding of designed inhibitory tracers to focal adhesion kinase as well as the effect of structural modifications, such as altering chain length on inhibitory

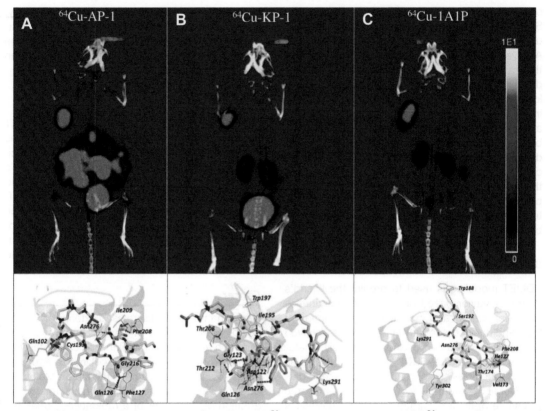

Fig. 4. Top) Small animal PET/CT images of 3 probes. (*A*) ^{64}Cu-AP-1 (SUV= 4.6 0.8) and (*B*) ^{64}Cu-KP-1 (SUV= 3.2 0.2) were developed with a new chelator and labeling approach compared with (*C*) [64]Cu-1A1P (SUV= 2.8 0.4), a probe with a first generation chelator. Tumor uptake was only modestly affected by chelator modification, as predicted by molecular docking of each probe in lower panel. However, the biodistribution of the probe was completely altered as shown in PET images. (*Adapted from* Cai Z, Ouyang Q, Zeng D, et al. 64Cu-labeled somatostatin analogues conjugated with cross-bridged phosphonate-based chelators via strain-promoted click chemistry for PET imaging: in silico through in vivo studies. *J Med Chem.* 2014;57(14):6019-6029;with permission. (Figures available at link: https://pubs.acs.org/doi/10.1021/jm500416f. Further permission related to the material excerpted should be directed to the publisher.).)

potency of designed compounds.[69–71] Similar approach was used for targeting gamma glutamyl transferase and human farnesyl pyrophosphate synthase.[72,73]

Central Nervous System

Developing radiopharmaceuticals for imaging different receptors, enzymes, and pathologic aggregates in the central nervous system has been of great interest and an area of intense research. In addition to specificity for the target, a potent radiopharmaceutical for central nervous system imaging has to cross the blood–brain barrier and wash out from the non-target tissue fairly rapidly, posing an additional challenge. Therefore, the use of in silico methods has gained a lot of attention in central nervous system radiopharmaceutical development. Novel PET tracers for cerebral

adenosine receptors (AR), phosphodiesterase 2A (PDE2A), and serotonin transporter were among the first attempts of using in silico models in central nervous system radiopharmaceutical design.[14,41,74]

PDE2A is expressed mainly in limbic area and basal ganglia and could be of importance for cognitive function through modulating the signal transduction by regulating cyclic guanasine monophosphate and cyclic adenosine monophosphate levels. Therefore, the development of selective PDE2A PET ligands has been of interest using the in silico models. For this purpose, a large database of successful and failed central nervous system PET tracers was created and screened to identify favorable ADMET properties for central nervous system PET imaging. Using these ADMET features enabled researchers to easily narrow down a library of more than 1000 PDE2A inhibitors to fewer than 10 compounds. Next, a SAR model was used to design more potent analogs from the identified lead compound before in vivo studies. As predicted by in silico models, the final compound demonstrated optimal performance in vivo.[14] A similar approach was used to design promising radiotracers for PDE4B and nociceptin opioid peptide receptor.[75,76]

AR is distributed widely in the brain and involved in different signaling pathways. Therefore, AR PET imaging can be useful for diagnosis and treatment monitoring in a broad range of psychiatric, neurovegetative diseases and Parkinson's disease. A number of [11]carbon (^{11}C)-labeled tracers and a [18]fluorine (^{18}F)-labeled AR tracer have been developed using in silico methods.[77] For instance, ^{18}F-FESCH, which is specific for AR subtype 2A (AR$_{2A}$) receptor has been developed using silico metabolite analysis. This tracer showed high binding affinity for AR$_{2A}$ and favorable pharmacokinetics in preclinical studies. PET imaging of rat brains showed this tracer is accurate for mapping AR$_{2A}$ expression in the brain.[41,78] In silico methods, although very powerful, are not always predictive of in vivo behavior of radiopharmaceuticals. Most recently, using quantitative SAR and molecular docking ^{18}F-TOZ1 was developed based on the structure of tozadenant, an AR$_{2A}$ antagonist with excellent binding affinity. Despite its ability to pass the blood–brain barrier and high brain uptake, AR$_{2A}$ specific binding was insufficient.[79]

When placing a chelator for radiometal labeling of a lead molecule to image enzymes or cell surface receptors, molecular docking is a useful tool to predict if it affects the binding site or adversely affects the binding affinity. Examples are radiotracers developed for imaging cholinesterase, for imaging Alzheimer's disease or histamine receptor type 1.[37,39]

Pathologic aggregates, such as tau protein, amyloid β and α-synuclein aggregates, have been extensively investigated in the pathophysiology of neurodegenerative diseases.[80–82] The complexity of their structure and different molecular isoforms can make tracer design challenging for these targets.[3,83] With the microscopic structure of more aggregates now being discovered, in silico design can accelerate developing high-affinity radiotracers for PET imaging of neurodegenerative diseases.[84,85] In addition, off-target binding of these tracers to other targets such as monoamine oxidase B can be predicted by molecular docking approaches.[84,86,87] Such information can help to optimize the binding specificity of the next generation of PET radiopharmaceuticals for central nervous system imaging. Combining different modeling methods to design a merged workflow can improve the ultimate accuracy of modeled data.[81] Further optimization of the modeling strategy and variable definition is required to ensure maximal correlation of modeled predictions with in vivo performance.[88] For instance, when different simulation approaches were used to predict the binding affinity of styrylbenzoxazole-based tracers for amyloid β, it highlighted the shortcomings of some of the model predictions; molecular dynamics, a complex approach that incorporates particle movements in the model, had higher accuracy than conventional docking models, whereas quantum mechanical methods significantly improved prediction accuracy compared with both. Despite greater accuracy, the downside of molecular dynamics and quantum mechanical models is the increased complexity and cost of simulations.[81]

Infection and Inflammation

Developing noninvasive imaging probes to detect infection has been gaining more attention in recent years, because structural imaging modalities are insensitive for the detection of the site of infection at an early stage. Antibacterial antibiotics are attractive compounds for developing radiotracers because they are specific for bacterial targets, allowing for the distinction between bacterial infection and inflammation, and they have a favorable tissue biodistribution for reaching the infected tissue. In addition, their minimal interaction with eukaryotic cells and wash out from normal tissue makes them desirable for infection imaging.[89,90] Because the structure of the antibiotics is usually available, a chemical similarity search and SAR modeling can be used to screen the libraries of antibiotic analogs that have an appropriate binding affinity for imaging purposes. SBDD methods can also be used as the structure of antibiotics' target is commonly known.[89] Ordonez and colleagues[91] screened commercially available libraries of random radiolabeled small molecules to identify potential substrates involved in bacterial metabolism or interacting with bacteria but with minimal mammalian cell interaction. The identified molecules demonstrated high level of in vitro accumulation in a wide range of bacterial species. Candidate compounds were then labeled with ^{18}F and successfully identified infection from sterile inflammation in vivo in murine models.[91]

Molecular docking has also been used for designing the inflammation PET tracer, ^{68}Ga-Siglec-9, which targets vascular adhesion protein-1. Siglec-9 was identified by phage display as a ligand for vascular adhesion protein-1.

Molecular docking aided to assess the binding of Siglec-9 to vascular adhesion protein-1 before proceeding with in vivo experiments.[92]

Other

SAR models were used to predict the in vivo performance of 3 potential radiopharmaceuticals for lung perfusion scan, namely, ^{99m}Tc-hexoprenaline, a β_2 adrenergic agonist; ^{99m}Tc-zolmitriptan, a selective serotonin receptor agonist; and ^{131}I-dapoxetine, a selective serotonin reuptake inhibitor. Lungs are the reservoirs for zolmitriptan and dapoxetine. In the case of hexoprenaline, the most energetically favored confirmation required addition of ^{99m}Tc to a moiety essential for appropriate interaction of hexoprenaline with its target. Hence, poor in vivo binding was predicted for this radiotracer. In contrast, the position of ^{131}I in dapoxetine and ^{99m}Tc in zolmitriptan did not affect vital sites for tracer–target interaction, and appropriate target binding was predicted. In vivo experiments in mice confirmed modeled predictions for all 3 radiopharmaceuticals.[59,93]

SUMMARY

In silico approaches are novel tools that guide conventional in vitro and in vivo radiopharmaceutical design experiments and accelerate novel radiopharmaceuticals' bench to bedside translation if used and interpreted appropriately. Various examples of successful incorporation of in silico approaches in radiopharmaceutical design and confirmed validation of modeled data in vivo in a wide range of diseases highlights the additional value of AI integration in this field. However, successful modeling depends on careful inclusion of appropriate variables in the model, the modeling approach, choice of software, and availability of accurate structure of the ligands and targets. Thus, developing a systematic workflow could help to incorporate computational modeling in the routine radiopharmaceutical design process and overcome the current challenges of this valuable technology.

CLINICS CARE POINTS

- AI can greatly use the advances in structural chemistry to accelerate the design of a broad range of radiopharmaceuticals for clinical use.
- In silico approaches can markedly shorten the time frame and decrease the cost associated

with radiopharmaceutical development to make them more accessible for noninvasive imaging and therapy in a wide range of targets.

- AI methods have been particularly helpful for central nervous system radiotracer design, where the blood–brain barrier poses an additional challenge for the radiopharmaceutical to reach its target.
- Currently, a well-established systematic approach for incorporating in silico methods in the radiopharmaceutical design workflow is lacking.
- AI is complementary to the conventional radiopharmaceutical design methods and does not replace them.
- In vivo studies and clinical trials are required to confirm the usefulness of in silico designed radiopharmaceuticals.

DISCLOSURE

Dr P. Heidari funding source: fund number K08 CA249047.

REFERENCES

1. Lau J, Rousseau E, Kwon D, et al. Insight into the development of PET radiopharmaceuticals for oncology. Cancers 2020;12(5):1312.
2. Fani M, Maecke HR. Radiopharmaceutical development of radiolabelled peptides. Eur J Nucl Med Mol Imaging 2012;39(Suppl 1):S11–30.
3. Saint-Aubert L, Lemoine L, Chiotis K, et al. Tau PET imaging: present and future directions. Mol Neurodegener 2017;12(1):19.
4. Tornesello AL, Buonaguro L, Tornesello ML, et al. New insights in the design of bioactive peptides and chelating agents for imaging and therapy in oncology. Molecules 2017;22(8):1282.
5. George GPC, Pisaneschi F, Nguyen Q-D, et al. Positron emission tomographic imaging of CXCR4 in cancer: challenges and promises. Mol Imaging 2015;14(1). 7290.2014.00041.
6. Nguyen QD, Aboagye EO. Imaging the life and death of tumors in living subjects: preclinical PET imaging of proliferation and apoptosis. Integr Biol (Camb) 2010;2(10):483–95.
7. Vermeulen K, Vandamme M, Bormans G, et al. Design and challenges of radiopharmaceuticals. Semin Nucl Med 2019;49(5):339–56.
8. Alonso H, Bliznyuk AA, Gready JE. Combining docking and molecular dynamic simulations in drug design. Med Res Rev 2006;26(5):531–68.
9. Chandrasekaran B, Abed SN, Al-Attraqchi O, et al. Chapter 21 - computer-aided prediction of

pharmacokinetic (ADMET) properties. In: Tekade RK, editor. Dosage form design parameters. Cambridge, Massachusetts, USA: Academic Press; 2018. p. 731–55.

10. Jean-Quartier C, Jeanquartier F, Jurisica I, et al. In silico cancer research towards 3R. BMC Cancer 2018;18(1):408.

11. Doke SK, Dhawale SC. Alternatives to animal testing: a review. Saudi Pharm J 2015;23(3):223–9.

12. Kleynhans J, Kruger HG, Cloete T, et al. In silico modelling in the development of novel radiolabelled peptide probes. Curr Med Chem 2020;27(41):7048–63.

13. Zhang L, Villalobos A. Strategies to facilitate the discovery of novel CNS PET ligands. EJNMMI Radiopharm Chem 2017;1(1):13.

14. Zhang L, Villalobos A, Beck EM, et al. Design and selection parameters to accelerate the discovery of novel central nervous system Positron Emission Tomography (PET) ligands and their application in the development of a novel phosphodiesterase 2A PET ligand. J Med Chem 2013;56(11):4568–79.

15. Chang M. Artificial intelligence for drug development, precision medicine, and healthcare. 1st edition. Chapman and Hall/CRC, Boca Raton, Florida, USA: CRC Press; 2020.

16. Ilem Ozdemir D, Asikoglu M. Radio imaging and diagnostic applications. Ed. Senyigit T., Ozcan I., Ozer O. Nanotechnology in progress: pharmaceutical applications. Asian J Pharm Sci.2012;16(1):24-46.

17. Schmidt BJ, Papin JA, Musante CJ. Mechanistic systems modeling to guide drug discovery and development. Drug Discov Today 2013;18(3–4):116–27.

18. Emine Selin Demir EO, Ekinci M, Gundogdu EA, et al. Computational study of radiopharmaceuticals. In: Stefaniu A, editor. Molecular docking and molecular dynamics. London, United Kingdom: IntechOpen; 2019. p. 79–90.

19. Honarparvar B, Govender T, Maguire GE, et al. Integrated approach to structure-based enzymatic drug design: molecular modeling, spectroscopy, and experimental bioactivity. Chem Rev 2014;114(1):493–537.

20. Brandt M, Cardinale J, Aulsebrook ML, et al. An overview of PET radiochemistry, part 2: radiometals. J Nucl Med 2018;59(10):1500–6.

21. Davis MI, Bennett MJ, Thomas LM, et al. Crystal structure of prostate-specific membrane antigen, a tumor marker and peptidase. Proc Natl Acad Sci U S A 2005;102(17):5981–6.

22. Wu B, Chien EY, Mol CD, et al. Structures of the CXCR4 chemokine GPCR with small-molecule and cyclic peptide antagonists. Science 2010;330(6007):1066–71.

23. Makrynitsa GI, Lykouras M, Spyroulias GA, et al. In silico drug design. John Wiley & Sons, Ltd: Chichester, United Kingdom: eLS. 2018; p. 1–7.

24. Yu W, MacKerell AD Jr. Computer-aided drug design methods. Methods Mol Biol 2017;1520:85–106.

25. Meng XY, Zhang HX, Mezei M, et al. Molecular docking: a powerful approach for structure-based drug discovery. Curr Comput Aided Drug Des 2011;7(2):146–57.

26. Kitchen DB, Decornez H, Furr JR, et al. Docking and scoring in virtual screening for drug discovery: methods and applications. Nat Rev Drug Discov 2004;3(11):935–49.

27. Grinter SZ, Zou X. Challenges, applications, and recent advances of protein-ligand docking in structure-based drug design. Molecules 2014;19(7):10150–76.

28. Ain QU, Aleksandrova A, Roessler FD, et al. Machine-learning scoring functions to improve structure-based binding affinity prediction and virtual screening. Wiley Interdiscip Rev Comput Mol Sci 2015;5(6):405–24.

29. Li H, Sze K-H, Lu G, et al. Machine-learning scoring functions for structure-based drug lead optimization. WIREs Comput Mol Sci 2020;10(5):e1465.

30. Ant Colony Optimization and Swarm Intelligence, 5th International Workshop, ANTS 2006, Brussels, Belgium, September 4–7, 2006, Proceedings. 2006.

31. Pereira JC, Caffarena ER, Dos Santos CN. Boosting docking-based virtual screening with deep learning. J Chem Inf Model 2016;56(12):2495–506.

32. Fu Y, Wu X, Chen Z, et al. A new approach for flexible molecular docking based on swarm intelligence. Math Probl Eng 2015;2015:540186.

33. Batool M, Ahmad B, Choi S. A structure-based drug discovery paradigm. Int J Mol Sci 2019;20(11):2783.

34. Somarowthu S, Ondrechen MJ. POOL server: machine learning application for functional site prediction in proteins. Bioinformatics 2012;28(15):2078–9.

35. Huang B. MetaPocket: a meta approach to improve protein ligand binding site prediction. Omics 2009;13(4):325–30.

36. Muhammed MT, Aki-Yalcin E. Homology modeling in drug discovery: overview, current applications, and future perspectives. Chem Biol Drug Des 2019;93(1):12–20.

37. Gniazdowska E, Koźmiński P, Halik P, et al. Synthesis, physicochemical and biological evaluation of tacrine derivative labeled with technetium-99m and gallium-68 as a prospective diagnostic tool for early diagnosis of Alzheimer's disease. Bioorg Chem 2019;91:103136.

38. Motaleb MA, El-Safoury DM, Abd-Alla WH, et al. Radiosynthesis, molecular modeling studies and biological evaluation of (99m)Tc-Ifosfamide complex as a novel probe for solid tumor imaging. Int J Radiat Biol 2018;94(12):1134–41.

39. Sanad MH, Ibrahim AA. Preparation and biological evaluation of 99mTc N-histamine as a model for

brain imaging: in silico study and preclinical evaluation. Radiochimica Acta 2018;106(3):229–38.

40. Khedr M, Rashed HM, Farag H, et al. Rational design of some substituted phenyl azanediyl (bis) methylene phosphonic acid derivatives as potential anticancer agents and imaging probes: computational inputs, chemical synthesis, radiolabeling, biodistribution and gamma scintigraphy. Bioorg Chem 2019;92:103282.

41. Khanapur S, Paul S, Shah A, et al. Development of [18F]-labeled pyrazolo[4,3-e]-1,2,4- triazolo[1,5-c] pyrimidine (SCH442416) analogs for the imaging of cerebral adenosine A2A receptors with positron emission tomography. J Med Chem 2014;57(15): 6765–80.

42. Scott DE, Coyne AG, Hudson SA, et al. Fragment-based approaches in drug discovery and chemical biology. Biochemistry 2012;51(25):4990–5003.

43. Kumar A, Voet A, Zhang KY. Fragment based drug design: from experimental to computational approaches. Curr Med Chem 2012;19(30):5128–47.

44. Yang S-Y. Pharmacophore modeling and applications in drug discovery: challenges and recent advances. Drug Discov Today 2010;15(11):444–50.

45. Katsila T, Spyroulias GA, Patrinos GP, et al. Computational approaches in target identification and drug discovery. Comput Struct Biotechnol J 2016;14: 177–84.

46. Vlachakis D, Fakourelis P, Megalooikonomou V, et al. DrugOn: a fully integrated pharmacophore modeling and structure optimization toolkit. PeerJ 2015;3: e725.

47. Stumpfe D, Bajorath J. Similarity searching. WIREs Comput Mol Sci 2011;1(2):260–82.

48. Boudreau RJ, Efange SM. Computer-aided radiopharmaceutical design. Invest Radiol 1992;27(8): 653–8.

49. Li H, Sutter J, Hoffmann R. HypoGen: an automated system for generating 3D predictive pharmacophore models. In: Güner OF, editor. Pharmacophore perception, development, and use in drug design. International University Line Publications, La Jolla, CA, USA, 2000. p. 171-187.

50. Martin YC. DISCO: What We Did Right and What We Missed. In: Güner OF, editor. Pharmacophore perception, development, and use in drug design. International University Line Publications, La Jolla, CA, USA, 2000. p. 49-68

51. Dixon SL, Smondyrev AM, Knoll EH, et al. PHASE: a new engine for pharmacophore perception, 3D QSAR model development, and 3D database screening: 1. Methodology and preliminary results. J Comput Aided Mol Des 2006;20(10):647–71.

52. Güner O, Clement O, Kurogi Y. Pharmacophore modeling and three dimensional database searching for drug design using catalyst: recent advances. Curr Med Chem 2004;11(22):2991–3005.

53. Wolber G, Seidel T, Bendix F, et al. Molecule-pharmacophore superpositioning and pattern matching in computational drug design. Drug Discov Today 2008;13(1–2):23–9.

54. Macalino SJ, Gosu V, Hong S, et al. Role of computer-aided drug design in modern drug discovery. Arch Pharm Res 2015;38(9):1686–701.

55. Zhang S. Computer-aided drug discovery and development. Methods Mol Biol 2011;716:23–38.

56. Lešnik S, Štular T, Brus B, et al. LiSiCA: a software for ligand-based virtual screening and its application for the discovery of butyrylcholinesterase inhibitors. J Chem Inf Model 2015;55(8):1521–8.

57. Ghasemi F, Mehridehnavi A, Pérez-Garrido A, et al. Neural network and deep-learning algorithms used in QSAR studies: merits and drawbacks. Drug Discov Today 2018;23(10):1784–90.

58. Martin YC, Kofron JL, Traphagen LM. Do structurally similar molecules have similar biological activity? J Med Chem 2002;45(19):4350–8.

59. Rashed HM, Ibrahim IT, Motaleb MA. 99mTc-hexoprenaline and 131I-dapoxetine: preparation, in silico modeling and biological evaluation as promising lung scintigraphy radiopharmaceuticals. J Radioanal Nucl Chem 2017;314(2):1297–307.

60. van de Waterbeemd H, Gifford E. ADMET in silico modelling: towards prediction paradise? Nat Rev Drug Discov 2003;2(3):192–204.

61. Moroy G, Martiny VY, Vayer P, et al. Toward in silico structure-based ADMET prediction in drug discovery. Drug Discov Today 2012;17(1–2):44–55.

62. Norinder U, Bergström CA. Prediction of ADMET properties. ChemMedChem 2006;1(9):920–37.

63. Price EW, Orvig C. Matching chelators to radiometals for radiopharmaceuticals. Chem Soc Rev 2014;43(1):260–90.

64. Clark DE. In silico prediction of blood–brain barrier permeation. Drug Discov Today 2003;8(20):927–33.

65. Sun X, Li Y, Liu T, et al. Peptide-based imaging agents for cancer detection. Adv Drug Deliv Rev 2017;110-111:38–51.

66. Evans BJ, King AT, Katsifis A, et al. Methods to enhance the metabolic stability of peptide-based PET radiopharmaceuticals. Molecules 2020;25(10): 2314.

67. Bayoumi NA, Amin AM, Ismail NSM, et al. Radioiodination and biological evaluation of Cladribine as potential agent for tumor imaging and therapy. Radiochimica Acta 2015;103(11):777–87.

68. Cai Z, Ouyang Q, Zeng D, et al. 64Cu-labeled somatostatin analogues conjugated with cross-bridged phosphonate-based chelators via strain-promoted click chemistry for PET imaging: in silico through in vivo studies. J Med Chem 2014;57(14):6019–29.

69. Fang Y, Wang D, Xu X, et al. Synthesis, biological evaluation, and molecular dynamics (MD) simulation

studies of three novel F-18 labeled and focal adhesion kinase (FAK) targeted 5-bromo pyrimidines as radiotracers for tumor. Eur J Med Chem 2017;127: 493–508.

70. Wang D, Fang Y, Wang H, et al. Synthesis and evaluation of novel F-18-labeled pyrimidine derivatives: potential FAK inhibitors and PET imaging agents for cancer detection. RSC Adv 2017;7(36): 22388–99.

71. Fang Y, Wang D, Xu X, et al. Preparation, in vitro and in vivo evaluation, and molecular dynamics (MD) simulation studies of novel F-18 labeled tumor imaging agents targeting focal adhesion kinase (FAK). RSC Adv 2018;8(19):10333–45.

72. Khurana H, Meena VK, Prakash S, et al. Preclinical evaluation of a potential GSH Ester based PET/SPECT imaging probe DT(GSHMe)₂ to detect gamma glutamyl transferase over expressing tumors. PLoS One 2015;10(7):e0134281.

73. Sakr TM, Khedr MA, Rashed HM, et al. In silico-based repositioning of Phosphinothricin as a Novel Technetium-99m imaging probe with potential anticancer activity. Molecules 2018;23(2):496.

74. Wellsow J, Kovar KA, Machulla HJ. Molecular modeling of potential new and selective PET radiotracers for the serotonin transporter. Positron Emission Tomography. J Pharm Pharm Sci 2002;5(3): 245–57.

75. Zhang L, Drummond E, Brodney MA, et al. Design, synthesis and evaluation of [(3)H]PF-7191, a highly specific nociceptin opioid peptide (NOP) receptor radiotracer for in vivo receptor occupancy (RO) studies. Bioorg Med Chem Lett 2014;24(22): 5219–23.

76. Zhang L, Chen L, Beck EM, et al. The discovery of a novel phosphodiesterase (PDE) 4B-preferring radioligand for positron emission tomography (PET) imaging. J Med Chem 2017;60(20):8538–51.

77. Vuorimaa A, Rissanen E, Airas L. In vivo PET imaging of adenosine 2A receptors in neuroinflammatory and neurodegenerative disease. Contrast Media Mol Imaging 2017;2017:6975841.

78. Khanapur S, van Waarde A, Dierckx RA, et al. Preclinical evaluation and quantification of (18)F-Fluoroethyl and (18)F-fluoropropyl analogs of SCH442416 as radioligands for PET imaging of the adenosine A(2A) receptor in rat brain. J Nucl Med 2017;58(3):466–72.

79. Lai TH, Toussaint M, Teodoro R, et al. Synthesis and biological evaluation of a novel (18)F-labeled radiotracer for PET imaging of the adenosine A(2A) receptor. Int J Mol Sci 2021;22(3):1182.

80. Okamura N, Harada R, Ishiki A, et al. The development and validation of tau PET tracers: current status and future directions. Clin Transl Imaging 2018; 6(4):305–16.

81. Balamurugan K, Murugan NA, Ågren H. Multistep modeling strategy to improve the binding affinity prediction of PET tracers to Aβ42: case study with styrylbenzoxazole derivatives. ACS Chem Neurosci 2016;7(12):1698–705.

82. Uzuegbunam BC, Librizzi D, Hooshyar Yousefi B. PET radiopharmaceuticals for Alzheimer's disease and Parkinson's disease diagnosis, the current and future landscape. Molecules 2020;25(4):977.

83. Leuzy A, Chiotis K, Lemoine L, et al. Tau PET imaging in neurodegenerative tauopathies-still a challenge. Mol Psychiatry 2019;24(8):1112–34.

84. Lemoine L, Gillberg P-G, Svedberg M, et al. Comparative binding properties of the tau PET tracers THK5117, THK5351, PBB3, and T807 in postmortem Alzheimer brains. Alzheimers Res Ther 2017;9(1):96.

85. Murugan NA, Nordberg A, Ågren H. Different positron emission tomography tau tracers bind to multiple binding sites on the tau fibril: insight from computational modeling. ACS Chem Neurosci 2018;9(7):1757–67.

86. Murugan NA, Chiotis K, Rodriguez-Vieitez E, et al. Cross-interaction of tau PET tracers with monoamine oxidase B: evidence from in silico modelling and in vivo imaging. Eur J Nucl Med Mol Imaging 2019;46(6):1369–82.

87. Ng KP, Pascoal TA, Mathotaarachchi S, et al. Monoamine oxidase B inhibitor, selegiline, reduces (18)F-THK5351 uptake in the human brain. Alzheimers Res Ther 2017;9(1):25.

88. Shaw RC, Tamagnan GD, Tavares AAS. Rapidly (and successfully) translating novel brain radiotracers from animal research into clinical use. Front Neurosci 2020;14:871.

89. Mota F, Ordonez AA, Firth G, et al. Radiotracer development for bacterial imaging. J Med Chem 2020;63(5):1964–77.

90. Signore A, Artiko V, Conserva M, et al. Imaging bacteria with radiolabelled probes: is it feasible? J Clin Med 2020;9(8):2372.

91. Ordonez AA, Weinstein EA, Bambarger LE, et al. A systematic approach for developing bacteria-specific imaging tracers. J Nucl Med 2017;58(1): 144–50.

92. Aalto K, Autio A, Kiss EA, et al. Siglec-9 is a novel leukocyte ligand for vascular adhesion protein-1 and can be used in PET imaging of inflammation and cancer. Blood 2011;118(13):3725–33.

93. Rashed HM, Marzook FA, Farag H. 99m Tc-zolmitriptan: radiolabeling, molecular modeling, biodistribution and gamma scintigraphy as a hopeful radiopharmaceutical for lung nuclear imaging. Radiol Med 2016;121(12):935–43.

Potential Applications of Artificial Intelligence and Machine Learning in Radiochemistry and Radiochemical Engineering

E. William Webb, PhD, Peter J.H. Scott, PhD*

KEYWORDS

- Radiochemistry • Radiolabeling • Positron emission tomography
- Copper-mediated radiofluorination

KEY POINTS

- Selecting an appropriate radiolabeling strategy and optimizing it for a new radiotracer has historically been a resource-intensive task.
- Machine learning has potential as a fundamental tool for designing radiochemical syntheses.
- Efforts are underway to use machine learning for identification of optimal labeling strategies and radiochemistry reaction optimization.

INTRODUCTION

Radiochemistry for PET applications is a complex amalgam of different areas of expertise. The field combines fundamental organic chemistry and analytical sciences, all under the constraint of timely production for short-lived isotopes (^{11}C, ^{18}F, and ^{68}Ga) to meet medical demand with sufficient activity and purity. Taken as a whole, these constraints have barred all but a few small molecules from being studied in animals and/or being commercialized. Although the generation of novel molecules for further study is addressed elsewhere in this issue, the role of radiochemists in the radiotracer pipeline (**Fig. 1**) is to identify which site in the molecule is best for labeling, to determine what is the ideal strategy for labeling at that site, to optimize the chemistry to effectively produce the radiolabeled product compound, and finally, to develop an appropriate analytical technique to verify the identity and purity of the labeled molecule. To date, the main approach to achieving these ends has been through substantial trial and error, consuming a great deal of time (both human and instrument) and resources. As many of the tools used in artificial intelligence (AI) and machine learning (ML) become accessible to researchers, there is mounting potential to turn these tools to the problems encountered in the production of radiolabeled molecules for PET applications.[1] Although a commonly bandied "buzzword" meant to evoke a superhuman ability to understand a system, AI is simply the "intelligence" displayed by machines that emulates the "natural intelligence" of animals or humans through the application of mathematical and computer science algorithms for evaluating data ("machine learning") and executing decisions. These do not replace humans in the scientific process; rather, these can be thought of as convenient "experts" and tools to complement and enhance chemists in the field. In this perspective, the authors outline some of the potential applications of AI in the field of radiochemistry.

Department of Radiology, University of Michigan, Ann Arbor, MI 48109, USA
* Corresponding author.
E-mail address: pjhscott@umich.edu
Twitter: @Scott_LabUM (P.J.H.S.)

PET Clin 16 (2021) 525–532
https://doi.org/10.1016/j.cpet.2021.06.012

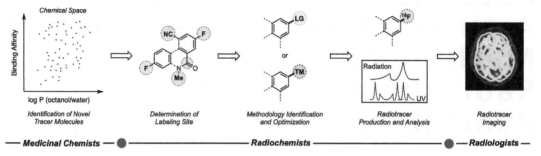

Fig. 1. Radiotracer development and production workflow and areas of radiochemist involvement.

HOW MACHINE LEARNING WORKS

There is some disagreement as to whether ML is a subfield of AI or a separate field that overlaps with some of the AI field.[2,3] Regardless of this disagreement, a functional definition is that AI is a nonbiological system that displays human-like intelligence through rules, whereas ML is represented by algorithms that learn from data and examples.[3] An AI could be developed by an expert to run through a set of encoded decisions (a series of if-then statements), similar to an expert's logical and experiential workflow. Following the encoding, an AI agent would then be capable of following the same logic for a novel input to determine a predicted output just as the expert would provide based on their logic and experience. Alternatively, ML could be used to develop a similar set of encoded decisions starting from data or examples using a variety of algorithms, just as the expert once learned.[3] The focus of this perspective is on the development of AIs in radiochemistry from data, without the intermediacy of an expert, and thus is most aptly described as ML for radiochemistry and radiochemical engineering.

ML has been traditionally broken into 3 categories: (1) supervised learning, in which the algorithms are presented with data containing example inputs (features) and corresponding desired outputs (labels); (2) unsupervised learning, in which the labels are not given, and algorithms discover underlying structure; and (3) reinforcement learning, in which an algorithm interacts with an environment and is provided with rewards to maximize or losses (penalties) to minimize.[3,4] Depending on the question under study by the researcher, the appropriate mode of ML may be different. For example, examining a large set of chest radiograph images using unsupervised learning techniques may identify certain characteristics consistent with a pathologic condition (perhaps an increase in localized densities or increased heart size) without knowing those attributes were a part of the diagnosis. Alternatively,

radiographic images labeled with a diagnosis may be used to train a supervised model to diagnose on the basis of an image. However, for the purposes of radiochemical engineering and radiochemistry, supervised and reinforcement learning methods are the most easily applicable.

Whatever the approach and the problem under study, care must be taken to verify that the model generalizes.[4] With small data sets and a large number of features, overfitting can readily occur in supervised learning.[4,5] This functionally tests whether the model can "memorize" rather than correctly perform the desired function. In unsupervised learning contexts, clustering and attribute features can be identified simply because of the original data set. Testing an additional data set composed of similar data to verify that the same features are recognized prevents making assertions that will not hold.[5,6]

IDENTIFICATION OF OPTIMAL SITE AND STRATEGY FOR LABELING

After identifying an appropriate target molecule, a key part of radiochemistry is to distinguish next which site is optimal for labeling from a metabolic stability perspective and radiochemical accessibility.[7] Automated retrosynthetic analysis dates back to proposals by Corey and colleagues[8,9] in the late 1960s, and as accessibility has risen with hardware capabilities, additional implementations of ML and AI as applied to retrosynthetic analysis have seen an upswing.[10] Schematically, older versions of the programs developed for automated retrosynthetic analysis sought to "disconnect" molecules according to template reactions that were encoded by an expert.[10,11] For example, in 2'-methoxyphenyl-(N-2'-pyrinyl)-p-fluoro-benzamidoethylpiperazine (MPPF) an amide bond may be retrosynthetically broken down into an acyl chloride and an amine according to one template, whereas another template breaks down the molecule into an amide and an electrophile, whereas still another may break the same amide bond into a palladium-catalyzed carbonylation-amination (**Fig. 2A**). The program iteratively applies these templates to the building blocks produced by each disconnection until arriving at a set of building block molecules that are commercially available or unable to be disconnected into simpler species using the set of templates. This produces an entire "tree" of routes that converge on the target molecule (**Fig. 2B**). However, this "tree" contains some effective routes and some ineffective routes.[10] To identify the most viable path for synthetic efforts, the various routes need to be ranked by some criteria. The various retrosynthetic routes may be scored by "greenness," by length of route, commercial availability of building block materials, or some other criterion developed alongside the program.[10–12] More recent advances have used ML and reaction databases to eliminate the need for an expert in the construction of template sets and more sophisticated scoring systems that measure the feasibility of the forward reactions to determine the viability of a given retrosynthetic route.[10]

In contrast to typical, multistep organic synthesis, radiochemists are specifically focused on just one step: the incorporation of the radioisotope, ideally as the last step in the synthetic pathway. This last step is further complicated as different radiolabeling strategies may require completely different starting materials, conditions, workup, or purification strategies, all of which must be completed while limiting radiation exposure, using standardized equipment, and incorporating sufficient activity for transport to the scanning suite and completion of the imaging study. For example, apply a retro-*radio*-synthetic approach to [^{11}C]UCB-J as a prospective compound for labeling (**Fig. 2C**).[13] Any of the aryl fluorides

(highlighted in green) could potentially undergo effective labeling via S_NAr[14] or a transition metal-mediated radiofluorination with [^{18}F]fluoride.[15] Alternatively, at another site, an iodopyridyl moiety could be labeled with [^{11}C]MeLi,[16] whereas the used strategy of methylation with [^{11}C]MeI of a pyridyl trifluoroborate[13] offers still another labeling chemistry (highlighted in red). *Ab initio*, the selection of which strategy to pursue is an extremely difficult problem. An S_NAr approach would necessitate the formation of any of several highly reactive electrophiles, whereas using a transition-metal–mediated approach, such as copper-mediated radiofluorination, may not tolerate *ortho*-fluorine substitution.[14,15] Taken altogether, this obligates either a brute force approach to radiosynthesis, testing all possible methodologies presented in the literature and variations thereof in a limited throughput manner, or testing the most easily accessed methodology, which, even if modestly successful, may not be optimal. If either of those approaches fail to provide sufficient activity in a timely fashion, all too often the target molecule is discarded as "unlabelable."

Just as ML provides additional tools for retrosynthetic analysis, ML has potential as a fundamental tool for constructing a retro-radiosynthesis tool. Similar to traditional retrosynthetic analysis tools, template reactions for radiolabeling can be developed. However, the difference between traditional retrosynthetic tools and any potential tool for retro-radio-synthesis is in the scoring function defined for radiochemistry. Any program for this purpose will seek to maximize feasibility, activity, and specific activity while minimizing time for the all-important radiolabeling step and metabolic breakdown[7,17,18] rather than the economics or "greenness" of the route.

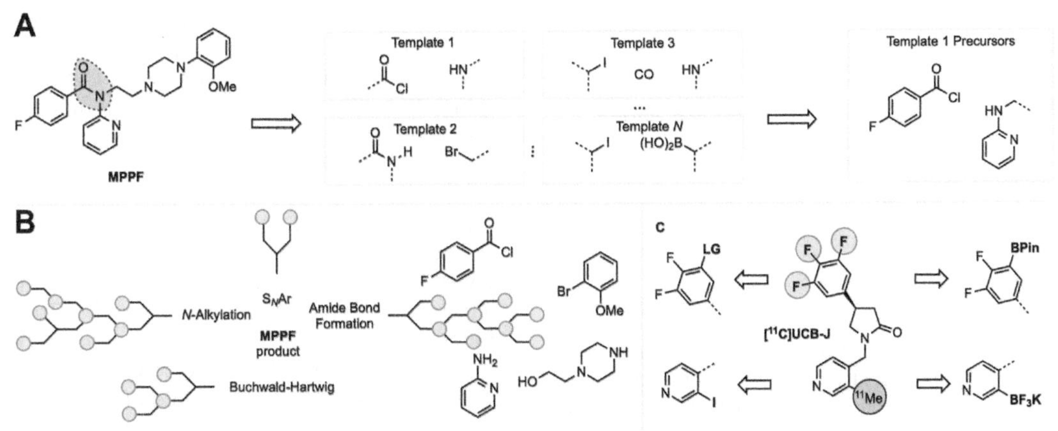

Fig. 2. (*A*) Template-based retrosynthetic analysis of a complex molecule. (*B*) Exhaustive deconstruction and generation of multiple potentially viable routes. (*C*) Retro-radio-synthetic analysis of [^{11}C]UCB-J.

Foundationally, this will require a change in the way radiochemistry methodology development is conducted. Methodologies will need to be conducted with the intent of translation of the corresponding data set into an ML model that can be further augmented as additional methodologies are developed.[10] For this to occur, substrate scopes, the main data sets of methodologies, must be redefined. This redefinition of substrate scope evaluations must include the following:

1. Not just successful reactions but also unsuccessful reactions
2. Substrates that span the chemical space of accessible *or* pertinent substrates
3. "Clean" data

Only by following these constraints can robust ML models be developed to define the feasibility of any proposed reaction. Reaction chemical space is complex, and although two substrates may "seem" similar to a radiochemist, they may perform radically different for a given methodology. As demonstrated by Taylor and colleagues,[19] two seemingly similar aryl boronic acid pinacol esters undergo labeling with extremely different efficacy (**Fig. 3A**). Without actively conducting this

experiment, it would be difficult to predict this effect, as humans would identify these two substrates as near in chemical space. In contrast, with appropriate featurization, most ML algorithms could identify whether these two substrates are neighbors in feature space or not. Given a novel substrate that could potentially be reactive, unreactive model substrates may be nearer in *n*-dimensional chemical feature space than successful scope substrates (**Fig. 3B**). This would lead to the prediction that the novel substrate is more likely to perform similarly to poor performing substrates, but without substrate scopes that contain these unsuccessful substrates such a comparison is unable to be made by models. Unfortunately, the inclusion of ineffective substrates in the literature remains a rarity, except in the case of clearly instructive examples.

Unsuccessful substrates help define the radiolabeling reaction efficiency surface (**Fig. 3B**). To best define that surface, substrates would be selected to fully span and represent the whole of chemical space. However, spanning chemical space is a daunting and, in truth, impossible prospect. The number of molecules theoretically accessible in small molecule chemical space is more than 10^{60} molecules.[20] Even when the set of methodology input molecules is reduced to only those functionally pertinent, such as aryl boronate derivatives for a Chan-Lam coupling,[21] and then reducing further to the set of commercially available (as an approximate estimation of actual accessibility), brings one into a regime $\sim 10^6$ molecules. This is still beyond the synthetic accessibility of most laboratories that lack high-throughput experimentation equipment. Because this scale remains synthetically out of reach to most laboratories, two approaches have become commonplace: additive screening with a model reaction[22] and identification of representative sets[23,24] (**Fig. 3C**). Additive screening is able to readily identify functional groups that act as poisons using a single analytical method but fail to capture the effect those functional groups may have when more proximate to the reactive center.[19,22,23] For the identification of representative libraries, after property calculations are performed on a large number of potential molecules, the set may be reduced through principal components analysis[23] or via finding the most diverse small set using the Kennard-Stone Algorithm.[25,26] These informer sets may not include all potential functionality and may also be combined with additive screening to provide an information-rich data set for model construction.[24] To date, a standardized set of representative functional group molecules for additive screening has not been demonstrated,

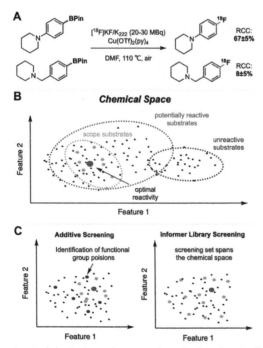

Fig. 3. (A) Similar substrates that display drastically different activity.[19] (B) Literature bias of methodology scope toward highly reactive substrates around optimal reactivity rather than potentially reactive or unreactive substrates. (C) Comparison of how different screening strategies span chemical space.

but the introduction of a common set would provide a better evaluation of differences between literature methodologies. By attempting to span a wider range of chemical space algorithmically, ML models will demonstrate higher generalizability to novel molecules, in particular, for the substrates of labeling interest.

"Clean" data are, unfortunately, the most ambiguous and potentially most important part for the construction of ML data sets for predicting labeling efficiency. There are few standardized and tabulated data of radiochemical reactions and conditions that are fit to be parsed and mined for AI development. Even the wider organic chemistry field notes the absence of tabulated reaction data.[10] Minute variations in multiple variables that are not clearly annotated in the literature can combine to produce a very large "hidden" variable. Differences in amount of precursor, amount of activity used, the preparation of that activity, or even amounts of different counterions all may have an effect on labeling efficiency. In a supervised learning problem when two data sets that share a common point are combined, without clear annotation of these differences, one input may map to two outputs in the training set. This will increase the error rate of the model simply because of this "hidden" difference. To achieve so-called "clean" data, as many variables as possible need to be annotated and consistent across all experiments. With data sets designed for ML, the major hurdle for implementation and use of ML can be overcome and the potential of AI for radiolabeling chemistry realized.

REACTION OPTIMIZATION

After determining an appropriate target and labeling strategy, radiochemistry becomes an optimization problem, in both reaction development and analytical chemistry. For optimization of a specific reaction, chemist-led or design-of-experiment approaches have been most prevalently applied.[27] Fully automated systems have the brute-force capability to conduct many more experiments than a chemist; however, a chemist's intuition may be more efficient in identifying the best experiment to run for optimization.[28,29] Although a chemist's instinct and flexibility may be invaluable, it cannot be parallelized and is dependent on the chemist who, although perhaps an expert on one type of reaction, may not be an expert on the specifically needed reaction. In the case whereby the chemist is not an expert, a large number of variable conditions may be readily identified from the literature, leading to an exponentially increasing number of potential experiments ("the curse of dimensionality").

As a complement to chemical intuition and to speed navigation of this high dimensional optimization problem, efforts have been undertaken to automate the decision-making process of a chemist so that an optimal set of conditions can be identified in a minimal number of experiments. These algorithms are most similar to a reinforcement learning approach: an initial environment is defined, and on the basis of the outcome of those experiments, additional experiments are selected to maximize (optimize) a reward function (**Fig. 4**).

For a continuous, single objective variable system optimization, for example, identifying optimal amounts of reactants or chromatography gradients, various algorithms have been demonstrated, such as the Nelder-Mead simplex method, Stable Noisy Optimization by Branch and Fit, and gradient descent optimization.[29,30] However, chemistry is rife with categorical variables as well as continuous variables. For these, alternative approaches, like mixed integer linear programming, as demonstrated by the Jensen lab,[28–31] Bayesian optimization,[32,33] or Deep Reinforcement Optimization,[34] may be used to optimize across mixed variables. Even multiple objective optimizations have been demonstrated to be feasible.[33]

Taken as a whole, the opportunities for optimization algorithms in radiochemistry are plentiful. Ideal analytical methods that most efficiently and effectively characterize the target molecule can be found in an automated fashion; optimization of reaction conditions can be treated as a multi-objective

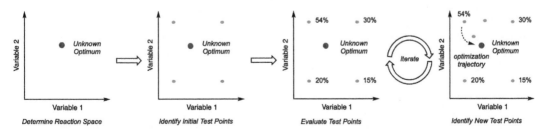

Fig. 4. Algorithmic and automated optimization.

maximization problem for yield, purity, molar activity, and ease of purification. The high degree of automation currently used in radiochemistry will facilitate the implementation of these techniques. However, further efforts will be needed to adapt fully automated systems (both hardware and software) into a radiochemical optimization workflow. At present, standard automated synthesis boxes that are commercially available (both cassette-based modules and fixed tube systems)[35] balance current good manufacturing practice (cGMP) features and flexibility for production of various different radiotracers, but are poorly adapted to sequential, fully automated testing. With appropriate equipment and software application programming interfaces (API), implementation of AI into the workflow for radiochemistry methodology and tracer development becomes accessible to general radiochemistry laboratories.

PRODUCTION AND OTHER CONCERNS

The workflow of radiochemistry extends past identification and development of a tracer to long-term, repeated production.[36] In the course of long-term production, additional issues may arise that impact effective production. These range from maintenance of automated equipment like cyclotrons and synthesis boxes to changes in the quality of production reagents. Provided a problem in these areas can be defined and reduced to several input factors (for example, electrical current use or coolant temperature may provide alarms for cyclotron maintenance) or sufficient tabulated data collected for unsupervised-learning and identification of underlying patterns, the potential for implementing ML in other areas may be readily realized.

SUMMARY

Radiochemistry, as a field, has readily embraced automated technology to solve various problems, including radiation safety and cGMP compliance. For both radiochemistry and radiochemical engineering, ML and AI offer an additional, powerful tool for evaluating data. This tool will be applied with increasing regularity and offers many time- and cost-saving advantages over traditional resource-intensive laboratory approaches. This perspective sheds light on the potential problems to which ML may be applied, and how to begin approaching those problems. This article is far from exhaustive, and the only limit as to what problems are fit for ML and AI is how well scientists and engineers can define their problems to apply these techniques.

CLINICS CARE POINTS

- ML/AI programs and models are not infallible and must be undergo adequate robustness testing via external validation and at all points in model development, appropriate controls to prevent information leakage and bias must be in place. These include use of cross-validation and external validation datasets to prevent information leak and appropriately large and varied datasets to prevent bias. Any developed models or programs must demonstrate real world performance prior to implementation.

- A number of "black box" algorithms exist but for medical applications and cGMP, development of non-"black box"-models is paramount for transparency, standardization, quality control, trustworthiness and long-term security.

ADDITIONAL RESOURCES

Given the rapidly developing nature of artificial intelligence and machine learning, references quickly become outdated. There are several readily accessible manuals for beginning to construct the coding framework for ML models from O'Reilly Publishers and others. These should remain effective provided the program language in vogue (presently Python, R, or Matlab) does not update. For further concepts and updated applied research on chemistry and AI, the Web sites of the following professors will likely provide the most up-to-date information: Prof. Alán Aspuru-Guzik, Prof. Connor W. Coley, Prof. Klavs F. Jensen, Prof. Abigail G. Doyle, Prof. Leroy Cronin, Prof. Timothy A. Cernak, and Prof. Scott E. Denmark.

ACKNOWLEDGMENTS

This work was supported by the NIH (Award Number R01EB021155). The authors gratefully thank Dr. J.S. Wright, Dr. A.F. Brooks, and K. Cheng, as well as Prof. Melanie S. Sanford and her group members for helpful discussions.

DISCLOSURE

The authors declare that they have no conflicts of interest relating to the subject matter of the present review.

REFERENCES

1. Webb EW, Wright JS, Sharninghausen LS, et al. Machine learning for translation of published methodologies. J Nucl Med 2021;62 (Suppl. 1):13.

2. Garbade MJ. Clearing the confusion: AI vs machine learning vs deep learning differences. 2018. Available at: https://towardsdatascience.com/clearing-the-confusion-ai-vs-machine-learning-vs-deep-learning-differences. Accessed February 23, 2021.

3. Raschka S. Introduction to machine learning and deep learning 2020. Available at: https://sebastianraschka.com/blog/2020/intro-to-dl-ch01.html. Accessed February 23, 2021.

4. Géron A. The landscape of machine learning. In: Hands-on machine learning with scikit-learn, Keras, and Tensorflow: concepts, tools, and techniques to build intelligent systems. Sebastopol (CA): O'Reilly; 2019. p. 1–33.

5. Roberts M, Driggs D, Thorpe M, et al. Common pitfalls and recommendations for using machine learning to detect and prognosticate for COVID-19 using chest radiographs and CT scans. Nat Mach Intell 2021;3(3):199–217.

6. US Food and Drug Administration (FDA). Proposed Regulatory Framework for Modifications to Artificial Intelligence/Machine Learning (AI/ML)-Based Software as a Medical Device (SaMD)-Discussion Paper and Request for Feedback. US Food Drug Adm. 2019:1-20. Available at: https://www.fda.gov/files/medical%20devices/published/US-FDA-Artificial-Intelligence-and-Machine-Learning-Discussion-Paper.pdf. Accessed July 23, 2021.

7. Liang SH, Vasdev N. Total radiosynthesis: thinking outside "the box. Aust J Chem 2015;68(9):1319–28.

8. Corey EJ, Long AK, Rubenstein SD. Computer-assisted analysis in organic synthesis. Science 1985;228(4698):408–18.

9. Corey EJ. General methods for the construction of complex molecules. Pure Appl Chem 1967;14(1):19–38.

10. Coley CW, Green WH, Jensen KF. Machine learning in computer-aided synthesis planning. Acc Chem Res 2018;51(5):1281–9.

11. Szymkuć S, Gajewska EP, Klucznik T, et al. Computer-assisted synthetic planning: the end of the beginning. Angew Chem Int Ed Engl 2016;55(20):5904–37.

12. Coley CW, Rogers L, Green WH, et al. Computer-assisted retrosynthesis based on molecular similarity. ACS Cent Sci 2017;3(12):1237–45.

13. Nabulsi NB, Mercier J, Holden D, et al. Synthesis and preclinical evaluation of 11C-UCB-J as a PET tracer for imaging the synaptic vesicle glycoprotein 2A in the brain. J Nucl Med 2016;57(5):777–84.

14. Cole E, Stewart M, Littich R, et al. Radiosyntheses using fluorine-18: the art and science of late stage fluorination. Curr Top Med Chem 2014;14(7):875–900.

15. Wright JS, Kaur T, Preshlock S, et al. Copper-mediated late-stage radiofluorination: five years of impact on preclinical and clinical PET imaging. Clin Transl Imaging 2020;8(3):167–206.

16. Helbert H, Antunes IF, Luurtsema G, et al. Cross-coupling of [11C]methyllithium for 11C-labelled PET tracer synthesis. Chem Commun 2021;57(2):203–6.

17. Miller PW, Long NJ, Vilar R, et al. Synthesis of 11C, 18F, 15O, and 13N radiolabels for positron emission tomography. Angew Chem Int Ed Engl 2008;47(47):8998–9033.

18. Djoumbou-Feunang Y, Fiamoncini J, Gil-de-la-Fuente A, et al. A comprehensive computational tool for small molecule metabolism prediction and metabolite identification. J Cheminform 2019;11(1):1–25.

19. Taylor NJ, Emer E, Preshlock S, et al. Derisking the Cu-mediated 18F-fluorination of heterocyclic positron emission tomography radioligands. J Am Chem Soc 2017;139(24):8267–76.

20. Virshup AM, Contreras-García J, Wipf P, et al. Stochastic voyages into uncharted chemical space produce a representative library of all possible drug-like compounds. J Am Chem Soc 2013;135(19):7296–303.

21. Chen JQ, Li JH, Dong ZB. A review on the latest progress of Chan-Lam coupling reaction. Adv Synth Catal 2020;362(16):3311–31.

22. Collins KD, Glorius F. Intermolecular reaction screening as a tool for reaction evaluation. Acc Chem Res 2015;48(3):619–27.

23. Kutchukian PS, Dropinski JF, Dykstra KD, et al. Chemistry informer libraries: a chemoinformatics enabled approach to evaluate and advance synthetic methods. Chem Sci 2016;7(4):2604–13.

24. Ahneman DT, Estrada JG, Lin S, et al. Predicting reaction performance in C–N cross-coupling using machine learning. Science 2018;360(6385):186–90.

25. Kennard ARW, Stone LA. Computer aided design of experiments. Technometrics 2016;11(1):137–48.

26. Zahrt AF, Henle JJ, Rose BT, et al. Prediction of higher-selectivity catalysts by computer-driven workflow and machine learning. Science 2019;363(6424):eaau5631.

27. Bowden GD, Pichler BJ, Maurer A. A design of experiments (DoE) approach accelerates the optimization of copper-mediated 18F-fluorination reactions of arylstannanes. Sci Rep 2019;9(1):1–10.

28. Reizman BJ, Wang Y-M, Buchwald SL, et al. Suzuki–Miyaura cross-coupling optimization enabled by automated feedback. React Chem Eng 2016;1:658–66.

29. Baumgartner LM, Coley CW, Reizman BJ, et al. Optimum catalyst selection over continuous and discrete process variables with a single droplet microfluidic reaction platform. React Chem Eng 2018;3(3):301–11.

30. Reizman BJ, Jensen KF. Feedback in flow for accelerated reaction development. Acc Chem Res 2016; 49(9):1786–96.

31. Reizman BJ, Jensen KF. Simultaneous solvent screening and reaction optimization in microliter slugs. Chem Commun 2015;51(68):13290–3.

32. Shields BJ, Stevens J, Li J, et al. Bayesian reaction optimization as a tool for chemical synthesis. Nature 2021;590:89.

33. Schweidtmann AM, Clayton AD, Holmes N, et al. Machine learning meets continuous flow chemistry: automated optimization towards the Pareto front of multiple objectives. Chem Eng J 2018;352:277–82.

34. Zhou Z, Li X, Zare RN. Optimizing chemical reactions with deep reinforcement learning. ACS Cent Sci 2017;3(12):1337–44.

35. Bruton L, Scott PJH. Automated synthesis modules for PET radiochemistry. In: Kilbourn MR, Scott PJH, editors. Handbook of radiopharmaceuticals: methodology and applications. 2nd edition. Hoboken: Wiley; 2021. p. 437–56.

36. Thompson S, Kilbourn MR, Scott PJH. Radiochemistry, PET imaging, and the internet of chemical things. ACS Cent Sci 2016;2(8):497–505.

The Evolution of Image Reconstruction in PET
From Filtered Back-Projection to Artificial Intelligence

Kuang Gong, PhD, Kyungsang Kim, PhD, Jianan Cui, PhD, Dufan Wu, PhD, Quanzheng Li, PhD*

KEYWORDS

• Image reconstruction • Artificial intelligence • Deep neural network

KEY POINTS

- Image reconstruction plays an essential role in PET image generation, with various methods developed through analytical or iterative approaches.
- Deep learning methods have found various applications in medical imaging. They can be utilized for PET image reconstruction through different approaches.
- More evaluations based on clinical data sets and comparisons with current state-of-the-art methods are needed to better understand the advantages and shortcomings of the deep learning approaches.

INTRODUCTION

PET is a nuclear-medicine imaging technique that can provide functional images revealing physiologic processes in vivo. By providing a quantitative measurement of the tracer uptake, PET has wide clinical applications. The most common applications are oncology-related[1–3] for tumor diagnosis,[4] cancer staging,[5] assessment of treatment response,[6] and recurrence monitoring.[7] In neurology, PET has steadily drawn attention owing to its ability for noninvasive examination of brain function,[8] thus providing more information for the diagnosis of dementia,[8–10] movement disorders,[11] epilepsy,[12,13] and stroke.[14] In cardiology, myocardial blood flow and myocardial metabolism can be evaluated based on PET.[15,16]

Although PET has many applications, there are still some limitations that compromise its precision: the absorption of photons in the body causes signal attenuation; the dead-time limit of system components leads to the loss of the count rate; the scattered and random events received by the detector introduce additional noise; and the characteristics of the detector limit the spatial resolution.[17–19] In addition, another limitation is the low signal-to-noise ratio (SNR) caused by the scan-time limit and dose concern. Frames with short intervals are preferred in dynamic PET for higher temporal resolution, and low-count protocols are proposed to reduce the radiation exposure.[20] Both of them decrease the detected count rate and increase the noise level.

The collected raw data are transformed to PET images with reconstruction algorithms, which are of vital importance for PET, as well-designed reconstruction algorithms can correct the physics artifacts and improves estimation accuracy of the tracer biodistribution. The early PET reconstruction methods, such as the filtered back-projection (FBP) algorithm,[21] are analytical approaches based on an idealized mathematical model. Iterative approaches[22–25] were developed

Department of Radiology, Center for Advanced Medical Computing and Analysis, Gordon Center for Medical Imaging, Massachusetts General Hospital, Harvard Medical School, Boston, MA, USA
* Corresponding author.
E-mail address: li.quanzheng@mgh.harvard.edu

PET Clin 16 (2021) 533–542
https://doi.org/10.1016/j.cpet.2021.06.004

that made it possible to consider physical factors during image reconstruction. More reconstruction approaches were later proposed to reduce the scan time or dose based on the theory of compressed sensing and sparse representation.[26]

Nowadays, deep learning–based methods have injected new vitality into the field of image reconstruction.[27–30] As early as 1991, Floyd[31] introduced the concept of neural network in single-photon emission computed tomography (SPECT) image reconstruction. Recently, with the appearance of large, high-quality data sets and parallel GPU computing, deep learning–based methods have enormous growth, especially in the field of computer vision,[32] which have been gradually introduced into the area of medical imaging and applied to PET image reconstruction.

Compared with the traditional reconstruction methods in which the models are designed based on mathematical characterizations, deep learning–based reconstruction methods are data-driven models that can learn intrinsic information and features from big data sets.[33] The deep learning–based reconstruction methods have shown empirical performance improvement over traditional reconstruction methods. However, further evaluations and investigations are needed to better understand and characterize the deep learning–based reconstruction methods. In addition, it should be noted that PET images have lower SNR compared to natural images and images from other imaging modalities, e.g., magnetic resonance (MR) and computed tomography (CT). Thus, obtaining high-quality PET images as the training labels is one challenge to be further addressed.

In this article, the authors provide a review of the evolution of image reconstruction methods in PET. The structure of this article is as follows. We first give an overview of traditional reconstruction methods for PET imaging. Five different ways that deep learning-based methods can aid PET reconstruction are later described in details.

TRADITIONAL PET IMAGE RECONSTRUCTION

For PET image reconstruction, a sinogram (or list-mode) with radial, angular, and axial variables is generated by counting coincident events between pairs of detectors. In the analytical reconstruction, although the FBP[34] is the standard algorithm in tomographic reconstruction, it is not routinely used in PET reconstruction owing to the low SNR. Particularly, slice rebinning and presubtraction of scatter, random, and normalization counts can degrade the resolution and SNR. Instead, the iterative reconstruction plays an important role in PET image reconstruction. Maximum likelihood expectation maximization (MLEM)[35] and its accelerated version, ordered subset expectation maximization (EM),[23] are the most widely used iterative algorithms. The MLEM/OSEM is based on the maximum-likelihood approach where a statistical match between the PET data and the physical model is used to find the image most likely to have resulted in the data. No prior information were considered in the MLEM/OSEM framework. The fitting can be unstable if the data are noisy, which can produce a high-frequency check-shaped artifact.[36]

In PET reconstruction, noise suppression is crucial for clinical use. To address the noise issue, penalized iterative reconstruction, also known as maximum a posteriori reconstruction, has been intensively studied. Mumcuoglu and colleagues[37] proposed a penalized iterative reconstruction framework with a quadratic smoothness penalty, and Qi and colleagues[38] have applied it to the commercial scanner. The quadratic penalty is a prior assuming that intensities of neighboring pixels are smoothly varying, which could greatly suppress the noise. However, edges and small features could be oversmoothed. Therefore, advanced penalty functions, providing not only noise reduction but also resolution preservation, have been investigated in the penalized iterative reconstruction framework. Total variation[39] is one of the most popular penalty functions in tomographic imaging, which reduces the noise and enhances the edge structure. However, it can produce staircase artifacts and be sensitive to the pixel-based intensity variation. To improve the performance, patch-based penalty functions have been developed, which use structural self-similarity, and are robust to noise while preserving the image resolution and geometric features. Wang and Qi[40] developed the unified framework using patch-based nonlocal means penalty, which improved the image quality and guaranteed the convergence because of its convexity. Kim and colleagues[41] developed the nonconvex patch-based low-rank method based on the matrix completion algorithm in the compressed sensing theory,[42] where the objective function was alternatively optimized by the convex-concave procedure method. By using the high-resolution computed tomographic (CT) and MR images, anatomic priors have been used in the penalty function. Bowsher anatomic prior[43] is the most popular method, which has improved the PET image quality using high-resolution images. Wang and Qi[44] proposed an alternative framework by incorporating penalty function into the Poisson log-likelihood, referred to as the kernel method, which simplifies the implementation by merging the kernel representation into the MLEM algorithm. Nutys and colleagues[45] developed a relative difference penalty (RDP) function where the prior penalizes relative differences rather than absolute differences. The RDP function has been used in the penalized PET image reconstruction (known as Q.Clear) recently introduced by GE healthcare.[46]

Besides handcrafted sparse transformation, dictionary learning has also been investigated in PET reconstruction by learning the transformation from data. Patch-based dictionaries are learned from prior images using K-SVD and kept fixed or optimized simultaneously with the PET images during iterative reconstruction.[47–49] Sudarshan and colleagues[50] used the same coefficients but different dictionary atoms for joint PET-MR reconstruction. Xie and colleagues[51] used a convolutional dictionary learned from prior images, which is faster than the patch-based approach. Yu and colleagues[52] considered the kinetic parametric images as dictionary atoms for joint reconstruction of activity and kinetic parametric images in dynamic PET. Compared with traditional penalty functions, the learning-based penalties can give better results because of more information extracted from the populational data sets. Interested readers can read more details about iterative PET image reconstruction and different penalty functions in previous review papers.[53-56]

DEEP LEARNING–BASED PET IMAGE RECONSTRUCTION

Deep neural networks (DNNs)-based denoising methods have been demonstrated effective to improve PET image quality through image-to-image or sinogram-to-sinogram mapping, which can be achieved through supervised learning, transfer learning, or unsupervised learning approaches.[57–76] Apart from denoising, DNNs can also be used for PET image reconstruction, aiding the process of sinogram-to-image translation. Compared with image denoising, combining DNNs with PET image reconstruction has two benefits. Firstly, the neural network have more information to utilize from the raw sinogram data. Secondly, because of the constraints from PET physics, the potential pitfalls owing to mismatches between training and testing data can be mitigated. There are several different approaches to combine DNNs with image reconstruction, which are further discussed later.

Direct Sinogram-to-Image Mapping

One approach based on the strong representation power of DNNs is to directly generate PET images from the sinograms, without the analytical/iterative image reconstruction process nor PET system modeling. One rationale of this approach is that PET system modeling is based on approximations and is far from perfect, which can be replaced by an implicit mapping learned through large and high-quality training data sets. The other advantage is its fast inference speed as no image reconstruction process is needed.

Several researchers have explored this direction. DeepPET proposed by Häggström and colleagues[77] used an encoder-decoder network to directly generate the PET image from the whole sinogram. Simulation and real data studies were used to show the improvements of the DeepPET approach. Liu and colleagues[78] proposed a conditional generative adversarial network (GAN)-based approach, where the generator was based on a U-net structure, and the evaluation with the Zubal head phantom demonstrated its effectiveness. Hu and colleagues[79] proposed a Wasserstein generative adversarial network (WGAN)-based approach, named DPIR-Net. The loss function contained the WGAN loss, the VGG-based perceptual loss, and the mean-squared error loss. Simulations based on forward-projected patient images and in vivo mouse data sets from the scanner with depth-of-interaction capability were conducted in the evaluation. Kandarpa and colleagues[80] proposed a multistep GAN-based direct reconstruction framework, named DUG-RECON. It contains 3 components: a U-net performing the sinogram-domain denoising, a double U-net–based generator mapping from sinogram to image, and finally, a Resi-Net implementing image-domain superresolution. Both CT and PET data sets were used in the evaluation. The widespread adoption of time-of-flight (TOF) information in clinical PET scanners has been a major advancement of PET hardware, which leads to substantially improved SNR. Recently, Whiteley and colleagues[81] proposed a FastPET framework to directly generate TOF images from view-grouped histo-images without the image reconstruction process, which has fewer memory requirements and network parameters, as sinograms were not input to the network directly. It processed the list-mode data based on the most likely annihilation position (MLAP) histogrammer, which estimated the most likely voxel along the line of response. Clinical data sets of various tracers were used to demonstrate the effectiveness of this method.

One challenge of the direct mapping approach is that the network complexity should be large enough to enable 3-dimensional (3D) mapping from sinogram to image. Correspondingly, it needs

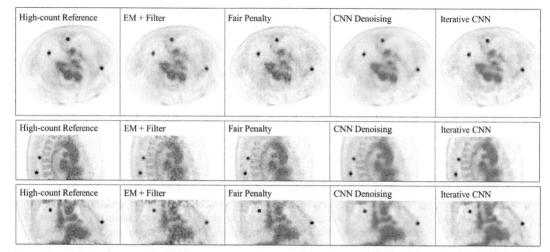

Fig. 1. Three views of one clinical data set processed using different methods. EM+filter stands for the method of applying Gaussian post filtering on the results from the MLEM algorithm. Fair Penalty stands for fair penalty function-based penalized PET image reconstruction. CNN denoising stands for directly using the trained 3D Unet to perform PET image denoising. The iterative CNN method stands for the method proposed in Gong, K., et al., Iterative PET image reconstruction using convolutional neural network representation. IEEE transactions on medical imaging, 2018. 38(3): p. 675-685.

a large number of high-quality training images to learn the mapping accurately. Because of this, more evaluations of its robustness using clinical data sets are needed.

Combining Deep Neural Networks with Iterative Reconstruction

Apart from direct mapping from sinogram to image, several works have been proposed to embed the DNN into the traditional iterative image reconstruction framework. For PET image reconstruction, the mean of the measured data $\bar{y}$ can be written as

$$\bar{y} = Px + r, \tag{1}$$

where P is the PET system model, x is the image of the unknown PET tracer bio-distribution, and r stands for the mean of randoms and scatters. Gong and colleagues[82] proposed using the convolutional neural network (CNN) to represent the unknown image x as

$$x = f(\mathbf{z}; \theta), \tag{2}$$

where $\mathbf{z}$ is the network input, θ stands for the network parameter, and f represents the network mapping function. θ was obtained by a supervised pretraining process. Based on this DNN representation, the original system model can be rewritten as

$$\bar{y} = Pf(\mathbf{z}; \theta) + r. \tag{3}$$

Based on the distribution of measured PET raw data, the image reconstruction process of finding the optimum x will be changed to estimate the network input z as

$$\hat{\mathbf{z}} = \text{argmax}_{\mathbf{z}} L(\mathbf{y}|f(\mathbf{z}; \theta)). \tag{4}$$

Here y is the PET measurements, L indicates the log-likelihood function, and the argmax operation represents finding the optimum variable that maximize the log-likelihood function. Accordingly, the final reconstructed image will be $\hat{x}=f(\hat{z}; \theta)$. During image reconstruction, the trained network can act as a constraint, so that the final estimated PET image will not only fit to the PET data, but also be similar to the high-quality network output. **Fig. 1** shows the results based on one clinical dataset, which demonstrates the superiority of the proposed method compared with the DNN denoising approach as well as other state-of-the-art methods. Apart from using the CNN as a manifold constraint, Xie and colleagues[83] proposed using a GAN with an additional attention operation as the image representation to further improve the results. An additional constraint of enforcing the network input following the PET system model was added to make the training more robust. Oncology data sets and simulations were conducted, and comprehensive comparisons with the kernel method in this work further demonstrated the effectiveness of this DNN-representation approach.

Instead of using DNN as an image representation, Kim and colleagues[84] proposed embedding the network output into the penalty function. One challenge of directly embedding the network output into the penalty function without further network-parameter/network-input optimization is that the network output obtained from the populationally pretrained network may not fit the testing PET data. To address this issue, a local linear function, inspired by the guided image filter,[85] was introduced to further modify the network output during each iterative update. This idea is similar to fine-tuning the network during each iteration to match the iterative update.

In summary, the advantages of combining DNN with the iterative reconstruction framework is that the system model and raw data are combined with the learned DNN during the testing time to reduce the potential mismatches between testing and training data sets. In addition, existing optimization algorithms/packages can be reutilized in this approach. The challenge of this approach is that the penalty parameter still needs to be adjusted,[84] and additional computation is needed when updating the network input.[82,83]

Unrolled Neural Network-Based Image Reconstruction

Pioneered by the Learned ISTA framework,[86] many unrolled networks have been developed for inverse problems. One advantage of applying unrolled neural networks to PET image reconstruction is that during both network training and testing, PET physics is considered. In the approach of combining deep learning and iterative reconstruction described in the section "Combining Deep Neural Networks with Iterative Reconstruction," PET physics is only considered during the testing time.

Several unrolled neural networks have been developed for PET image reconstruction using different optimization algorithms, network structures, and training strategies. Lim and colleagues applied a BCD-Net[87] to PET image reconstruction. To reduce the computational requirements, the unrolled neural network was trained module by module to be memory efficient. Inspired by the ADMM-Net,[88] Gong and colleagues[89] proposed an MAPEM-Net for PET image reconstruction. The data-fidelity module was constructed based on the popular MAPEM reconstruction algorithm.[90] A 3D U-net was used to find a spatially smooth solution near the MAPEM update. For both the BCD-Net and the MAPEM-Net, different network parameters were used for different unrolled modules. Mehranian and Reader[91] further proposed the FBSEM-Net framework where the forward-backward splitting algorithm was used for the

optimization of the data-fidelity term. Unlike the BCD-Net and the MAPEM-Net, the same network structure and parameters were used for each unrolled module to reduce the network parameters. Apart from low-dose PET images, the MR prior image was supplied as an additional input channel to provide extra spatial information.

One big challenge of unrolled neural networks for PET image reconstruction is its implementation difficulty. PET raw data are large, and the forward/backward projection is time-consuming. In addition, the PET data-fidelity item cannot be solved analytically (iterative updates are needed), and multiple unrolled blocks are needed to fully use the data-fidelity item. Training module by module as shown in Chun and Fessler[87] is one practical solution to reduce the GPU memory requirement. Further comparisons of the end-to-end and module-by-module training and also proposing more efficient structures are needed for this unrolled-neural-networks approach.

Unsupervised Learning-Based Image Reconstruction

The abovementioned approaches are all based on supervised learning whereby high-quality training labels are available. For low-dose/faster-scanning applications, full-dose PET datasets can be utilized as training labels. However, if we want to further improve the image quality of full-dose PET, obtaining higher-quality PET data as training labels is not easy. One solution is utilizing simulated datasets to pre-train the network. Accuracy of the physical modeling during simulation can affect the final results. Another soluiton is unsupervised deep learning. Inspired by the deep image prior (DIP) framework,[92] Gong and colleagues[93] proposed a DIPRecon framework to train the neural network based on the statistical distribution of PET raw data, where high-quality training labels are not needed. The basic idea is using a DNN to represent the unknown image, the same as shown in equation (2). The network input, fixed during reconstruction, is the high-resolution prior image z_a from the same patient, which is widely available in current PET/CT or PET/MR scanners. Through this representation, the image reconstruction problem was transferred to the network optimization problem: the network parameters θ were iteratively updated to minimize the data fidelity term. The whole image reconstruction process can be summarized in 2 steps as

$$\hat{\theta} = \text{argmax}_{\theta} L(f(\theta|z_a), y), \quad \hat{x} = f(\hat{\theta}|z_a).$$

Fig. 2 shows the results of simulation and clinical data sets. It can be observed that the

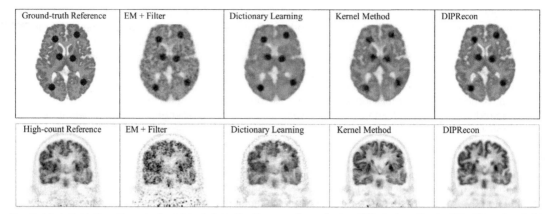

Fig. 2. The simulation (*top row*) and real data (*bottom row*) results for different methods. EM+filter stands for the method of applying Gaussian post filtering on the results from the MLEM algorithm. Dictionary learning stands for the method proposed in Chen S, Liu H, Shi P, et al. Sparse representation and dictionary learning penalized image reconstruction for positron emission tomography. Phys Med Biol 2015;60(2):807-23. Kernel method stands for the method proposed in Wang G, Qi J. PET image reconstruction using kernel method. IEEE Trans Med Imaging 2015; 34(1):61-71. The DIPRecon method stands for the method proposed in Gong, K., et al., PET image reconstruction using deep image prior. IEEE transactions on medical imaging, 2019. 38(7): p. 1655 – 1665.

DIPRecon framework can better recover the cortical details while also reducing the image noise. It should be noted that the network in the DIP framework is trained from scratch. If the network is pre-trained based on other datasets/tasks and further fine-tuned inside the DIP framework, the results should be further improved.

For dynamic PET imaging, the scanning time is long. Considering patient comfort and safety, it is not feasible to further increase the scanning time or radiation dose. Unsupervised deep learning is thus one solution for dynamic PET image denoising/reconstruction. Gong and colleagues[94] further extended the DIPRecon to direct PET Patlak parametric image reconstruction, where the input is the patient's prior image, and the output is the Patlak slope and intercept images. The PET Patlak model was represented as a convolutional layer inside the network. Yokota and colleagues[95] proposed using DIP for dynamic PET denoising. The reconstructed PET images were factorized to a spatial matrix and a temporal matrix. Each component of the spatial matrix component was represented by a U-net. Unsupervised deep learning can make deep learning more affordable in various applications. Further evaluations and comparisons with state-of-the-art methods are needed to understand its potentials. Novel ways of constructing the unsupervised learning-based framework for PET image reconstruction are exciting, should be encouraged, and deserve further explorations.

Joint Image Reconstruction and Other Tasks

Apart from purely deep learning–based image reconstruction, there are works focusing on achieving better image reconstruction with other tasks, such as image segmentation and motion correction. Lim and colleagues[96] proposed a joint reconstruction and segmentation network, where the pretrained segmentation network was embedded into the unrolled neural network to provide the edge information. In addition, the reconstructed PET image aided by the edge information (derived from the segmentation network) can further improve the image segmentation performance. Regarding motion correction, Li and colleagues[97] proposed a joint motion-estimation and image-reconstruction framework to improve gated PET image reconstruction. The motion estimation network was similar to the structure used in the VoxelMorph framework.[98] Zhou and colleagues[99] proposed a motion correction and image denoising network, named MDPET, for gated low-dose PET imaging denoising, where the joint denoising and motion correction were implemented based on a temporal siamese pyramid network through using both spatial and temporal information. These prior works combined the denoising network with a registration/segmentation network for specific tasks, which are encouraging and deserve further exploring.

SUMMARY

Compared with other imaging modalities, the image quality of PET imaging is worse, and further improvements are in urgent need. In recent years, because of the initial success in computer vision, tremendous and encouraging research related to deep learning applications in PET image enhancements have been seen, which opens new paths for

PET image reconstruction research, such as direct mapping from sinogram to image, unrolled neural networks, and joint reconstructions with segmentation/registration. In addition, research is actively on-going about how to combine traditional iterative image reconstruction with deep learning approaches. More evaluations based on clinical data sets and comparisons with current state-of-the-art methods are needed to better understand the advantages and shortcomings of each reconstruction approach.

CLINICS CARE POINTS

- Deep learning methods are being developed for PET image reconstruction and show better performance than state-of-the-art methods.

- More evaluations based on clinical data sets are needed to further evaluate and better understand the deep learning approaches.

DISCLOSURE

This work was supported by the National Institutes of Health under grants R21AG067422, R03EB030280, RF1AG052653 and P41EB022544.

REFERENCES

1. Strauss LG, Conti PS. The applications of PET in clinical oncology. J Nucl Med 1991;32(4):623–50.
2. Kubota K. From tumor biology to clinical PET: a review of positron emission tomography (PET) in oncology. Ann Nucl Med 2001;15(6):471–86.
3. Belhocine T, Spaepen K, Dusart M, et al. 18FDG PET in oncology: the best and the worst (review). Int J Oncol 2006;28(5):1249–61.
4. Sundin A, Eriksson B, Bergström M, et al. PET in the diagnosis of neuroendocrine tumors. Ann N Y Acad Sci 2004;1014(1):246–57.
5. Fischer B, Lassen U, Mortensen J, et al. Preoperative staging of lung cancer with combined PET-CT. N Engl J Med 2009;361(1):32–9.
6. Ben-Haim S, Ell P. 18F-FDG PET and PET/CT in the evaluation of cancer treatment response. J Nucl Med 2009;50(1):88–99.
7. Lei L, Wang X, Chen Z. PET/CT imaging for monitoring recurrence and evaluating response to treatment in breast cancer. Adv Clin Exp Med 2016; 25(2):377–82.
8. Herholz K. PET studies in dementia. Ann Nucl Med 2003;17(2):79–89.
9. Jagust W, Reed B, Mungas D, et al. What does fluorodeoxyglucose PET imaging add to a clinical diagnosis of dementia? Neurology 2007;69(9):871–7.
10. Herholz K, Salmon E, Perani D, et al. Discrimination between Alzheimer dementia and controls by automated analysis of multicenter FDG PET. Neuroimage 2002;17(1):302–16.
11. Ruottinen HM, Partinen M, Hublin C, et al. An FDOPA PET study in patients with periodic limb movement disorder and restless legs syndrome. Neurology 2000;54(2):502–4.
12. PET and SPECT in epilepsy: a critical review. Epilepsy \& Behav 2009;15(1):50–5.
13. Sarikaya I. PET studies in epilepsy. Am J Nucl Med Mol Imaging 2015;5(5):416–30.
14. Werner P, Saur D, Zeisig V, et al. Simultaneous PET/MRI in stroke: a case series. J Cereb Blood Flow Metab 2015;35(9):1421–5.
15. Plein S, Sivananthan M. The role of positron emission tomography in cardiology. Radiography 2001;7(1):11–20.
16. Schwaiger M, Ziegler S, Nekolla SG. PET/CT: challenge for nuclear cardiology. J Nucl Med 2005; 46(10):1664–78.
17. Meikle SR, Badawi RD. Quantitative techniques in PET. In: Positron emission tomography. London: Springer; 2005. p. 93–126.
18. Iriarte A, Marabini R, Matej S, et al. System models for PET statistical iterative reconstruction: a review. Comput Med Imaging Graph 2016;48:30–48.
19. Efthimiou N. New challenges for PET image reconstruction for total-body imaging. PET Clin 2020; 15(4):453–61.
20. Catana C. The dawn of a new era in low-dose PET imaging. 2019. DOI: https://doi.org/10.1148/radiol. 2018182573.
21. Shepp LA, Logan BF. The Fourier reconstruction of a head section. IEEE Trans Nucl Sci 1974;21(3):21–43.
22. Vardi Y, Shepp LA, Kaufman L. A statistical model for positron emission tomography. J Am Stat Assoc 1985;80(389):8–20.
23. Hudson HM, Larkin RS. Accelerated image reconstruction using ordered subsets of projection data. IEEE Trans Med Imaging 1994;13(4):601–9.
24. Green PJ. Bayesian reconstructions from emission tomography data using a modified EM algorithm. IEEE Trans Med Imaging 1990;9(1):84–93.
25. Qi J, Leahy RM, Cherry SR, et al. High-resolution 3D Bayesian image reconstruction using the microPET small-animal scanner. Phys Med Biol 1998;43(4): 1001–13.
26. Malczewski K. PET image reconstruction using compressed sensing. In: 2013 signal processing: algorithms, architectures, arrangements, and applications (SPA). IEEE; 2013. p. 176–81.
27. Reader AJ, Corda G, Mehranian A, et al. Deep learning for PET image reconstruction. IEEE Trans Radiat Plasma Med Sci 2020;5(1):1–25.

28. Ravishankar S, Ye JC, Fessler JA. Image reconstruction: from sparsity to data-adaptive methods and machine learning. Proc IEEE Inst Electr Electron Eng 2020;108(1):86–109.

29. Gong K, Berg E, Cherry SR, et al. Machine learning in PET: from photon detection to quantitative image reconstruction. Proc IEEE 2019;108(1):51–68.

30. Wang G, Ye JC, Mueller K, et al. Image reconstruction is a new frontier of machine learning. IEEE Trans Med Imaging 2018;37(6):1289–96.

31. Floyd CE. An artificial neural network for SPECT image reconstruction. IEEE Trans Med Imaging 1991; 10(3):485–7.

32. Voulodimos A, Doulamis N, Doulamis A, et al. Deep learning for computer vision: a brief review. Comput Intell Neurosci 2018;2018:7068349.

33. Zhang H-M, Dong B. A review on deep learning in medical image reconstruction. J Operations Res Soc China 2020;1–30.

34. Feldkamp LA, Davis LC, Kress JW. Practical cone-beam algorithm. J Opt Soc Am A 1984;1(6):612–9.

35. Shepp LA, Vardi Y. Maximum likelihood reconstruction for emission tomography. IEEE Trans Med Imaging 1982;1(2):113–22.

36. Bailey DL, Maisey MN, Townsend DW, et al. Positron emission tomography, vol. 2. London: Springer; 2005.

37. Mumcuoglu EÜÜ, Leahy RM, Cherry SR. Bayesian reconstruction of PET images: methodology and performance analysis. Phys Med Biol 1996;41(9): 1777–807.

38. Jinyi Qi J, Leahy RM, Chinghan Hsu fnm, et al. Fully 3D Bayesian image reconstruction for the ECAT EXACT HR+. IEEE Trans Nucl Sci 1998;45(3): 1096–103.

39. Panin VY, Zeng GL, Gullberg GT. Total variation regulated EM algorithm [SPECT reconstruction]. IEEE Trans Nucl Sci 1999;46(6):2202–10.

40. Wang G, Qi J. Penalized likelihood PET image reconstruction using patch-based edge-preserving regularization. IEEE Trans Med Imaging 2012; 31(12):2194–204.

41. Kim K, Son YD, Bresler Y, et al. Dynamic PET reconstruction using temporal patch-based low rank penalty for ROI-based brain kinetic analysis. Phys Med Biol 2015;60(5):2019–46.

42. Candès EJ, Recht B. Exact matrix completion via convex optimization. Found Comput Math 2009; 9(6):717–72.

43. Bowsher JE, Johnson VE, Turkington TG, et al. Bayesian reconstruction and use of anatomical a priori information for emission tomography. IEEE Trans Med Imaging 1996;15(5):673–86.

44. Wang G, Qi J. PET image reconstruction using kernel method. IEEE Trans Med Imaging 2015; 34(1):61–71.

45. Nuyts J, Beque D, Dupont P, et al. A concave prior penalizing relative differences for maximum-a-posteriori reconstruction in emission tomography. IEEE Trans Nucl Sci 2002;49(1):56–60.

46. Ahn S, Ross SG, Asma E, et al. Quantitative comparison of OSEM and penalized likelihood image reconstruction using relative difference penalties for clinical PET. Phys Med Biol 2015;60(15):5733.

47. Zhang W, Gao J, Yang Y, et al. Image reconstruction for positron emission tomography based on patch-based regularization and dictionary learning. Med Phys 2019;46(11):5014–26.

48. Chen S, Liu H, Shi P, et al. Sparse representation and dictionary learning penalized image reconstruction for positron emission tomography. Phys Med Biol 2015;60(2):807–23.

49. Tang J, Yang B, Wang Y, et al. Sparsity-constrained PET image reconstruction with learned dictionaries. Phys Med Biol 2016;61(17):6347–68.

50. Sudarshan VP, Egan GF, Chen Z, et al. Joint PET-MRI image reconstruction using a patch-based joint-dictionary prior. Med Image Anal 2020;62:101669.

51. Xie N, Gong K, Guo N, et al. Penalized-likelihood PET image reconstruction using 3D structural convolutional sparse coding. IEEE Trans Biomed Eng 2020. https://doi.org/10.1109/TBME.2020.3042907.

52. Yu H, Chen S, Chen Y, et al. Joint reconstruction of dynamic PET activity and kinetic parametric images using total variation constrained dictionary sparse coding. Inverse Probl 2017;33(5):055011.

53. Reader AJ, Zaidi H. Advances in PET image reconstruction. PET Clinics 2007;2(2):173–90.

54. Bai B, Li Q, Leahy RM. Magnetic resonance-guided positron emission tomography image reconstruction. Semin Nucl Med 2013;43(1):30–44.

55. Qi J, Leahy RM. Iterative reconstruction techniques in emission computed tomography. Phys Med Biol 2006;51(15):R541.

56. Tong S, Alessio AM, Kinahan PE. Image reconstruction for PET/CT scanners: past achievements and future challenges. Imaging Med 2010;2(5):529.

57. Xiang L, Qiao Y, Nie D, et al. Deep auto-context convolutional neural networks for standard-dose PET image estimation from low-dose PET/MRI. Neurocomputing 2017;267:406–16.

58. Xu J, Gong E, Pauly J, et al. 200x Low-dose PET reconstruction using deep learning. arXiv preprint arXiv:1712.04119, 2017.

59. Wang Y, Yu B, Wang L, et al. 3D conditional generative adversarial networks for high-quality PET image estimation at low dose. Neuroimage 2018;174: 550–62.

60. Gong K, Guan J, Liu CC, et al. PET image denoising using a deep neural network through fine tuning. IEEE Trans Radiat Plasma Med Sci 2019;3(2):153–61.

61. Chen KT, Gong E, de Carvalho Macruz FB, et al. Ultra–low-dose 18F-florbetaben amyloid PET imaging

using deep learning with multi-contrast MRI inputs. Radiology 2018;180940.

62. Liu C-C, Qi J. Higher SNR PET image prediction using a deep learning model and MRI image. Phys Med Biol 2019;64(11):115004.

63. Yang B, Fontaine K, Carson R, et al. Brain PET dose reduction using a shallow artificial neural network. J Nucl Med 2018;59(supplement 1):99a.

64. Kaplan S, Zhu Y-M. Full-dose PET image estimation from low-dose PET image using deep learning: a pilot study. J digital Imaging 2018;32(5):773–8.

65. Yang B, Ying L, Tang J. Artificial neural network enhanced Bayesian PET image reconstruction. IEEE Trans Med Imaging 2018;37(6):1297–309.

66. Cui J, Gong K, Guo N, et al. PET image denoising using unsupervised deep learning. Eur J Nucl Med Mol Imaging 2019;46(13):2780–9.

67. da Costa-Luis CO, Reader AJ. Micro-networks for robust MR-guided low count PET imaging. IEEE Trans Radiat Plasma Med Sci 2020;5(2):202–12.

68. Song TA, Chowdhury SR, Yang F, et al. Super-resolution PET imaging using convolutional neural networks. IEEE Trans Comput Imaging 2020;6:518–28.

69. Sanaat A, Shiri I, Arabi H, et al. Deep learning-assisted ultra-fast/low-dose whole-body PET/CT imaging. Eur J Nucl Med Mol Imaging 2021;48(8):2405–15.

70. Lu W, Onofrey JA, Lu Y, et al. An investigation of quantitative accuracy for deep learning based denoising in oncological PET. Phys Med Biol 2019;64(16):165019.

71. Chan C, Zhou J, Yang L, et al. Noise to noise ensemble learning for PET image denoising. in 2019 IEEE Nuclear Science Symposium and Medical Imaging Conference (NSS/MIC). 26 Oct.-2 Nov. 2019. IEEE. Manchester, UK.

72. Hashimoto F, Ohba H, Ote K, et al. Dynamic PET image denoising using deep convolutional neural networks without prior training datasets. IEEE Access 2019;7:96594–603.

73. Zhou L, Schaefferkoetter JD, Tham IWK, et al. Supervised learning with cyclegan for low-dose FDG PET image denoising. Med Image Anal 2020;65:101770.

74. Klyuzhin IS, Cheng JC, Bevington C, et al. Use of a tracer-specific deep artificial neural net to denoise dynamic PET images. IEEE Trans Med Imaging 2020;39(2):366–76.

75. Sun H, Peng L, Zhang H, et al. Dynamic PET image denoising using deep image prior combined with regularization by denoising. IEEE Access 2021;9:52378–92.

76. Angelis GI, Fuller OK, Gillam JE, et al. Denoising non-steady state dynamic PET data using a feed-forward neural network. Phys Med Biol 2021;66(3):034001.

77. Häggström I, Schmidtlein CR, Campanella G, et al. DeepPET: a deep encoder-decoder network for directly solving the PET image reconstruction inverse problem. Med Image Anal 2019;54:253–62.

78. Liu Z, Chen H, Liu H. Deep learning based framework for direct reconstruction of PET images. in International Conference on Medical Image Computing and Computer-Assisted Intervention. October 13-17, 2019. Springer Shenzhen, China.

79. Hu Z, Xue H, Zhang Q, et al. DPIR-Net: direct PET image reconstruction based on the Wasserstein generative adversarial network. IEEE Trans Radiat Plasma Med Sci 2020;5(1):35–43.

80. Kandarpa VS, Bousse A, Benoit D, et al. DUG-RECON: a framework for direct image reconstruction using convolutional generative networks. IEEE Trans Radiat Plasma Med Sci 2020;5(1):44–53.

81. Whiteley W, Panin V, Zhou C, et al. FastPET: near real-time reconstruction of PET histo-image data using a neural network. IEEE Trans Radiat Plasma Med Sci 2020;5(1):65–77.

82. Gong K, Guan J, Kim K, et al. Iterative PET image reconstruction using convolutional neural network representation. IEEE Trans Med Imaging 2018;38(3):675–85.

83. Xie Z, Baikejiang R, Li T, et al. Generative adversarial network based regularized image reconstruction for PET. Phys Med Biol 2020;65(12):125016.

84. Kim K, Wu D, Gong K, et al. Penalized PET reconstruction using deep learning prior and local linear fitting. IEEE Trans Med Imaging 2018;37(6):1478–87.

85. He K, Sun J, Tang X. Guided image filtering. IEEE Trans pattern Anal Machine Intelligence 2012;35(6):1397–409.

86. Gregor K, LeCun Y. Learning fast approximations of sparse coding. in Proceedings of the 27th International Conference on Machine Learning. June 21-24, 2010. Haifa, Israel.

87. Chun Y, Fessler JA. Deep BCD-net using identical encoding-decoding CNN structures for iterative image recovery. in 2018 IEEE 13th Image, Video, and Multidimensional Signal Processing Workshop (IVMSP). 10-12 June 2018. Aristi Village, Greece.

88. Sun J, Li H, Xu Z. Deep ADMM-Net for compressive sensing MRI. Adv Neural Inf Process Syst 2016.

89. Gong K, Wu D, Kim K, et al. MAPEM-Net: an unrolled neural network for fully 3D PET image reconstruction. in 15th International Meeting on Fully Three-Dimensional Image Reconstruction in Radiology and Nuclear Medicine. June 2-6, 2019. International Society for Optics and Photonics. Philadelphia, United States

90. Pierro De. A.R., A modified expectation maximization algorithm for penalized likelihood estimation in emission tomography. IEEE Trans Med Imaging 1994;14(1):132–7.

91. Mehranian A, Reader AJ. Model-based deep learning PET image reconstruction using forward-backward splitting expectation maximisation. IEEE Trans Radiat Plasma Med Sci 2020;5(1):54–64.

92. Ulyanov D, Vedaldi A, Lempitsky V. Deep image prior. In Proceedings of the IEEE conference on computer vision and pattern recognition 2018 (pp. 9446-9454).

93. Gong K, Catana C, Qi J, et al. PET image reconstruction using deep image prior. IEEE Trans Med Imaging 2019;38(7):1655–65.

94. Gong K, Catana C, Qi J, et al. Direct patlak reconstruction from dynamic PET using unsupervised deep learning. in 15th International Meeting on Fully Three-Dimensional Image Reconstruction in Radiology and Nuclear Medicine. June 2-6, 2019. International Society for Optics and Photonics. Philadelphia, United States.

95. Yokota T, Kawai K, Sakata M, et al. Dynamic pet image reconstruction using nonnegative matrix factorization incorporated with deep image prior. in Proceedings of the IEEE/CVF International Conference on Computer Vision. October 27 to November 2, 2019. Seoul, Korea.

96. Lim H, Dewaraja YK, Fessler JA. Joint low-count PET/CT segmentation and reconstruction with paired variational neural networks. In: Medical imaging 2020: Physics of medical imaging, vol. 11312. International Society for Optics and Photonics; 2020. p. 113120U. https://doi.org/10.1117/12.2543252.

97. Li T, Zhang M, Qi W, et al. Deep learning based joint PET image reconstruction and motion estimation. J Nucl Med 2020;61(supplement 1):11.

98. Balakrishnan G, Zhao A, Sabuncu MR, et al. VoxelMorph: a learning framework for deformable medical image registration. IEEE Trans Med Imaging 2019;38(8):1788–800.

99. Zhou B, Tsai YJ, Chen X, et al. MDPET: a unified motion correction and denoising adversarial network for low-dose gated PET. IEEE Trans Med Imaging 2021. https://doi.org/10.1109/TMI.2021.3076191.

Artificial Intelligence–Based Data Corrections for Attenuation and Scatter in Position Emission Tomography and Single-Photon Emission Computed Tomography

Alan B. McMillan, PhD*, Tyler J. Bradshaw, PhD

KEYWORDS

- Artificial intelligence • Deep learning • Attenuation correction • Scatter correction • PET • SPECT

KEY POINTS

- Promising artificial intelligence (AI) techniques are being used to improve attenuation and scatter correction for PET and single-photon emission computed tomography (SPECT) imaging.
- AI-based attenuation correction can provide high-quality synthetic computed tomography scans from other available images such as MR imaging or uncorrected PET images to improve the capability of PET and SPECT.
- AI-based scatter correction can accelerate PET reconstruction.
- AI methods can be used to estimate both attenuation and scatter simultaneously.

INTRODUCTION

Both PET and single-photon emission computed tomography (SPECT) reconstructions require several corrections to yield high-quality quantitative images. These corrections include correction for random coincidences, detector dead-time, detector normalization, scattered coincidences (commonly referred to as scatter correction), and attenuation.[1] For the correction of scatter and attenuation, the tendency of electrons within the underlying tissue is to induce Compton scattering due to electron interaction of PET or SPECT photons. This results in undetected annihilation events (attenuation) or the detection of anomalous coincidences (scatter). The likelihood of a photon interacting with a medium increases with both the distance traveled as well as the electron density of the underlying tissue and material through which the photons travel. Therefore, to accurately estimate attenuation and scatter, an additional image that provides linear attenuation coefficients of the material is needed. Historically this has necessitated the use of an external radioactive source to obtain transmission images on a PET system,[2] and more recently has relied on the use of CT to obtain this information for PET/computed tomography (CT) and SPECT/CT. The more recent development of PET/MR has complicated this matter, where MR images are not routinely capable of identifying bone with positive contrast, making a direct conversion of MR data into a linear attenuation coefficients challenging.[1]

Scattered coincidences typically account for 30% to 50% of the detected coincidence events in a PET scan. Scatter correction algorithms,

Department of Radiology, University of Wisconsin, 3252 Clinical Science Center, 600 Highland Avenue, Madison, WI 53792, USA
* Corresponding author.
E-mail address: amcmillan@uwhealth.org
Twitter: @alan_b_mcmillan (A.B.M.); @tybradshaw11 (T.J.B.)

PET Clin 16 (2021) 543–552
https://doi.org/10.1016/j.cpet.2021.06.010
1556-8598/21/© 2021 Elsevier Inc. All rights reserved.

such as the single-scatter simulation method, require knowledge of the local activity concentration in addition to the attenuation coefficients of the object to estimate the likelihood of scattered coincidences. As the local activity concentration is only known after image reconstruction with scatter correction, iterative methods are typically required and can be time-consuming to compute. Although a full review of scatter corrections is not possible here, several reviews are dedicated to this problem.[3–5]

In the past several years, there has been a great effort to develop algorithms that use artificial intelligence (AI), that is, machine learning and deep learning techniques, to aid in the processing and reconstruction of medical imaging data. These techniques hold much promise in solving some of the quantitative challenges related to scatter and attenuation, particularly when additional transmission or CT imaging is unavailable or undesired in the attempt to reduce patient ionizing radiation exposure, or when patient motion degrades the effectiveness of the CT image, or for other reasons. Particularly in the development of PET/MR systems, where CT is not possible, there has been a particularly intense focus on the development of machine learning–based techniques that have demonstrated strong preliminary performance. AI-based approaches, unlike other algorithms, "learn" to perform the task at hand, which in this case is the production of a CT-like image. AI techniques often use the concept of supervised learning, where examples of input images, such as an MR imaging scan, are paired with training labels that represent the desired output image, such as a CT. Through a complex process of backpropagation and iterative training,[6,7] these algorithms are able to learn the relationships between features of the input data and the desired output. More recently, deep learning–based techniques, and in particular convolutional neural networks, have received substantial interest compared with more conventional machine learning–based techniques.

ARTIFICIAL INTELLIGENCE–BASED METHODS

A block diagram of an AI-based workflow for AI-based attenuation and/or scatter correction is shown in **Fig. 1**. Here an MR input image is paired with a CT image from the same patient to create a database of image pairs. On successful spatial registration of these 2 datasets, a deep learning network is used to train a model that synthesizes a CT-like image from only an MR imaging input. Once fully trained, the model is able to yield synthetic CT images that would be appropriate inputs into a conventional PET reconstruction pipeline.

The performance of any given AI-based approach is going to depend on the type and structure of the underlying model that is used. Although numerous types of models or networks could be used for a given application, the literature suggests that several types of specific model architectures are particularly effective. For example, most AI-based approaches use convolutional neural networks (CNNs). CNNs consist of multiple layers of synthetic neurons that learn the convolution kernels and sample weights to encode various features in both the input and desired output images.[6,7] There are many CNN-based architectures that have been developed, but 2 specific architectures have been the most studied for attenuation and scatter correction, shown in **Fig. 2**. The first is the UNet, which is nearly ubiquitous in its application to image processing in a wide range of fields.[7] This model uses a combination of essentially 2 models, one to encode the features of the input image, and another to decode the learned features into the desired output image. A key feature of the UNet is the sharing of learned features between the encoding and decoding side of the network, which improves model performance. Another popular model structure is the generative adversarial network (GAN). A GAN consists of 2 separate models, one model as a generator, which is used to synthesize the output, and a second model, a discriminator, which is used to determine the quality of the synthesized output from the generator.[8] Essentially, the generator is trained such that it can create a synthesized image (eg, a synthetic CT image) for which the discriminator cannot determine whether the generated image is real or fake. The discriminator learns from real examples and is trained to identify the fake images from the generator. The advantage of GAN-based approaches is that they can produce more realistic-looking outputs. Some types of GANs do not require spatially registered input-output pairs, which can be challenging to acquire, thus greatly reducing the burden of having paired datasets with multimodality image registration.

Evaluation Metrics

The performance of a trained algorithm in synthesizing CT images is typically evaluated using various metrics that compare the model's synthetic CT image with the original CT from the same patient. Common metrics to assess quality include root mean square error (RMSE), mean absolute error (MAE), structural similarity index (SSIM), peak signal to noise ratio (PSNR), and Dice coefficient (DC). In addition, the PET or SPECT images reconstructed using the synthetic

AI-based Attenuation Correction

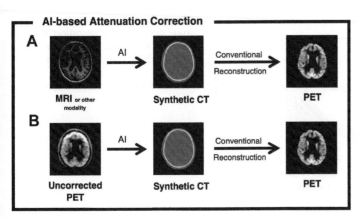

A   MRI or other modality → AI → Synthetic CT → Conventional Reconstruction → PET

B   Uncorrected PET → AI → Synthetic CT → Conventional Reconstruction → PET

AI-based Scatter Correction

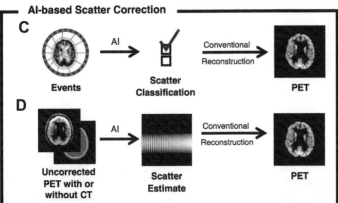

C   Events → AI → Scatter Classification → Conventional Reconstruction → PET

D   Uncorrected PET with or without CT → AI → Scatter Estimate → Conventional Reconstruction → PET

AI-based Attenuation and Scatter Correction

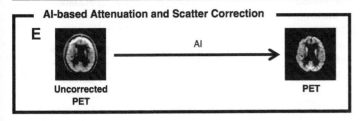

E   Uncorrected PET → AI → PET

Fig. 1. AI-based workflows for attenuation and scatter correction in PET (similar approaches are analogous for SPECT), depicting the use of (*A*) an MR image or other images to create a synthetic CT to be used in a conventional reconstruction pipeline; (*B*) an uncorrected PET image to create a synthetic CT to be used in a conventional reconstruction pipeline; (*C*) a classification system to determine scattered coincidence; (*D*) an uncorrected PET image with or without a CT to estimate scatter; and (*E*) an uncorrected PET image to synthesize a corrected PET image, incorporating both attenuation and scatter correction.

CT can be compared with the same image reconstructed using the ground truth CT. The final bias in the reconstructed image can then be quantified. Each of these metrics have their own relative strengths and weaknesses and thus the evaluation of a single model's performance should use multiple metrics. There exist no standard approaches for the assessment of attenuation and scatter algorithms, so investigators typically report using 1 or more of the aforementioned metrics. Unfortunately, this can make it difficult to compare results between different approaches.

Root mean square error (RMSE) is a measure of the square root of the average squared difference between the synthesized CT and the original CT calculated for each voxel in the image, using the following equation:

$$RMSE(\hat{y}, y) = \sqrt{\frac{\sum(\hat{y} - y)^2}{n}} \quad (1)$$

, where $\hat{y}$ is the synthesized CT, y is the original CT, and n is the number of voxels. RMSE values are often calculated separately for soft tissue regions and bone and have units that match the original image, in this case Hounsfield units (HU). High-performing approaches typically have RMSE values of 100 HU or less.[9–11]

Mean absolute error (MAE) is similar to the RMSE except that it is the absolute error rather than the squared error as calculated using the following equation:

$$MAE(\hat{y}, y) = \sqrt{\frac{\sum|\hat{y} - y|}{n}} \quad (2)$$

A UNet

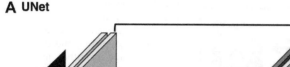
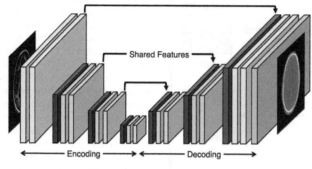

Shared Features

← Encoding → ← Decoding →

Fig. 2. (*A*) Layout of a UNet architecture depicting an encoding and decoding structure. (*B*) Layout of a GAN architecture depicting a generator to synthesize images and a discriminator to assess the quality.

B GAN

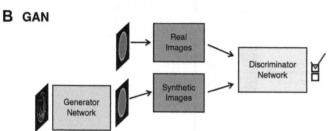

Real Images

Synthetic Images

Generator Network

Discriminator Network

MAE also yields error in units that match the original image. One limitation of the MAE approach is that if errors are centered around zero, the values of MAE may be much smaller than RMSE. Both RMSE and MAE can be sensitive to the cropping of the images: if images contain large amounts of surrounding air, this can have the effect of decreasing the average error, as models can often predict surrounding air with near perfect accuracy.

Structural similarity index (SSIM) is another measure of the image quality widely used throughout the computer vision literature. SSIM yields a metric on a scale that ranges between −1 and 1, where an SSIM 1 represents a perfect recovery of the original image. SSIM can be calculated using the following equations:

$$SSIM(\hat{y}, y) = \frac{\left(2\mu_{\hat{y}}\mu_y + c_1\right)\left(2\sigma_{\hat{y}y} + c_2\right)}{\left(\mu_{\hat{y}}^2 + \mu_y^2 + c_1\right)\left(\sigma_{\hat{y}}^2 + \sigma_y^2 + c_2\right)}$$ (3)

$$c_1 = (K_1 L)^2$$

$$c_2 = (K_2 L)^2$$

, where $\mu_{\hat{y}}$, μ_y, $\sigma_{\hat{y}}^2$, σ_y^2, $\sigma_{\hat{y}y}$ are the average, variance, and covariance of $\hat{y}$ and y, respectively. K_1 and K_2 are constants equal to 0.01 and 0.03. L is equal to the dynamic range (ie, the range from the smallest to largest pixel value) in the image.

Peak signal-to-noise ratio (PSNR) is a measure of relative power of the relative difference or noise in an image compared with its reference, and can be calculated using the following equation:

$$PSNR = 10\log_{10}\left(L^2 / MSE\right)$$ (4)

Dice coefficient (DC) is measure of overlap between discrete regions of a segmented image, where a coefficient of 1 means perfect overlap. This metric is frequently used to determine the ability of AI approaches to estimate specific regions, such as air, soft tissue, and bone. DC can be calculated using the following equation:

$$DC = (2 * TP)/(2 * TP + FN + FP)$$ (5)

where *TP* is the number of true positives, *FN* is the number of false negatives, and *FP* is the number of false positives in a segmented image relative to the reference. DC is often used to assess the quality of bone estimate in brain attenuation correction approaches. For studies in the brain, DC of 0.8 or greater in bone typically identifies a very good performing synthetic CT approach.

The end goal of CT synthesis is to use the CT for attenuation and scatter correction and create nuclear medicine images with minimum bias. Thus, reconstruction bias is an important metric that compares the end result of a given attenuation or scatter correction approach with the conventional approach. Bias is typically represented as a percentage of error within a given region or over the entire image. Reconstruction image bias is typically calculated as follows:

$$Bias(\widehat{y}, y) = \frac{y - \widehat{y}}{y} \times 100\% \qquad (6)$$

Reconstruction bias averaged over the entire image can hide errors or biases occurring in small regions of high importance, such as tumors. These regions should be quantified and compared.

ARTIFICIAL INTELLIGENCE–BASED ATTENUATION CORRECTION

For AI-based attenuation correction methods, the AI algorithm synthesizes a CT-like image that can then be used in place of a CT within a conventional reconstruction pipeline. The input for the algorithm is typically an MR image (as used for simultaneous PET/MR imaging), as shown in **Fig. 1**A, or the underlying uncorrected PET or SPECT image itself, as shown in **Fig. 1**B. The goal of the AI algorithm is not necessarily to create a diagnostic image, but one that is a sufficiently realistic image and minimizes the reconstruction bias in the final image. One shortcoming of most published AI approaches is that the models are typically trained to be tuned to identifying one anatomic region, such as the brain, chest, or pelvis, and are generally not applicable to the whole body. Although this does not necessarily limit these algorithms for their intended use, it does require that separate approaches be developed for each individual body part. As the feasibility of anatomic-specific algorithms for attenuation correction has already been well established, future approaches should focus on whole-body corrections, such that a uniform approach can be used regardless of the anatomy being scanned.

Several recent reviews have compared the performance of the increasing number of AI-based approaches proposed for synthetic CT generation.[9–11] In **Table 1**, we highlight several approaches evaluated in different body regions, including the brain, chest, and pelvis, for both PET and SPECT. Due to the rapid pace of innovation in this area, these results are likely to be soon joined by new and better-performing approaches. However, these results demonstrate that high-performing approaches already exist that appear to provide sufficient quantitative results without the need for the acquisition of a CT. Note that approaches that include a joint estimation of attenuation and scatter (see **Fig. 1**E) are listed in **Table 3**.

In the future, AI-based approaches may even exceed the capability of existing CT approaches, for example, in the case of motion, where it might not be feasible to acquire additional CT imaging due to physiologic and/or bulk patient movement. It could also improve dynamic imaging over long periods (or dual time point imaging) without needing to reacquire a CT. It appears that it may be feasible to leverage an AI-based approach to construct a motion-compensated synthetic CT or even a multiphase CT, directly from the underlying PET or SPECT data. Although there exist some potential limitations with AI-based approaches, it is likely that these approaches will gain greater clinical acceptance in the near future. Furthermore, the development of AI-based approaches for synthetic CT images to aid in attenuation correction is highly synergistic with the development of MR-only radiotherapy.[28] In this application, the valuable soft tissue contrast of MR imaging is useful in the delineation of tumors, yet MR imaging is challenged in the direct synthesis of CT-like images. Therefore, there has also been great interest in developing synthetic CT technology using AI in the radiotherapy. Developments for both improved diagnostic imaging capability in PET and SPECT as well as for radiotherapy are expected to be mutually beneficial, as the underlying techniques and AI models are highly similar.

ARTIFICIAL INTELLIGENCE SCATTER CORRECTION

AI-based approaches to scatter correction promise to increase the overall speed of image reconstruction due to the often time-consuming nature of estimating scatter correction. In addition, AI may allow for more accurate scatter estimation, potentially replacing single-scatter simulation with an AI model that approximates multiscatter events by using training data from Monte Carlo modeling. For example, as shown in **Fig. 1**C, one proposed approach for accelerating scatter uses the position and energy level of each coincidence event to predict whether an event can be categorized as originating from scatter or not.[29] Most approaches attempt to estimate the scatter profile directly from given inputs of activity as shown in **Fig. 1**D. A summary of recent approaches to improve scatter correction (not including methods that jointly estimate scatter and attenuation) are listed in **Table 2**.

Given that attenuation information is necessary to perform scatter estimation, and both are unknown without a CT image, many recent approaches have attempted to use AI approaches to determine *both* attenuation and scatter, particularly using only uncorrected PET and SPECT images as inputs. The example workflow is shown in **Fig. 1**E and a summary of these methods are listed in **Table 3**.

Table 1
Artificial intelligence–based approaches for attenuation correction

Application	Approach	Advance	Quantitative Comparison vs Acquired CT	Reference
Brain perfusion SPECT	CNN	Enable correction for SPECT-only scanners	PSNR 62.2 dB, SSIM 0.9995	Sakaguchi et al,[12] 2021
Brain PET (FDG)	CNN, UNet	Enable correction for PET-only scanners	Dice coefficients of 0.80 ± 0.02 for air, 0.94 ± 0.01 for soft tissue, and 0.75 ± 0.03 for bone, MAE of 111 ± 16 HU, PET reconstruction bias <1%	Liu et al,[13] 2018
Brain PET/MR (FDG)	CNN	Synthesize CT from T1 MR imaging for PET/MR imaging	Dice coefficient of 0.936 ± 0.011 for soft tissue, and 0.803 ± 0.021 for bone, PET reconstruction bias −0.7% ± 1.1%	Liu et al,[14] 2017
Brain PET/MR (FDG)	CNN, GAN	Synthesize CT from T1 MR imaging for PET/MR imaging	Dice coefficient of 0.77 ± 0.07 for bone, PET reconstruction bias <4%	Arabi et al,[15] 2019
Brain PET/MR (FDG)	CNN, GAN	Synthesize CT from T1 MR imaging for PET/MR imaging	Dice coefficient of 0.74 ± 0.05 for bone, PET reconstruction bias <0.025 SUV	Gong et al,[16] 2020
Brain PET/MR (FDG)	CNN, UNet	Synthesize CT from T1 MR imaging for PET/MR imaging	Dice coefficient of 0.81 ± 0.03 for bone, PET RMSE 253.5, PET reconstruction bias <1%	Blanc-Durand et al,[17] 2019
Brain PET/MR (FDG)	CNN, UNet	Synthesize CT from T1 and ZTE MR imaging for PET/MR imaging	Dice coefficient of 0.86 ± 0.03 for bone, PET reconstruction bias <0.02 SUV	Gong et al,[18] 2018
Brain PET/MR (FDG)	CNN, UNet	Synthesize CT from UTE MR imaging for PET/MR imaging	Dice coefficient of 0.96 ± 0.006 for soft tissue, 0.88 ± 0.01 for bone, PET reconstruction bias <1%	Jang et al,[19] 2018
Brain PET/MR (FET)	CNN, UNet	Synthesize CT from UTE MR imaging for PET/MR imaging	PET reconstruction bias <1%	Ladefoged et al,[20] 2019

(continued on next page)

Table 1
(continued)

Application	Approach	Advance	Quantitative Comparison vs Acquired CT	Reference
Myocardial perfusion SPECT	CNN	Enable correction for SPECT-only scanners	MAE 3.60% ± 0.85% in whole body, 1.33% ± 3.80% in the left ventricle	Shi et al,[21] 2020
Myocardial perfusion SPECT	CNN	Enable correction for SPECT-only scanners	Mean segmental errors 0.49 ± 4.35%, mean absolute segmental errors 3.31 ± 2.87%	Yang et al,[22] 2021
Myocardial perfusion SPECT	GAN	Enable correction for SPECT-only scanners	RMSE 0.141 ± 0.0768, PSNR 36.382 ± 3.74 dB, SSIM 0.995 ± 0.0043	Torkaman et al,[23] 2021
Pelvis PET/MR (68Ga-PSMA)	CNN, GAN	Synthesize CT from T1 MR imaging for PET/MR imaging	PET reconstruction bias <2.2%	Pozaruk et al,[24] 2021
Pelvis PET/MR (FDG)	CNN	Synthesize CT from T1 and T2 MR imaging for PET/MR imaging	Dice coefficient of 0.98 ± 0.01 for soft tissue, 0.79 ± 0.03 for cortical bone, PET reconstruction bias 4.9%	Bradshaw et al,[25] 2018
Pelvis PET/MR (FDG)	CNN, UNet	Synthesize CT from T1 MR imaging for PET/MR imaging	PET reconstruction bias <4%	Torrado-Carvajal et al,[26] 2019
Whole-body PET (FDG)	CNN, GAN	Enable correction for PET-only scanners	PET reconstruction bias −0.8% ± 8.6%	Armanious et al,[27] 2020

Abbreviations: CNN, convolutional neural network; CT, computed tomography; GAN, generative adversarial network; MAE, mean absolute error; PSNR, peak signal to noise ratio; RMSE, root mean square error; SPECT, single-photon emission computed tomography; SSIM, structural similarity index.

CHALLENGES AND OPPORTUNITIES FOR ARTIFICIAL INTELLIGENCE APPROACHES

The implementation of AI is not without challenges. There are numerous issues that must be addressed with regard to the application of AI in medical imaging, and many of those issues affect the techniques described herein. Generalization, or the ability of a developed model to be applied to a wide range of input data, and bias, or the tendency of the developed models to favor only certain situations, are important challenges in the field of AI.[39] For the applications of AI in attenuation and scatter correction, these biases affect the generalizability of a model and are thus critical to understand and address. Although bias can be unintentional, it can have significant effects on the performance of models in the field compared with the tightly constrained environment of a research laboratory.

Areas of bias relevant to the techniques described herein are related to the application, population, and equipment used to develop a given AI model. If the model is applied to datasets that differ greatly in any of these categories, then the model may give spurious outputs that fall outside of the reported performance specifications. An example of application bias would be the use of an AI model for CT synthesis designed for brain imaging being applied to the pelvis. If the model was developed using only brain imaging data, it cannot be expected to perform well in other body regions. In addition, if the model was trained with a particular MR imaging sequence but applied using a different MR imaging sequence, performance may be degraded.

Table 2
Artificial intelligence–based approaches for scatter correction

Application	Approach	Advance	Reference
PET	Machine learning to classify events as true or scattered coincidences	Potential for scatter correction being performed before imaging reconstruction	Prats et al,[29] 2019
PET	Cascade of CNNs to estimate Monte Carlo–based approach	Improved speed relative to Monte Carlo methods	Qian et al,[32] 2017
PET/MR	CNN to estimate single-scatter simulation (SSS)	Significant increase in reconstruction speed	Berker et al,[30] 2018
SPECT	CNN to improve filtered back-projection images to approximate Monte Carlo–based approach	>200x faster than Monte Carlo method	Dietze et al,[33] 2019
SPECT, Y-90 bremsstrahlung imaging	CNN to estimate scatter projections	>120x faster than Monte Carlo method	Xiang et al,[31] 2020

Abbreviations: CNN, convolutional neural network; SPECT, single-photon emission computed tomography.

Another source of bias is related to the population of which the model is trained and applied to. Patients with different or abnormal anatomy of types that were not included within the training data could cause the model to give unexpected outputs. Therefore, training datasets must incorporate the type of data that is expected to be applied to the model or population-specific biases (eg, female and male, adult and pediatric, implants and amputations) will lead to unpredictable performance of model. There exist many recent demonstrations of this type of bias in AI in popular media outlets.

Finally, the specific equipment used may have a direct impact on the output of a given model. A given model may ultimately be specific to aspects of the equipment from which the images came, including, but not limited to the choice of vendor or site-specific protocols. Although this may be

Table 3
Artificial intelligence–based approaches for simultaneous attenuation and scatter correction

Application	Approach	Quantitative Comparison vs. Acquired CT	Reference
Brain PET (FDG, FDOPA, Flortaucipir, Flutemetamol)	CNN	PET reconstruction bias <9%	Arabi et al,[34] 2020
Brain PET (FDG)	CNN, UNet	PET reconstruction bias −4.2% ± 4.3%	Yang et al,[35] 2019
Whole-body PET (68Ga-PSMA)	CNN	MAE 0.91 ± 0.29 SUV, SSIM 0.973 ± 0.034, PSNR 48.17 ± 2.96 dB, PET reconstruction bias −2.46% ± 10.10%	Mostafapour et al,[36] 2021
Whole-body PET (FDG)	CNN	PET reconstruction bias −1.72 ± 4.22%	Shiri et al,[37] 2020
Whole-body PET (FDG)	CNN	NRMSE 0.21 ± 0.05 SUV, SSIM 0.98 ± 0.01, PSNR 36.3 ± 3.0 dB	Yang et al,[38] 2020
Whole-body PET (FDG)	CNN, GAN	MAE of <110 HU, PET reconstruction bias <1%, PSNR >42 dB	Dong et al,[15] 2019

Abbreviations: CNN, convolutional neural network; CT, computed tomography; GAN, generative adversarial network; HU, Hounsfield unit; MAE, mean absolute error; NRMSE, normalized root mean square error; PSNR, peak signal to noise ratio; SPECT, single-photon emission computed tomography; SSIM, structural similarity index.

advantageous to a single medical imaging equipment vendor, the ability of an AI model to be applied to multiple scanner systems is likely to be more impactful and lead to greater standardization of these powerful new methods. The key to enabling greater generalization lies in the development of multisite and multivendor trials, where models are trained on data originating from different sites and equipment from different vendors. The use of federated learning techniques,[40] where training is distributed to different sites, without requiring the transfer of individual images, is gaining traction as a valuable method to reduce site-specific bias and increase generalizability of developed models.

SUMMARY

AI technology holds great promise to improve methods related to quantitative PET and SPECT imaging. The ability of AI-based approaches to obviate the need for an additional CT or transmission image greatly improves the capability of existing equipment and potentially reduces the cost of future systems. Integrating AI into scatter correction also leads to the ability to improve quantification as well as patient throughput by accelerating these necessary corrections. It can only be expected that these methods will continue to improve in the future and further increase capability.

CLINICS CARE POINTS

- Many AI-based approaches to improve attenuation correction for PET and SPECT have been demonstrated in the literature, and will likely make their way to the clinic soon.

- AI-based methods for scatter correction can improve the reconstruction time, potentially improving throughput.

- AI-based approaches can be subject bias based on the data used to train the model. Care should be taken when these methods are applied to different populations and patients with abnormal anatomy for which the AI model has not been trained to use.

FUNDING

Research reported in this publication was supported by the National Institute of Biomedical Imaging and Bioengineering of the National Institutes of Health under award number R01EB026708.

DISCLOSURE

The Department of Radiology at the University of Wisconsin receives support from GE Healthcare.

REFERENCES

1. Lee TC, Alessio AM, Miyaoka RM, et al. Morphology supporting function: attenuation correction for SPECT/CT, PET/CT, and PET/MR imaging. Q J Nucl Med Mol Imaging 2016;60(1):25–39.
2. Bailey DL. Transmission scanning in emission tomography. Eur J Nucl Med 1998;25(7):774–87.
3. Watson CC, Casey ME, Michel C, et al. Advances in scatter correction for 3D PET/CT. In: IEEE Symposium Conference Record Nuclear Science, 16-22 Oct 2004.Rome, Italy;Vol 5:3008-3012.
4. Zaidi H, Montandon M-L. Scatter compensation techniques in PET. PET Clin 2007;2(2):219–34.
5. Hutton BF, Buvat I, Beekman FJ. Review and current status of SPECT scatter correction. Phys Med Biol 2011;56(14):R85–112.
6. Torres-Velázquez M, Chen W-J, Li X, et al. Application and construction of deep learning networks in medical imaging. IEEE Trans Radiat Plasma Med Sci 2021;5(2):137–59.
7. Bradshaw TJ, McMillan AB. Anatomy and Physiology of Artificial Intelligence in PET Imaging. PET Clin. Published online. doi: 10.1016/j.cpet.2021.06.003.
8. Sorin V, Barash Y, Konen E, et al. Creating artificial images for radiology applications using generative adversarial networks (GANs) - a systematic review. Acad Radiol 2020;27(8):1175–85.
9. Lee JS. A review of deep-learning-based approaches for attenuation correction in positron emission tomography. IEEE Trans Radiat Plasma Med Sci 2021;5(2):160–84.
10. Wang T, Lei Y, Fu Y, et al. Machine learning in quantitative PET: a review of attenuation correction and low-count image reconstruction methods. Phys Med 2020;76:294–306.
11. Spadea MF, Maspero M, Zaffino P, Seco J. Deep learning-based synthetic-CT generation in radiotherapy and PET: a review. 2021.
12. Sakaguchi K, Kaida H, Yoshida S, et al. Attenuation correction using deep learning for brain perfusion SPECT images. Ann Nucl Med 2021.
13. Liu F, Jang H, Kijowski R, et al. A deep learning approach for 18F-FDG PET attenuation correction. EJNMMI Phys 2018;5(1):24.
14. Liu F, Jang H, Kijowski R, et al. Deep learning MR imaging–based attenuation correction for PET/MR imaging. Radiology 2017;170700.
15. Arabi H, Zeng G, Zheng G, et al. Novel adversarial semantic structure deep learning for MRI-guided attenuation correction in brain PET/MRI. Eur J Nucl Med Mol Imaging 2019;46(13):2746–59.

16. Gong K, Yang J, Larson PE, et al. MR-based attenuation correction for brain PET using 3D cycle-consistent adversarial network. IEEE Trans Radiat Plasma Med Sci 2020;5(2):185–92.

17. Blanc-Durand P, Khalife M, Sgard B, et al. Attenuation correction using 3D deep convolutional neural network for brain 18F-FDG PET/MR: comparison with Atlas, ZTE and CT based attenuation correction. PLoS One 2019;14(10):e0223141.

18. Gong K, Yang J, Kim K, et al. Attenuation correction for brain PET imaging using deep neural network based on Dixon and ZTE MR images. Phys Med Biol 2018;63(12):125011.

19. Jang H, Liu F, Zhao G, et al. Technical Note: deep learning based MRAC using rapid ultrashort echo time imaging. Med Phys 2018.

20. Ladefoged CN, Marner L, Hindsholm A, et al. Deep learning based attenuation correction of PET/MRI in pediatric brain tumor patients: evaluation in a clinical setting. Front Neurosci 2018;12:1005.

21. Shi L, Onofrey JA, Liu H, et al. Deep learning-based attenuation map generation for myocardial perfusion SPECT. Eur J Nucl Med Mol Imaging 2020;47(10):2383–95.

22. Yang J, Shi L, Wang R, et al. Direct attenuation correction using deep learning for cardiac SPECT: a feasibility study. J Nucl Med 2021.

23. Torkaman M, Yang J, Shi L, et al. Direct image-based attenuation correction using conditional generative adversarial network for SPECT myocardial perfusion imaging. Proc Spie– Int Soc Opt Eng 2021;11600.

24. Pozaruk A, Pawar K, Li S, et al. Augmented deep learning model for improved quantitative accuracy of MR-based PET attenuation correction in PSMA PET-MRI prostate imaging. Eur J Nucl Med Mol Imaging 2021;48(1):9–20.

25. Bradshaw TJ, Zhao G, Jang H, et al. Feasibility of deep learning-based PET/MR attenuation correction in the pelvis using only diagnostic MR images. Tomogr Ann Arbor Mich 2018;4(3):138–47.

26. Torrado-Carvajal A, Vera-Olmos J, Izquierdo-Garcia D, et al. Dixon-VIBE deep learning (DIVIDE) pseudo-CT synthesis for pelvis PET/MR attenuation correction. J Nucl Med 2018.

27. Armanious K, Hepp T, Küstner T, et al. Independent attenuation correction of whole body [18F]FDG-PET using a deep learning approach with Generative Adversarial Networks. EJNMMI Res 2020;10(1):53.

28. Jonsson J, Nyholm T, Söderkvist K. The rationale for MR-only treatment planning for external radiotherapy. Clin Transl Radiat Oncol 2019;18:60–5.

29. Prats J, Larroza A, Oliver S, et al. PET scatter correction using machine learning techniques. In: 2019 IEEE Nuclear Science Symposium and Medical Imaging Conference (NSS/MIC). IEEE; Manchester, UK. 26 Oct.-2 Nov. 2019:1-3.

30. Berker Y, Maier J, Kachelrieß M. Deep Scatter Estimation in PET: Fast Scatter Correction Using a Convolutional Neural Network. In: 2018 IEEE Nuclear Science Symposium and Medical Imaging Conference Proceedings (NSS/MIC). ydney, NSW, Australia; 10-17 Nov. 2018:1-5.

31. Xiang H, Lim H, Fessler JA, et al. A deep neural network for fast and accurate scatter estimation in quantitative SPECT/CT under challenging scatter conditions. Eur J Nucl Med Mol Imaging 2020; 47(13):2956–67.

32. Qian H, Rui X, Ahn S. Deep learning models for PET scatter estimations. In: 2017 IEEE Nuclear Science Symposium and Medical Imaging Conference (NSS/MIC). IEEE; Atlanta, Georgia. 21-28 Oct. 2017:1-5.

33. Dietze MMA, Branderhorst W, Kunnen B, et al. Accelerated SPECT image reconstruction with FBP and an image enhancement convolutional neural network. EJNMMI Phys 2019;6(1):14.

34. Arabi H, Bortolin K, Ginovart N, et al. Deep learning-guided joint attenuation and scatter correction in multitracer neuroimaging studies. Hum Brain Mapp 2020;41(13):3667–79.

35. Yang J, Park D, Gullberg GT, et al. Joint correction of attenuation and scatter in image space using deep convolutional neural networks for dedicated brain 18F-FDG PET. Phys Med Biol 2019;64(7):075019.

36. Mostafapour S, Gholamiankhah F, Dadgar H, et al. Feasibility of deep learning-guided attenuation and scatter correction of whole-body 68Ga-PSMA PET studies in the image domain. Clin Nucl Med 2021.

37. Shiri I, Arabi H, Geramifar P, et al. Deep-JASC: joint attenuation and scatter correction in whole-body 18F-FDG PET using a deep residual network. Eur J Nucl Med Mol Imaging 2020;47(11):2533–48.

38. Yang J, Sohn JH, Behr SC, et al. CT-less direct correction of attenuation and scatter in the image space using deep learning for whole-body FDG PET: potential Benefits and pitfalls. Radiol Artif Intell 2021;3(2):e200137.

39. Kaushal A, Altman R, Langlotz C. Geographic distribution of US cohorts used to train deep learning algorithms. JAMA 2020;324(12):1212–3.

40. Rieke N, Hancox J, Li W, et al. The future of digital health with federated learning. NPJ Digit Med 2020;3:119.

Artificial Intelligence-Based Image Enhancement in PET Imaging
Noise Reduction and Resolution Enhancement

Juan Liu, PhD[a,1], Masoud Malekzadeh, MS[b,1], Niloufar Mirian, MSc[a],
Tzu-An Song, MS[b], Chi Liu, PhD[a,*], Joyita Dutta, PhD[b,c,*]

KEYWORDS

- PET • Artificial intelligence • Deep learning • Denoising • Deblurring • Super-resolution

KEY POINTS

- This paper reviews deep learning methods for PET image enhancement, specifically for noise reduction and resolution recovery.
- It comprehensively surveys neural network models (network architecture, loss functions, training schemes), quantitative evaluation metrics, and task-based performance assessment.
- It also explores emerging deep learning approaches for PET image enhancement, including transfer learning, federated learning, data harmonization, reinforcement learning, and network interpretability.
- Lastly, the paper outlines challenges associated with the development and deployment of deep learning techniques for PET image enhancement, examines the clinical impact of these methods, and discusses future research directions in this field.

INTRODUCTION

PET is a noninvasive molecular imaging modality that is increasingly popular in oncology, neurology, cardiology, and other fields.[1–3] Accurate quantitation of PET radiotracer uptake is vital for disease diagnosis, prognosis, staging, and treatment evaluation. The key confounding factors compromising PET image quality and quantitative accuracy are high noise and low spatial resolution. The high noise issue could be further accentuated in scenarios where the radiotracer dose is reduced to decrease a patient's radiation exposure or the scan time is decreased, possibly with the intent of increasing throughput or decreasing patient discomfort. A variety of physical and algorithmic factors contribute to the resolution limitations of PET, including the noncollinearity of the emitted photon pairs, finite crystal size, crystal penetration and intercrystal scatter of the detected photons, positron range, and within- or postreconstruction smoothing. The low resolution of PET images manifests as partial volume effects, which lead to the spillover of estimated activity across different regions of interest (ROIs). Collectively, the high noise and low resolution in PET images could lead to the overestimation or underestimation of

[a] Department of Radiology and Biomedical Imaging, Yale School of Medicine, New Haven, CT, USA;
[b] Department of Electrical and Computer Engineering, University of Massachusetts Lowell, 1 University Avenue, Ball 301, Lowell, MA 01854, USA; [c] Gordon Center for Medical Imaging, Massachusetts General Hospital and Harvard Medical School, Boston, MA, USA
[1] Equal contribution.
* Corresponding authors.
E-mail addresses: chi.liu@yale.edu (C.L.); dutta.joyita@mgh.harvard.edu (J.D.)

PET Clin 16 (2021) 553–576
https://doi.org/10.1016/j.cpet.2021.06.005

standardized uptake values (SUVs) in an ROI and inaccurate lesion delineation or detection.

A variety of within- and postreconstruction approaches have been developed to denoise and/or deblur PET images. Among within-reconstruction approaches, regularization using a quadratic penalty and early iteration termination are some of the most rudimentary techniques to tackle image noise,[4–6] whereas point spread function modeling in the image or sinogram domain is a common approach to improve resolution.[7,8] Many penalized likelihood reconstruction approaches have been proposed to improve the noise and resolution characteristics of the reconstructed images.[9] Among postreconstruction PET image enhancement approaches, Gaussian filtering is the most commonly used denoising technique and is built into the reconstruction software for most clinical and small animal PET scanners. Given the resolution loss associated with Gaussian filters, many edge-preserving alternatives have been proposed for PET image denoising. These include bilateral,[10,11] anisotropic diffusion,[12,13] wavelet-domain,[14–17] frequency-domain,[18] and nonlocal[19–21] filters. Although several penalized deconvolution approaches have been proposed for resolution enhancement,[22,23] the most popular resolution recovery approaches in PET are simple partial volume correction techniques that rely on a segmented anatomic template.[24–26] Some denoising approaches and nearly all deblurring approaches use high-resolution anatomic information based on structural magnetic resonance (MR) imaging or computed tomography (CT) scans.

With the advent of a new era in computing largely dominated by deep learning and artificial intelligence (AI), the fields of medical image reconstruction and processing have been revolutionized by the availability of a new generation of AI-powered image enhancement tools. This review focuses on AI-based approaches for PET image enhancement that have been developed in recent years and discusses new developments and emerging technologies in this arena. Because AI-based reconstruction techniques are the subject of Kuang Gong and colleagues' article, "The Evolution of Image Reconstruction in PET: From Filtered Back-Projection to Artificial Intelligence," in this Special Issue, this article focuses exclusively on AI-based postreconstruction PET image enhancement. We should note here that, although within-reconstruction image enhancement techniques tend to have improved bias variance characteristics compared with their postreconstruction counterparts, the latter category of methods is attractive for 2 main reasons. First, because these techniques do not require access to raw sinogram or list mode data, they cater to a wider base of users who only have access to the final reconstructed images. Second, data size is a major factor affecting the accuracy of AI models and most large image repositories and databases contain only the reconstructed images but no raw data, making it more practical to train AI models that receive image domain inputs.

It should be noted that most large data repositories that enable robust training and validation of AI-based image enhancement models are acquired over multiple hospitals and imaging centers. For these multisite studies, intersite differences in scanner models and image acquisition protocols (including radiotracer dosage, scan duration, and image reconstruction parameters) could lead to significant variability in image characteristics. As a result, many image enhancement techniques are motivated by the need for data harmonization across multiple data sources so as to enable collective use. This review discusses emerging PET image enhancement techniques that are particularly useful for data harmonization. A major bottleneck toward the robust training and validation of AI models for medical imaging modalities like PET is the need for centralized curation of data, which is mired in patient privacy regulations and data ownership concerns. Federated learning, which involves the sharing of deep learning models across institutions in place of data sharing, offers a promising path to circumvent the data sharing bottleneck and facilitate AI practice in the medical domain. We also discuss emerging trends in federated learning as it relates to PET.

In the Summary of existing methods, we tabulate and discuss recently published AI-based PET image enhancement approaches, including both supervised and unsupervised techniques. In Emerging approaches and novel applications, we highlight several active areas of research that are of direct relevance to PET image enhancement. Finally, in the Conclusion, we discuss future directions, identify barriers, and conclude the paper.

SUMMARY OF EXISTING METHODS

The PET image denoising and deblurring problems both involve the retrieval or restoration of a clean image from its corrupt counterpart. For the denoising problem, the corrupt image is a low-count (also referred to as low-dose) image and the clean image is a higher dose image. For the deblurring problem, the corrupt image is a lower resolution counterpart of a higher resolution clean image. Unlike the model-based approaches used in conventional image processing where the denoising and

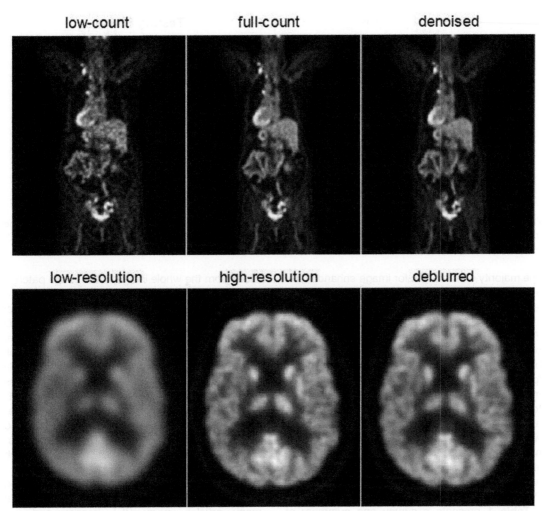

Fig. 1. Examples of corrupt (*left*), clean (*middle*), and enhanced (*right*) images for the denoising problem (*top*) and the deblurring problem (*bottom*). In the denoising example, a 3-dimensional (3D) U-net network was used to produce the denoised image from a 20% low-count image. In the deblurring example, a very deep convolutional neural network (CNN) was used to generate a high-resolution PET image similar to those produced by the Siemens HRRT dedicated brain scanner from a low-resolution one generated by the Siemens HR+.

deblurring problems are associated with very different models, the difference between AI-based image deblurring and denoising often lies in the data used for training. It should be noted here that, although a methodological dichotomy exists, in many practical scenarios, the objective may be to simultaneously deblur and denoise an image.

Fig. 1 provides examples of corrupt, clean, and restored/enhanced images for the denoising and deblurring problems. The images are all based on human PET imaging using the ^{18}F-fluorodeoxy-glucose (^{18}F-FDG) radiotracer. For both the denoising and deblurring examples, the enhanced images were produced by neural networks that received the corrupt image as its input.

The denoising and deblurring problems aim to compute an estimate, $\hat{x}$, of a clean image x from its corrupt counterpart y in the form of some explicit or implicit function, $\hat{x} = \mathcal{R}(y)$. Traditional image processing approaches compute the unknown image using either an analytical formula or a model-based iterative procedure. Unlike traditional analytical or iterative image processing methods, AI-based approaches for image enhancement learn the mapping from the corrupt to the clean image directly from the data. For a parametric model, this mapping is of the form $\hat{x} = f(y, w)$, where the vector w is a set of "weight" parameters for the neural network computed during the network training phase. This is achieved by minimizing a loss function.

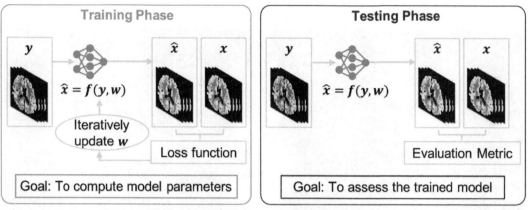

Fig. 2. A typical supervised learning setup for image enhancement with a training phase that computes the model parameters and requires paired clean and corrupt images and a testing phase that assesses the model's performance in an independent subset of paired images.

The majority of AI models for image enhancement are based on supervised learning. A supervised learning setup requires paired clean and corrupt images for network training, as illustrated in **Fig. 2**. After the training phase, the model is tested or validated on an independent subset of the data by comparing the enhanced images with the clean (ground truth) images using one or more evaluation metrics. Although supervised models are simpler to design and train, their need for paired clean and corrupt inputs limits their applicability to cases where clean counterparts of corrupt images may not be available. In contrast, unsupervised learning models obviate the need for paired inputs and are currently an active area of investigation for PET image enhancement.

Table 1 presents a survey and summary of some noteworthy AI-based image enhancement efforts for PET. In the following subsections, we discuss the supervised and unsupervised model architectures, loss functions, and evaluation metrics for several of the tabulated methods.

Supervised Learning Models and Network Architectures

Almost all AI-based PET image processing techniques, including both supervised and unsupervised techniques feature some convolutional layers in the neural network. CNNs, which contain convolutional layers and could also contain other layer types (eg, pooling or fully connected layers), have emerged as a vital family of image processing tools in the AI era and have been leveraged extensively for PET image enhancement.

Neural networks for image processing are often characterized as 2-dimensional (2D), 2.5-dimensional (2.5D), or 3D based on the input dimensionality. The 2D models receive as inputs 2D image slices from the whole image or 2D image patches (ie, a 2D slice from a subimage) in 1 or more orientations (ie, axial, coronal, or sagittal). A 2.5D model uses image "slabs," that is, sets of contiguous 2D slices, and carries some contextual information (ie, information on the local neighborhood of a voxel) unlike their 2D counterpart. Fully 3D models receive 3D whole images or 3D image patches as inputs and tend to outperform 2D and 2.5D models,[39,45] but have steep memory requirements. Gong and colleagues[43] proposed a mixed 2D and 3D encoder–decoder network to effectively synergize 2D and 3D features, which improved the fidelity of denoised images.

Many denoising approaches have exploited additional information from anatomic images. In many articles, noisy PET images and co-registered MR or CT images were provided to the network via distinct input channels.[28,57] Anatomically guided approaches have been reported to improve image quality and quantitative accuracy. However, some works mentioned the potential performance degradation that could stem from intermodality alignment errors.[53]

Many of the first supervised learning techniques for PET image denoising were based on CNNs with shallower architectures, that is, with relatively few layers. The CNN used by da Costa-Luis and coworkers, for example,[27] was based on only 3 layers. This network, termed μ-net, has relatively few unknown parameters and is well-adapted for settings with very limited training data. The μ-net was demonstrated to be more robust than deeper networks, which performed poorly in the validation phase owing to overfitting of the training data.[28] Later CNN implementations for PET image denoising use deeper architectures, such as the implementation by Gong and colleagues.[29] Many CNN-based PET denoising architectures have

Table 1
A summary of deep learning techniques for PET image enhancement

Task	Learning Style	Paper	Method and Architecture	Data and Radiotracer	Loss Function	Input and Output	Evaluation Metric
Denoising	Supervised	da Costa-Luis and Reader,[27] 2018; da Costa-Luis and Reader,[28] 2021	3D CNN 3 layers	^{18}F-FDG simulation and human data	L2 loss	Input: low-count PET images with and without resolution modeling, T1-weighted MR, and T1-guided NLM filtering of the resolution modeling reconstruction Output/training target: full-count PET	NRMSE Bias vs variance curves
		Gong et al,[29] 2019	CNN with residual learning 5 residual blocks	^{18}F-FDG simulation data, ^{18}F-FDG human data	L2 loss + perceptual loss	Input: low-count PET Output/Training target: full-count PET	CRC vs variance curves
		Xiang et al,[30] 2017	Deep auto-context CNN 12 convolutional layers	^{18}F-FDG human data	L2 loss + L2 norm weight regularization	Input: low-count PET, T1-weighted MR image Output/training target: full-count PET	NRMSE, PSNR
		Chen et al,[31] 2019	2D residual U-net	^{18}F- Florbetaben human brain data	L1 loss	Input: low-count PET, multicontrast MR images (T1-weighted, T2-weighted, T2 FLAIR) Output/training target: full-count PET	NRMSE, PSNR, SSIM
		Spuhler et al,[32] 2020	2D residual dilated CNN	^{18}F-FDG human data	L1 loss	Input: low-count PET Output/Training target: full-count PET	SSIM, PSNR, MAPE
		Serreno-Sosa et al,[33] 2020	2.5D U-net with residual learning and dilated convolution	^{18}F-FDG human brain data	–	Input: low-count PET Output/training target: full-count PET	SSIM, PSNR, MAPE
		Schaeffer-koetter	3D U-net	^{18}F-FDG human data	L2 loss		CRC

(continued on next page)

Table 1
(continued)

Task	Learning Style	Paper	Method and Architecture	Data and Radiotracer	Loss Function	Input and Output	Evaluation Metric
		et al,[34] 2020				Input: low-count PET Output/training target: full-count PET	
		Sano et al,[35] 2021	2D residual U-net	Proton-induced PET data from simulations and a human head and neck phantom study	L2 loss	Input: noisier low-count PET Output/training target: less noisy low-count PET	PSNR
		Wang et al,[36] 2019	GAN Generator: 3D U-net Discriminator: 4-convolution layer CNN	18F-FDG simulated data, 18F-FDG human brain data	L1 loss + adversarial loss	Input: low-count PET, T1-weighted MR image, fractional anisotropy and mean diffusivity images computed from diffusion MR image Output/training target: full-count PET	PSNR, SSIM
		Zhao et at,[37] 2020	CycleGAN Generator: multilayer CNN Discriminator: 4-convolution layer CNN	18F-FDG simulated data, 18F-FDG human data	L1 supervised loss + Wasserstein adversarial loss + cycle consistency loss + identity loss	Input: low-count PET Output/training target: full-count PET	NRMSE, SSIM, PSNR, learned perceptual image patch similarity, SUV bias
		Xue et al,[38] 2020	Least squares GAN Generator: 3D U-net like network with residual learning and self-attention modules Discriminator: 4-convolution layer CNN	18F-FDG human data	L2 loss + adversarial loss	Input: low-count PET Output/training target: full-count PET	PSNR, SSIM

Study	Architecture	Data	Loss function	Input/Output	Metrics
Wang et al,[39] 2018	cGANs with progressive refinement; Generator: 3D U-net; Discriminator: 4-convolution layer CNN	18F-FDG human brain data	L1 supervised loss + adversarial loss	Input: low-count PET; Output/training target: full-count PET	NMSE, PSNR, SUV bias
Kaplan et al,[40] 2019	GAN; Generator: 2D encoder–decoder with skip connection; Discriminator: 5-layer CNN	18F-FDG human data	L2 loss + gradient loss + total variation loss + adversarial loss	low-count PET; Output/training target: full-count PET	RMSE, MSSIM, PSNR
Zhou et al,[41] 2020	CycleGAN; Generator: multilayer 2D CNN; Discriminator: 6-layer CNN	18F-FDG human data	L1 supervised loss + Wasserstein adversarial loss + cycle consistency loss + identity loss	Input: low-count PET; Output/training target: full-count PET	NRMSE, SSIM, PSNR, SUV bias
Ouyang et al,[42] 2019	GAN; Generator: 2.5D U-net; Discriminator: 4-convolution layer CNN	18F-florbetaben human data	L1 loss + adversarial loss + task-specific perceptual loss	Input: low-count PET; Output/training target: full-count PET	SSIM, PSNR, RMSE
Gong et al,[43] 2021	GAN; Generator: hybrid 2D and 3D encoder-decoder; Discriminator: 6-layer CNN	18F-FDG human data	L2 loss + Wasserstein adversarial loss	Input: low-count PET; Output/training target: full-count PET	NRMSE, PSNR, Riesz transform-based feature similarity index, visual information fidelity

(continued on next page)

Table 1
(continued)

Task	Learning Style	Paper	Method and Architecture	Data and Radiotracer	Loss Function	Input and Output	Evaluation Metric
		Liu et al,[44] 2020	3D U-net Cross-tracer cross-protocol transfer learning	^{18}F-FDG human data, ^{18}F-FMISO human data, ^{68}Ga-DOTATATE data	L2 loss	Input: low-count PET Output/training target: full-count PET	NRMSE, SNR, SUV bias
		Lu et al,[45] 2019	Network comparison: Convolutional autoencoder, U-net, residual U-net, GAN, 2D vs 2.5D vs 3D	^{18}F-FDG human lung data	L2 loss	Input: low-count PET Output/training target: full-count PET	NMSE, SNR, SUV bias
		Ladefoged et al,[46] 2021	3D U-net	^{18}F-FDG human cardiac data	Huber loss	Input: low-count PET, CT Output/training target: full-count PET	NRMSE, PSNR, SUV bias
		Sanaat et al,[47] 2020	3D U-net	^{18}F-FDG human data	L2 loss	Input: low-dose PET image/sinogram Output/training target: standard-dose PET image/sinogram	RMSE, PSNR, SSIM, SUV bias
		He et al,[48] 2021	Deep CNN	^{18}F-FDG simulated brain data, ^{18}F-FDG dynamic data	L1 loss + gradient loss + total variation loss	Input: noisy dynamic PET, MR imaging Output/training target: composite dynamic images	RMSE, SSIM, CRC vs variance curves
		Wang et al,[49] 2021	Deep CNN	^{18}F-FDG human whole-body data	Attention-weighted loss	Input: low-count PET, T1-weighted LAVA MR image Output/training target: full-count PET	NRMSE, SSIM, PSNR, SUV bias

Study	Method/Architecture	Data	Loss	Input/Output	Metrics
...rafini et al,[50] 2021	3D CNN with residual learning	^{18}F-PE2I, ^{18}F-FET human data	L2 loss	Input: reconstructed Low-count PET, T1-weighted MR image. Output/training target: enhanced PET (based on anatomic guidance)	CNR, SSIM
Jeong et al,[51] 2021	GAN Generator: 2D U-net Discriminator: 3-layer CNN	^{18}F-FDG human brain data	L2 loss + adversarial loss	Input: low-count PET. Output/training target: full-count PET	NRMSE, PSNR, SSIM, SUV bias
Tsuchiya et al,[52] 2021	2D CNN with residual learning	^{18}F-FDG whole-body data	Weighted L2 loss	Input: low-count PET. Output/training target: full-count PET	SUV bias
Liu et al,[53] 2019	2D U-net with asymmetric skip connections	Simulated ^{18}F-FDG brain data	L2 loss	Input: filtered backprojection reconstructed PET, T1-weighted MR image. Output/training target: MLEM-reconstructed PET	MSE, CNR, bias-variance images
Sanaat et al,[54] 2021	CycleGAN Generator: 2D U-net like network Discriminator: 9-layer CNN ResNet 20 convolutional layers	^{18}F-FDG human data	CycleGAN: L1 loss + adversarial loss ResNet: L2 loss	Input: low-count PET. Output/training target: full-count PET	MSE, PSNR, SSIM, SUV bias
Chen et al,[55] 2021	2D U-net with residual learning	^{18}F-FDG human brain data	L1 loss	Input: low-count PET, multicontrast MRI (T1-weighted, T2-weighted, T2 FLAIR). Output/training target: full-count PET	RMSE, PSNR, SSIM
Katsari et al,[56] 2021	SubtlePET AI	^{18}F-FDG PET/CT human data	-	-	SUV bias Subjective image quality, lesion detectivity

(continued on next page)

Table 1
(*continued*)

Task	Learning Style	Paper	Method and Architecture	Data and Radiotracer	Loss Function	Input and Output	Evaluation Metric
	Unsupervised, weakly-supervised, or self-supervised	Cui et al,[57] 2019	Deep image prior 3D U-net	Simulation and human data from 2 radiotracers: Ga-PRGD2 (PET/CT) and ^{18}F-FDG (PET/MR)	L2 loss	Inputs: CT/MR image Output: denoised PET Training target: noisy PET	CRC vs variance curves
		Hashimoto et al,[58] 2019	Deep image prior 3D U-net	^{18}F-FDG simulated data, ^{18}F-FDG monkey data	L2 loss	Input: static PET Training target: noisy dynamic PET image Output: denoised dynamic PET image	PSNR, SSIM, CNR
		Hashimoto et al,[59] 2021	4D deep image prior Shared 3D U-net as feature extractor and reconstruction branch for each output frame	^{18}F-FDG simulated data and ^{18}F-FDG and ^{11}C-raclopride monkey data	Weighted L2 loss	Input: static PET Training target: 4D dynamic PET image Output: denoised dynamic PET image	Bias vs variance curves, PSNR, SSIM
		Wu et al,[60] 2020	Noise2Noise 3D CNN encoder–decoder	^{15}O-water human data	L2 denoising loss + L2 bias control loss + L2 content loss	Inputs: low-count PET images from one injection Output: denoised low-count PET Training target: low-count PET images from another injection	CRC
		Yie et al,[61] 2020	Noisier2Noise 3D U-net	^{18}F-FDG human data	L2 loss	Inputs: extreme low-count PET Output: denoised low-count PET Training target: low-count PET	PSNR, SSIM

Deblurring	Supervised	Song et al,[62] 2020	Very Deep CNN 20-layer CNN with residual learning	^{18}F-FDG simulation and human data	L1 loss	Input: low-resolution PET, T1-weighted MR image, spatial (radial + axial) coordinates; Output/training target: high-resolution PET	PSNR, SSIM
		Gharedaghi et al,[63] 2019	Very deep CNN 16-Layer CNN with residual learning	Human data, radiotracer unknown	L2 loss	Input: low-resolution PET; Output/training target: high-resolution PET	PSNR, SSIM
		Chen et al,[64] 2020	CycleGAN Model trained on simulation data and applied to clinical data	^{18}F-FDG simulated images for training and human images for validation	Adversarial loss + cycle consistency loss	Input: low-resolution PET; Output/training target: high-resolution PET	Visual examples only, no quantitative results
	Unsupervised, weakly supervised, or self-supervised	Song et al,[65] 2020	Dual GANs Generator: 8-layer CNN Discriminator: 12-layer CNN	FDG simulated images for pretraining and human images for validation	2 L2 adversarial losses + cycle consistency loss + total variation penalty	Input: low-resolution PET, T1-weighted MR image, spatial (radial + axial) coordinates; Output: high-resolution PET; Training target: unpaired high-resolution PET	PSNR, RMSE, SSIM

Abbreviations: 2D, 2-dimensional; 4D, 4-dimensional; cGAN, conditional generative adversarial network; CNR, contrast-to-noise ratio; CRC, contrast recovery coefficient; DTI, diffusion tensor imaging; FLAIR, fluid-attenuated inversion recovery; ^{18}F-FMISO, ^{18}F-fluoromisonidazole; GAN, generative adversarial network; MAPE, mean absolute percent error; MLEM, maximum likelihood expectation maximization; MSE, mean square error; MSSIM, mean structural similarity index measure; NLM, non-local means; NRMSE, normalized root mean square error; OSEM, ordered subsets expectation-maximization; PSNR, peak signal noise ratio; RFSIM, riesz-transform based feature similarity metric; RMSE, root mean square error; SNR, signal noise ratio; SSIM, similarity structure index metrics; SUV, standard uptake value; VIF, visual information fidelity.

benefitted from a residual learning strategy,[66] which involves learning the difference between the clean and the corrupt images instead of directly learning the clean image.[29] Dilated convolutions have also been shown to improve PET image denoising performance.[32,67]

Although most early image denoising efforts were based on pure CNNs, many recent architectural innovations have greatly boosted image denoising performance. A popular architecture widely used for many different image processing tasks today is the U-net, which was originally proposed for image segmentation.[68] The U-net architecture consists of a contracting path (resembling an encoder) that decreases input dimensionality followed by an expansive path (resembling a decoder) with multiple skip connections between the paths that enable feature concatenation to aid upsampling. U-net applications include supervised denoising models[34,35,42,45] as well as unsupervised models[57–59,61] to be discussed elsewhere in this article. A thorough comparison of different U-net formats—2D, 2.5D, and 3D—was conducted in an article by Lu and colleagues,[45] which showed that a fully 3D U-net leads to lower SUV bias than 2D or 2.5D alternatives. A detailed discussion of neural network architectures can be found in Fereshteh Yousefirizi and colleagues' article, "Towards High-Throughput AI-Based Segmentation in Oncological PET Imaging," of this Special Issue.

Generative adversarial networks (GANs)[69] have rapidly gained popularity in the PET image reconstruction and processing arenas. A GAN consists of 2 competing neural networks, a generator and a discriminator, that are simultaneously trained. For an image enhancement task, the generator seeks to produce synthetic versions of clean images, and the discriminator tries to distinguish between real and synthetic versions of the clean images. Upon completion of the training, the generator would be able to synthesize a highly realistic clean image from a corrupt image. Although many PET image enhancement efforts based on GANs are unsupervised, GANs have been successfully used in supervised settings to synthesize realistic clean PET images from their noisy counterparts and have been shown to outperform CNN-based alternatives.[41,42,54,64,65] Wang and colleagues[39] published a PET denoising technique based on 3D conditional GANs that uses an iterative refinement scheme for robust training. Ouyang and colleagues[42] proposed a GAN to denoise ultra-low-dose (1% of the standard dose) amyloid PET images and used a U-net for the generator, a feature matching adversarial loss to decrease artifacts in the synthetic images, and a task-specific perceptual loss to boost the presence of accurate neuropathological details in the images. In an article on PET image denoising by Xue and colleagues,[38] residual learning and self-attention were reported to improve GAN performance by preserving structural details and edges in the images. Gong and colleagues[43] used Wasserstein distances to boost GAN performance at the PET image denoising task and relied on task-specific initialization based on transfer learning to reduce the training time. Zhou and colleagues[70] used a Siamese adversarial network to recover high-dose respiratory-gated PET image volumes from their low-dose gated counterparts.

The CycleGAN,[71] a specialized configuration of 2 pairs of GANs originally proposed for domain translation, has found widespread use in image synthesis and processing. CycleGANs for PET image enhancement consist of 2 generator–discriminator pairs, with the first generator performing the mapping from the corrupt image domain to the clean image domain and the second generator performing the reverse mapping. A cycle consistency loss is introduced to ensure parity between the synthetic and the original corrupt images. Zhou and colleagues[41] proposed a Cycle-GAN for denoising low-dose oncological images that relies on the Wasserstein distance metric for the generator loss function to stabilize training and showed that this method leads to low bias in both the tumor and background tissues. **Fig. 3** shows the network architecture and sample denoised images from Zhou and colleagues.[41] Zhao and colleagues[37] also use the CycleGAN for low-dose PET image restoration. Sanaat and colleagues[54] compared CycleGAN with a residual network for one-eighth low-dose whole-body PET image denoising. The CycleGAN achieved better image quality than a residual network and led to similar performance in lesion detectability compared with full-dose images.

Similar to the denoising problem, solutions to the deblurring and super-resolution problems have been developed in the image processing and computer vision communities that rely on CNNs or more complex architectures like the U-net, GAN, or CycleGAN.[72–75] Specifically, for PET image enhancement, Song and colleagues[62] used a very deep CNN architectures with 20 layers. Alongside low-resolution PET, the network received high-resolution anatomic MR imaging inputs to facilitate resolution recovery. High-resolution PET image patches were used as targets for network training. To accommodate the spatially varying nature of PET image resolution, radial and axial locations for each input patch

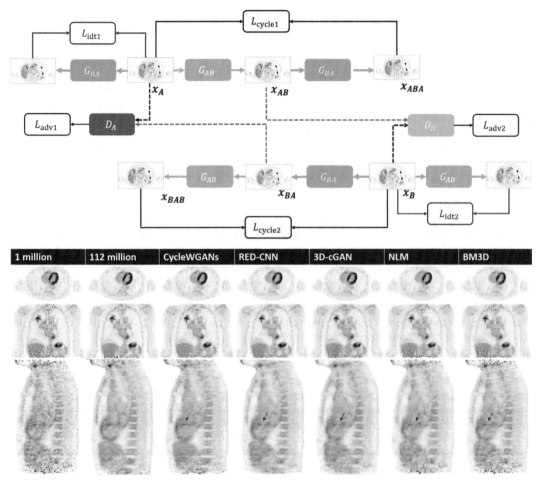

Fig. 3. Network architecture of a Wasserstein CycleGAN (referred to here as CycleWGAN) for supervised image denoising (*top*) and sample denoising results (*bottom*). (*Adapted from* Zhou, L., et al., *Supervised learning with cyclegan for low-dose FDG PET image denoising.* Medical Image Analysis, 2020. 65: p. 101770.)

were passed as additional inputs to the CNN. Training was performed in supervised mode for both simulation and clinical data, and it was shown that the very deep CNN with anatomic guidance outperforms penalized deconvolution as well as shallower CNNs.

Unsupervised, Weakly Supervised, and Self-Supervised Learning Models and Network Architectures

The techniques discussed in the previous section are all based on supervised learning and require clean target images corresponding with each corrupt image for network training. In clinical settings, such paired datasets are difficult to come by. For denoising, this process would require high-count images corresponding with each low-count image. Such image pairs can be generated by performing rebinning on high-count list-mode data,[32,76] but this step would require access to raw list-mode data. For the deblurring task, a supervised learning model would require a high-resolution image corresponding with each low-resolution image. This goal can be achieved either by performing 2 scans of the same subject, one on a state-of-the-art high-resolution scanner and another on a lower resolution scanner, or by artificially degrading a high-resolution PET image using the measured or estimated point spread function corresponding with the low-resolution input. These stringent data requirements limit the practical usefulness of supervised learning models. This factor has led to a steadily growing interest in unsupervised models for PET denoising and deblurring. It should be noted that the term *self-supervised* learning is often used to refer to some unsupervised techniques that learn the corrupt-to-clean mapping directly from the input image (e.g. from neighborhood information or population-level characteristics) without requiring a separate paired clean image. *Weakly supervised* methods, in contrast, rely on noisy or imprecise targets for supervision.

The Noise2Noise technique is a promising weakly supervised denoising approach that reconstructs a clean image from multiple independent corrupt observations.[77] This method was applied to multiple noise realizations of a PET image with similar counts by Chan and colleagues[78] to create a denoised PET image and was shown to be able to suppress noise while promoting a natural noise texture and reducing speckle and clustered noise. Wu and colleagues applied Noise2Noise for denoising ^{15}O-water dynamic PET images with a short half-life of only approximately 2 minutes, which tend to be extremely noisy, by using noisy time-frames from separate injections as the independent noise realizations required for the Noise2-Noise method.[60]

The Noise2Noise technique requires at least 2 noise realizations, which are not available for most clinical datasets, except for tracers with short half-lives that enables repeated scans with a low total patient dose, such as ^{15}O-water and ^{82}Rb. In comparison, the Noisier2Noise approach trains the network with noisy and noisier image pairs, where the noisier image is derived from a single noise realization with added synthetic noise based on a known statistical model.[79] Yie and colleagues[61] compared PET image denoising performance of Noisier2Noise with Noise2Noise and a supervised approach. Their Noisier2Noise model was trained using PET images acquired over 10-second time frames as the input and corresponding 40-second duration images as the target. It was compared with Noise2Clean (input: 40-second duration images, training target: 300-second duration images) and Noise2Noise (pairs of 40-second duration images used for network training). Their results show that, although Noise2-Noise and Noise2Clean demonstrate comparable denoising performance, Noisier2Noise is effective at noise suppression while maintaining the noise texture in the input.

The deep image prior is another very popular and versatile technique that is unsupervised and was originally demonstrated to be useful for a wide range of image restoration problems.[80] This method is founded on the idea that the intrinsic structure of a generator network is able to capture low-level image statistics and can be used to regularize an image without any learning. Cui and colleagues[57] used the deep image prior with a U-net based generator to denoise PET images in an unsupervised manner. Instead of providing a random input to the generator, they provided an anatomic image at the input and reported notable improvements in the contrast-to-noise ratio (CNR). Hashimoto and colleagues[59] use the deep image prior for dynamic PET imaging denoising and used a less noisy static PET image as the input to a U-net generator.

Unsupervised methods for PET image deblurring and partial volume correction are still emerging. Song and colleagues[65] reported a dual GAN architecture somewhat similar to the Cycle-GAN for self-supervised resolution recovery of PET images using unpaired low- and high-resolution image sets. **Fig. 4** shows the network architecture and sample denoised images from Song and colleagues.[65] The network received as inputs a low-resolution PET image, a high-resolution anatomic MR image, spatial information (axial and radial coordinates), and a high-dimensional feature set extracted from an auxiliary CNN that was trained separately in a supervised manner using paired simulation datasets.

Evaluation Metrics

Traditionally, PET image reconstruction and enhancement techniques are assessed by studying the tradeoff between 2 statistical measures—bias and variance. The normalized root-mean-square error is an error metric with broad application in many domains and is frequently used in the context of PET as well. In addition, the mean absolute percentage error, peak signal-to-noise ratio and structural similarity index, 2 image quality metrics popular in the computer vision community, are frequently used nowadays to evaluate AI-based PET image enhancement techniques. In addition, metrics like the contrast recovery coefficient, CNR, and SUV bias are also widely used. In the following, the ground truth and estimated images are denoted x and $\hat{x}$, respectively. We use the notations μ_x and σ_x, respectively, for the mean and standard deviation of x based on averaging over the voxels, with N being the number of voxels in the whole image or over 1 ROI.

1. Bias and variance: Many image enhancement techniques reduce noise in the images by adding bias. It is desirable to simultaneously achieve both low bias and low variance. When M noise realizations of the enhanced image are available, the bias and variance at the ith voxel can be computed as follows:

$$bias_i = \frac{1}{M} \sum_{k=1}^{M} \left(\hat{x}_i^k - x_i \right),$$

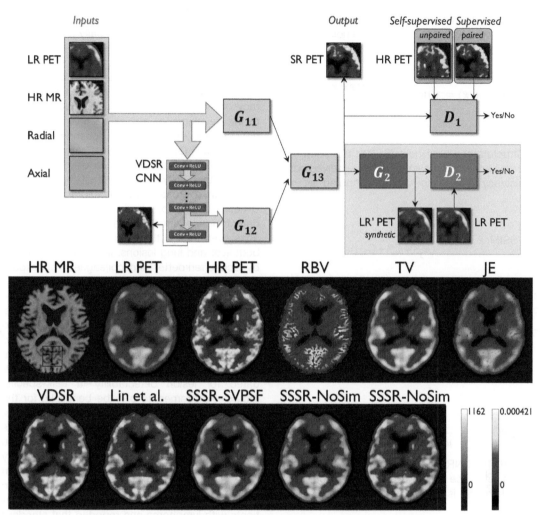

Fig. 4. Network architecture based on dual GANs for self-supervised image super-resolution (SSSR) (*top*) and sample deblurring results (*bottom*). HR, high-resolution; LR, low-resolution, JE, joint entropy; RBV, region-based voxel-wise; TV, total variation; VDSR, very deep super-resolution. (*Adapted* from Song, T.A., et al., PET image super-resolution using generative adversarial networks. Neural Netw, 2020. 125: p. 83-91.)

$$var_i = \frac{1}{M} \sum_{k=1}^{M} \left(\widehat{x}_i^k - \frac{1}{M} \sum_{j=1}^{M} \left(\widehat{x}_i^j \right) \right)^2,$$

where j and k are sample indices. To study the bias–variance tradeoff, the bias and variance (for all voxels or within an ROI) can be plotted against each other. Among a set of image reconstruction or enhancement techniques being compared, the method with the lowest lying bias–variance curve is preferred. This technique is very robust, but requires the knowledge of the ground truth and multiple noise realizations, both of which are feasible in simulations.

2. Normalized root-mean-square error (NRMSE): The NRMSE can be computed by normalizing the root-mean-square error by the mean:

$$NRMSE(\widehat{x}, x) = \frac{\sqrt{\frac{1}{N} \sum_{i=1}^{N} \left(\widehat{x}_i - x_i \right)^2}}{\mu_x}$$

3. Mean absolute percentage error (MAPE): The MAPE can be computed as:

$$MAPE(\widehat{x}, x) = \frac{1}{N} \sum_{i=1}^{N} \left| \frac{\widehat{x}_i - x_i}{x_i} \right|.$$

4. Peak signal-to-noise ratio (PSNR): PSNR is defined as the ratio of the maximum signal,

typically the maximum image voxel value that could be sensitive to noise, to the noise power:

$$PSNR(\widehat{x}, x) = 10 \log_{10}\left(\frac{max(x)^2}{\frac{1}{N}\sum_{i=1}^{N}\left(\widehat{x}_i - x_i\right)^2}\right)$$

5. Structural similarity index (SSIM): The SSIM[81] is a well-accepted measure of the perceived consistency of the image and is computed as:

$$SSIM(\widehat{x}, x) = \frac{(2\mu_{\widehat{x}}\mu_x + C_1)(2\sigma_{\widehat{x}x} + C_2)}{(\mu_{\widehat{x}}^2 + \mu_x^2 + C_1)(\sigma_{\widehat{x}}^2 + \sigma_x^2 + C_2)},$$

where C_1 and C_2 are parameters that are used to stabilize the division operation and $\sigma_{\widehat{x}x}$ is the covariance of the x and $\widehat{x}$.

6. Contrast recovery coefficient (CRC): The CRC for a target ROI $\mathscr{R}$ with respect to a reference region $\mathscr{R}_{ref}$ (eg, a tumor vs its background) is defined as follows:

$$CRC = \frac{\mu_x^{\mathscr{R}} - \mu_x^{\mathscr{R}_{ref}}}{\mu_x^{\mathscr{R}_{ref}}}.$$

7. CNR: The CNR for a target ROI $\mathscr{R}$ with respect to a reference region $\mathscr{R}_{ref}$ (eg, a tumor vs its background) is defined as follows:

$$CNR = \frac{\mu_x^{\mathscr{R}} - \mu_x^{\mathscr{R}_{ref}}}{\sqrt{\left[\left(\sigma_x^{\mathscr{R}}\right)^2 + \left(\sigma_x^{\mathscr{R}_{ref}}\right)^2\right]}}$$

To assess how well an enhanced image performs relative to the original corrupt image, some papers compute a CNR improvement ratio by taking the difference between the CNRs of the enhanced and original images and dividing it by the CNR of the original image.

8. SUV bias: The SUV is a semiquantitative metric that is used widely in clinical practice. The mean or the maximum SUV in an ROI $\mathscr{R}$ are both commonly used for ROI quantitation. To assess how well an enhanced image performs relative to the original corrupt image, the SUV change can be computed by taking the difference between the mean or maximum SUV of the enhanced and original images and dividing it by the corresponding number of the original image.

These metrics are all task-independent metrics that assess image quality globally or for an ROI. PET images are often acquired for a specific clinical task, for example, detection of a cancerous lesion. A general improvement in image quality may not always proportionally impact the accuracy of the final clinical task. This factor has led to the development of task-based image quality metrics that are application dependent. Liu and colleagues,[82] for example, investigated the impact of noise reduction achieved via deep learning on lesion detectability as a function of count statistics based on a cross-center phantom study. Their U-net–based denoiser substantially improved the detectability of small lesions in low-count PET images even though there was reduced contrast in both liver and lung lesions. In a study conducted by Schaefferkoetter and colleagues,[34] 3 experienced physicians ranked denoised PET images based on both subjective image quality and lesion detectability for different noise and count levels. Their U-net–based denoiser outperformed Gaussian filtering in terms of physician-assigned image quality ranks with the largest improvement reported for the lowest count images. When evaluated for lesion detectability—a task-specific metric—AI seemed to only be beneficial for the low-count images. For the standard count images, U-net and conventional Gaussian filtered images led to similar lesion detectability outcomes. Xu and colleagues[83] used an AI-based proprietary software package SubtlePET (which has been cleared by the US Food and Drug Administration) to enhance low-dose noisy PET images of patients with lymphoma and reported that standard count and AI-enhanced low count PET images led to similar lymphoma staging outcomes based on assessments by 2 physicians. Katsari and colleagues[56] also used SubtlePET to process ^{18}F-FDG PET/CT examinations obtained with 66% standard dose. Their results showed that there was no significant difference between AI-enhanced low-dose images and standard dose images in terms of lesion detectability and SUV-based lesion quantitation. Nai and colleagues[84] conducted a lesion detection study using a PET/CT protocol for lung screening based on 30% of the standard radiotracer dose. The study found that the AI-processed low-dose images achieved substantial image quality improvement and were able to preserve lesion detectability. Chen and colleagues[55] also found that AI-enhanced 1% dose PET images achieved comparable accuracy for amyloid status determination as standard dose images. Tsuchiya and colleagues[52] conducted a study involving ^{18}F-FDG PET datasets from 50 patients and reported AI-based image enhancement significantly improved tumor delineation and overall image quality and suppressed image noise compared with a conventional Gaussian filter. A more detailed description of task-based assessment of AI can be found in Abhinav K. Jha and colleagues' article, "Objective Task-Based Evaluation of Artificial Intelligence-Based Medical Imaging Methods: Framework, Strategies and Role of the Physician," of this Special Issue.

Loss Functions

The loss function plays an important role in network training. **Table 1** specifies the loss function(s) used in each listed article. The most common loss function used for image enhancement applications is the mean squared error loss, which is based on the L2 norm of the difference between the network output and the training target and is also referred to as the *L2 loss*. A common alternative is the *L1 loss*, which is based on the L1 norm and is less sensitive to outliers than the L2 loss. Some investigators have used an L2 or L1 loss term based on the difference between the gradients of the output and target as a way to better preserve structural information in images.[40,48] A number of loss functions compare probability distributions instead of individual datapoints. One such common measure from information theory widely used as a loss function in machine learning is the *Kullback-Leibler divergence*, which measures how one probability distribution diverges from a second expected probability distribution. Another common loss function, the *Jensen–Shannon divergence*, is based on the Kullback–Leibler divergence, but is a symmetric measure with an upper bound of 1. This divergence metric computed between the generator output and observed data distributions is commonly minimized for GAN training. The *Wasserstein distance*, also known as the earth mover's distance, has gained popularity as a loss function for many image enhancement problems. Several of the GAN-based denoising works discussed in this article and highlighted in **Table 1** rely on a Wasserstein loss function. The commonly used evaluation metric SSIM and its variant multiscale SSIM have also been used as a loss function in certain applications. Another notable loss function for many imaging applications, including PET, is the perceptual loss,[85] which is based on differences between high-level image feature representations extracted by a given network those from a pretrained CNN (mostly commonly a pretrained VGG16 network).[86] Perceptual loss has been shown to be very effective at improving the visual quality of images.

EMERGING APPROACHES AND NOVEL APPLICATIONS

The past trends in AI-based PET image enhancement have been presaged by related developments in the broader machine learning community. Some areas of emphasis in image processing and computer vision research today include the development of approaches that enable the collation and collective use of datasets across multiple centers to ensure higher volume and variety of training data and improved generalization of the resultant models. Another focal area in the machine learning field is the development of models that are interpretable. These efforts are only beginning to percolate through the medical imaging arena with relatively few applications demonstrated on PET imaging at this point. In the following subsections, we discuss some of these areas that are either beginning to impact PET imaging or are likely to do so in the near future.

Transfer Learning

Transfer learning involves training a model on one (usually larger) dataset and fine-tuning it for a related application using a different dataset.[87,88] Although transfer learning is not a new approach, it continues to find novel applications in the medical imaging field. It is particularly valuable in applications where the training data are limited, a scenario very commonly encountered in clinical settings. The image denoising technique by Gong and colleagues[29] described elsewhere in this article, for example, uses a model pretrained with simulation data and subsequently fine-tuned with real data. As can be seen from **Table 1**, the overwhelming majority of AI-based efforts in PET are based on the ^{18}F-FDG radiotracer. Smaller data sizes for non-FDG radiotracers and/or extremely long or short half-lives of some radioisotopes are impediments to the training of AI models based on radiotracers other than ^{18}F-FDG. Liu and colleagues[44] used transfer learning to extend denoising models trained on ^{18}F-FDG PET images to data based on 2 less-used tracers: ^{18}F-fluoromisonidazole (commonly referred to as FMISO) and ^{68}Ga-DOTATATE. They reported that fine-tuning greatly reduced NRMSE and ROI bias and improved the signal-to-noise ratio compared with cases with no transfer learning. Chen and colleagues[89] used transfer learning to generalize a deep learning model to overcome data bias in multisite PET/MR studies where there are disparities in acquisition protocols and reconstruction parameters. In this study, a U-net network was pretrained using data from a GE SIGNA scanner with time-of-flight capability and subsequently fine-tuned using the data from a Siemens mMR scanner.

Federated Learning

Data security and privacy issues are of great importance in the medical domain and pose a formidable barrier to the collation of large multi-center patient databases for the effective training and validation of AI models. Usually, in machine learning based on multisite data, the data from each location are uploaded to a centralized server and subsequently used for model training and validation. Federated learning is a novel and increasingly popular alternative to the traditional centralized learning paradigm and involves distributing the model training task across sites and eventually aggregating the results.[90] It allows collaborative and decentralized training of deep learning models without any patient data sharing. In federated learning, each site uses its local data to train the model and shares the trained model parameters with a centralized server which builds an aggregate model that is shared back with the individual sites. Federated learning has become a common trend in the medical imaging domain by enabling access to distributed data for training deep learning models while abiding by patient privacy regulations. Applications of federated learning in medical imaging are gradually emerging. Its usefulness has been demonstrated in the context of classification problems based on MR imaging and CT imaging. For example, Li and colleagues[91] used federated learning for MR imaging-based brain tumor segmentation. Additionally, Kumar and colleagues and Dou and colleagues used federated learning models for coronavirus disease 2019 detection using chest CT scans.[92,93] Although federated learning has not been investigated extensively for PET, the multisite transfer learning study by Chen and colleagues[89] involved model sharing across sites and compared finetuned models with directly trained models for site-specific datasets.

Data Harmonization

Data heterogeneity is a major bottleneck while processing multicenter medical imaging studies. Differences in image acquisition protocols (including scan time), scanner models, image reconstruction parameters, and postreconstruction processing could lead to substantial variability in image characteristics, for example, image size, field of view, spatial resolution, and noise. Scan time differences in acquisition protocols could lead to drastically different noise levels across sites. The collective processing of such image pools often involves aggressive Gaussian filtering that would render the lowest count images useable but oversmoothing the higher count images in the process. In many longitudinal multisite PET studies, some sites stick to lower resolution legacy scanners for temporal consistency, whereas others have access to state-of-the-art high-resolution scanners. In such scenarios, a common harmonization strategy involves degrading higher resolution images to match the spatial resolution of the lowest resolution images. The PET image denoising and deblurring techniques discussed in this review all have broad applicability for image harmonization because they enable improving the resolution and noise characteristics of the lowest quality images instead of degrading the highest quality images. The super-resolution techniques published by Song and colleagues[62,65] are useful for data harmonization because they focus on developing a mapping from a low-resolution image domain (of a legacy scanner) to a high-resolution image domain (of a state-of-the-art dedicated brain PET scanner).

Besides harmonization between images, PET is unique in that there is potential for using AI for within-image harmonization. Notably, the resolution of PET images is spatially variant with the resolution at the periphery typically much worse than that at the center of the image. Such resolution nonuniformities pose a severe challenge to PET quantitation. Over the years, the PET community has taken great interest in spatially variant regularization techniques that generate uniform resolution PET images.[94,95] AI-based PET image enhancement techniques that achieve uniform resolution are yet to be explored, but these methods may offer an accessible, purely postprocessing-based solution to a longstanding problem in PET.

Reinforcement Learning

There are 3 fundamental machine learning paradigms: supervised, unsupervised learning, and reinforcement learning. Although the first 2 have been discussed here at length, reinforcement learning is only beginning to be applied for image enhancement and restoration. In reinforcement learning, an artificial agent interacts with its environment through a series of actions intended to maximize the reward for a given task. Smith and colleagues[96] reported using reinforcement learning for PET image segmentation, where the main objective was to detect the location of a lesion by moving a bounding box in different directions in the image to maximize a cumulative reward. The reward function in this scenario was a measure of the agreement between the predicted location of the detected lesion that of the one predefined by radiologists. Although reinforcement learning has been used for image segmentation, its applications to image enhancement are gradually emerging. The pixelRL technique is one such approach, which was shown to work for a variety of image processing problems.[97] This method poses an image enhancement tasks as a multiagent reinforcement learning problem, where each pixel has an agent that can alter the pixel intensity by taking an action intended to maximize a reward. Other examples of reinforcement learning used for image enhancement include a superkernel approach proposed for image denoising[98] and the RL-Restore technique for image restoration.[99] Although medical image enhancement based on reinforcement learning is in a nascent stage, it is a most promising research direction for PET scanning. PET image enhancement, for example, could be formulated as a multiagent reinforcement learning problem where the intensity (i.e. the current state) of each voxel can be iteratively updated by means of an agent's action. The rewards can be defined as either image-based metrics or clinical task-based metrics. By defining rewards that are based on clinical tasks, it may be possible to integrate clinical decision-making with image enhancement, thereby making it easier to assess the clinical benefit of the image enhancement scheme.

Interpretability

The black box format of AI models sometimes makes them less attractive in a clinical setting where intuitive explanations are sought by the clinical end-users. Emerging interpretable or explainable AI techniques, therefore, have garnered high levels of interest in the clinic. Most interpretable AI tools for medical imaging have focused on image classification problems.[100–104] Current computer vision literature shows a rising trend in papers on interpretable AI models for image deblurring, particularly blind image deblurring. In this category, unrolled deep networks are notable. Unrolled deep networks incorporate a physical model based on with prior domain knowledge, which makes them fundamentally interpretable. They typically have efficient implementations free of the usual computational costs and inaccuracies associated with model inversion.[105–107] Although the unrolling methods explored so far in PET are in the context of image reconstruction, unrolled networks are equally promising for

postreconstruction PET image enhancement techniques like denoising and deblurring because they can incorporate knowledge of Poisson statistics (for image denoising) and measured spatially variant point spread functions (for image deblurring). Attention-based approaches have been used widely to create explainable AI models, and recently they have been applied to image super-resolution.[108] Manifold modeling in embedded space has been proposed as an interpretable alternative to the deep image prior, with broad applications in image denoising, super-resolution, and other inverse problems.[109] These methods are both highly relevant and easily extensible to PET imaging and, therefore, are likely to assume a more prominent role in PET image enhancement in the near future.

SUMMARY

The excitement around AI in the PET imaging field is no surprise given the promising early results for the ill-posed inverse problems that have plagued the field since its infancy. Most of the work discussed in this article demonstrate that AI-based approaches for PET image enhancement outperform conventional methods by a striking margin. Despite the rich variety in AI efforts for PET enhancement, a key challenge that we are facing today stems from the poor generalizability of most trained models. Data size and variability remain challenges to model training using medical image data and often lead to models that do not generalize well to diverse datasets. A decrease in performance is often observed when a trained network is applied to data from a different domain (ie, different scanner, different scanning protocol, different tracer, different reconstruction settings). For example, in PET denoising, when the AI model is trained on PET images with a specific noise level, it could have insufficient denoising in noisier PET images or overdenoising/oversmoothing in less noisy PET images. Specifically, in the context of PET scans, there is interest in models that perform well on images with resolution and noise characteristics that are very different from the training data. Although the recently proposed unsupervised denoising and deblurring models are significant steps to circumventing this challenge, there remains a performance gap between supervised and unsupervised approaches that needs to be bridged. Federated learning also offers the promise to surmount formidable barriers to data access and could lead to the development of more robust models, the performance of which can be replicated in data from multiple sites. Developments in this direction would be vital for engendering confidence in AI-based models and in ensuring the long-term success of AI in the PET imaging field.

Although the review focus on AI-based postreconstruction PET image enhancement, advanced sinogram denoising and PET image reconstruction techniques are vital to improve the image quality for postreconstruction image enhancement. Sanaat and colleagues[47] found that AI-based sinogram denoising outperformed AI-based image space denoising with higher image quality and lower SUV bias and variance. The integration of AI-based reconstruction and postreconstruction image enhancement has the potential to push advances in the performance of the underlying technology. Developments of intelligent image acquisition, reconstruction, analysis, detection, and diagnosis would release the superpower of AI.

Although AI models have shown high performance when adjudged solely based on image quality measures, the performance margins over traditional approaches get slimmer for task-based measures. Unlike the models discussed in this article, which receive corrupt images as inputs and create enhanced images at outputs, there also exist many end-to-end approaches that start with raw data, extract features, and directly output a clinical decision. Although this latter group of models are optimized for clinical tasks, these are mostly black box approaches that do not generate enhanced images. Interpretable image enhancement models that adopt an intermediate path that merges the image enhancement task with one or more clinical decision-making tasks could bridge the existing gap in knowledge and lead to goal-oriented image enhancement. Interpretability would also be vital for ensuring the wider adoptability of AI-based models in the clinic as it would address skepticism among clinicians about the black box nature of these models.

The community would also benefit from standardized datasets for benchmarking AI models for image enhancement. This feature would address the disjointedness of current efforts and allow approaches to be evaluated against a common standard. Although code sharing is an increasingly common practice in the PET community, the sharing of trained models would also be vital for the fair evaluation of emerging approaches. As in most other research areas, AI-based methods in the PET field today have appreciable momentum. There is reason to be hopeful that creative solutions to the aforementioned problems await us in the near future. With more diverse datasets, rigorous and reproducible validation standards, and innovative models that integrate with existing clinical pipelines, AI-based models for PET image enhancement could ultimately lead to improved diagnosis, prognosis, and treatment evaluation and increasingly personalized approaches to health care.

ACKNOWLEDGMENTS

J. Liu, N. Mirian, and C. Liu are supported by NIH grant R01EB025468. M. Malekzadeh, T.-A. Song, and J. Dutta are supported in part by NIH grants K01AG050711, R21AG068890, and R03AG070750.

DISCLOSURE

The authors have nothing to disclose.

REFERENCES

1. Bar-Shalom R, Valdivia AY, Blaufox MD. PET imaging in oncology. Semin Nucl Med 2000;30(3): 150–85.
2. Politis M, Piccini P. Positron emission tomography imaging in neurological disorders. J Neurol 2012; 259(9):1769–80.
3. Knaapen P, De Haan S, Hoekstra OS, et al. Cardiac PET-CT: advanced hybrid imaging for the detection of coronary artery disease. Neth Heart J 2010; 18(2):90–8.
4. Shepp LA, Vardi Y. Maximum likelihood reconstruction for emission tomography. IEEE Trans Med Imaging 1982;1(2):113–22.
5. Dutta J, Ahn S, Li Q. Quantitative statistical methods for image quality assessment. Theranostics 2013;3(10):741–56.
6. Leahy RM, Qi J. Statistical approaches in quantitative positron emission tomography. Stat Comput 2000;10(2):147–65.
7. Panin VY, Kehren F, Michel C, et al. Fully 3-D PET reconstruction with system matrix derived from point source measurements. IEEE Trans Med Imaging 2006;25(7):907–21.
8. Vargas PA, La Rivie're PJ. Comparison of sinogramand image-domain penalized-likelihood image reconstruction estimators. Med Phys 2011;38(8): 4811–23.
9. Tong S, Alessio AM, Kinahan PE. Image reconstruction for PET/CT scanners: past achievements and future challenges. Imaging Med 2010;2(5): 529–45.
10. Tomasi C, Manduchi R. Bilateral filtering for gray and color images. Sixth International conference on computer vision (IEEE cat. No.98CH36271), Bombay, India. January 7, 1998. pp.839–846.
11. Hofheinz F, Langner J, Beuthien-Baumann B, et al. Suitability of bilateral filtering for edge-preserving noise reduction in PET. EJNMMI Res 2011;1(1):23.

12. Perona P, Malik J. Scale-space and edge detection using anisotropic diffusion. IEEE Trans Pattern Anal Mach Intell 1990;12(7):629–39.

13. Antoine MJ, Travere JM, Bloyet D. Anisotropic diffusion filtering applied to individual PET activation images: a simulation study. In 1995 IEEE Nuclear Science Symposium and Medical Imaging Conference (NSS/MIC). San Francisco, United States. October 21–28, 1995. Vol. 3, pp.1465-1469.

14. Stefan W, Chen K, Guo H, et al. Wavelet-based denoising of positron emission tomography scans. J Sci Comput 2012;50(3):665–77.

15. Turkheimer FE, Aston JA, Banati RB, et al. A linear wavelet filter for parametric imaging with dynamic PET. IEEE Trans Med Imaging 2003;22(3):289–301.

16. Su Y, Shoghi KI. Wavelet denoising in voxel-based parametric estimation of small animal PET images: a systematic evaluation of spatial constraints and noise reduction algorithms. Phys Med Biol 2008; 53(21):5899–915.

17. Le Pogam A, Hanzouli H, Hatt M, et al. Denoising of PET images by combining wavelets and curvelets for improved preservation of resolution and quantitation. Med Image Anal 2013;17(8):877–91.

18. Arabi H, Zaidi H. Improvement of image quality in PET using post-reconstruction hybrid spatialfrequency domain filtering. Phys Med Biol 2018; 63(21):215010.

19. Buades A, Coll B, Morel J. A non-local algorithm for image denoising. In 2005 IEEE Computer Soc Conf Computer Vis Pattern Recognition (CVPR). San Diego, United States. June 20–26, 2005. Vol. 2, pp. 60-65.

20. Dutta J, LeahyRM LiQ. Non-localmeansdenoising of dynamic PET images. PLoS One 2013;8(12): e81390.

21. Chan C, Fulton R, Barnett R, et al. Postreconstruction nonlocal means filtering of whole-body PET with an anatomical prior. IEEE Trans Med Imaging 2014;33(3):636–50.

22. Kirov AS, Piao JZ, Schmidtlein CR. Partial volume effect correction in PET using regularized iterative deconvolution with variance control based on local topology. Phys Med Biol 2008;53(10):2577–91.

23. Song TA, Yang F, Chowdhury SR, et al. PET image Deblurring and superresolution with an MR based joint entropy prior. IEEE Trans Comput Imaging 2019;5(4):530–9.

24. Rousset OG, Ma Y, Evans AC. Correction for partial volume effects in PET: principle and validation. J Nucl Med 1998;39(5):904–11.

25. Thomas BA, Erlandsson K, Modat M, et al. The importance of appropriate partial volume correction for PET quantification in Alzheimer's disease. Eur J Nucl Med Mol Imaging 2011;38(6): 1104–19.

26. Müller-Gärtner HW, Links JM, Prince JL, et al. Measurement of radiotracer concentration in brain gray matter using positron emission tomography: MRI-based correction for partial volume effects. J Cereb Blood Flow Metab 1992;12(4):571–83.

27. Costa-Luis COD, Reader AJ. Convolutional micro-networks for MR-guided low-count PET image processing. In 2018 IEEE nuclear science symposium and medical imaging conference proceedings (NSS/MIC). Sydney, Australia. November 10–17, 2018. pp.1-4.

28. Costa-Luis COd, Reader AJ. Micro-Networks for robust MR-guided low count PET imaging. IEEE Trans Radiat Plasma Med Sci 2021;5(2):202–12.

29. Gong K, Guan J, Liu CC, et al. PET image denoising using a deep neural network through fine tuning. IEEE Trans Radiat Plasma Med Sci 2019;3(2): 153–61.

30. Xiang L, Qiao Y, Nie D, et al. Deep auto-context convolutional neural networks for standard-dose PET image estimation from low-dose PET/MRI. Neurocomputing 2017;267:406–16.

31. Chen KT, Gong E, de Carvalho Macruz FB, et al. Ultra-low-dose (18)F-florbetaben amyloid PET imaging using deep Learning with multi-contrast MRI inputs. Radiology 2019;290(3):649–56.

32. Spuhler K, Serrano-Sosa M, Cattell R, et al. Full-count PET recovery from lowcount image using a dilated convolutional neural network. Med Phys 2020;47(10):4928–38.

33. Serrano-Sosa M, Spuhler K, DeLorenzo C, et al. Denoising low-count PET images Using a dilated convolutional neural network for kinetic modeling. J Nucl Med 2020;61(supplement 1):437.

34. Schaefferkoetter J, Yan J, Ortega C, et al. Convolutional neural networks for improving image quality with noisy PET data. EJNMMI Res 2020;10(1): 105.

35. Sano A, Nishio T, Masuda T, et al. Denoising PET images for proton therapy using a residual U-net. Biomed Phys Eng Express 2021;7(2):025014.

36. Wang Y, Zhou L, Yu B, et al. 3D auto-context-based locality adaptive multi-modality GANs for PETsynthesis. IEEE Trans Med Imaging 2019;38(6): 1328–39.

37. Zhao K, Zhou L, Gao S, et al. Study of low-dose PET image recovery using supervised learning with CycleGAN. PLoS One 2020;15(9):e0238455.

38. Xue H, Teng Y, Tie C, et al. A 3D attention residual encoder–decoder least-square GAN for lowcount PET denoising. Nucl Instrum Methods Phys Res 2020;983:164638.

39. Wang Y, Yu B, Wang L, et al. 3D conditional generative adversarial networks for high-quality PET image estimation at low dose. Neuroimage 2018; 174:550–62.

40. Kaplan S, Zhu YM. Full-dose PET image estimation from low-dose PET image using deep learning: a pilot study. J Digit Imaging 2019;32(5):773–8.

41. Zhou L, Schaefferkoetter JD, Tham IW, et al. Supervised learning with CycleGAN for low-dose FDG PET image denoising. Med Image Anal 2020;65:101770.

42. Ouyang J, Chen KT, Gong E, et al. Ultra-low-dose PET reconstruction using generative adversarial network with feature matching and task-specific perceptual loss. Med Phys 2019;46(8):3555–64.

43. Gong Y, Shan H, Teng Y, et al. Parameter-transferred Wasserstein generative adversarial network (PT-WGAN) for low-dose PET image denoising. IEEE Trans Radiat Plasma Med Sci 2021;5(2):213–23.

44. Liu H, Wu J, Lu W, et al. Noise reduction with cross-tracer and cross-protocol deep transfer learning for low-dose PET. Phys Med Biol 2020;65(18):185006.

45. Lu W, Onofrey JA, Lu Y, et al. An investigation of quantitative accuracy for deep learning based denoising in oncological PET. Phys Med Biol 2019;64(16):165019.

46. Ladefoged CN, Hasbak P, Hornnes C, et al. Low-dose PET image noise reduction using deep learning: application to cardiac viability FDG imaging in patients with ischemic heart disease. Phys Med Biol 2021;66(5):054003.

47. Sanaat A, Arabi H, Mainta I, et al. Projection space implementation of deep learning-guided lowdose brain PET imaging improves performance over implementation in image space. J Nucl Med 2020;61(9):1388–96.

48. He Y, Cao S, Zhang H, et al. Dynamic PET image denoising with deep learning-based joint filtering. IEEE Access 2021;9:41998–2012.

49. Wang YJ, Baratto L, Hawk KE, et al. Artificial intelligence enables whole-body positron emission tomography scans with minimal radiation exposure. Eur J Nucl Med Mol Imaging 2021;48(9):2771–81.

50. Schramm G, Rigie D, Vahle T, et al. Approximating anatomically guided PET reconstruction in image space using a convolutional neural network. Neuroimage 2021;224:117399.

51. Jeong YJ, Park HS, Jeong JE, et al. Restoration of amyloid PET images obtained with short-time data using a generative adversarial networks framework. Sci Rep 2021;11(1):4825.

52. Tsuchiya J, Yokoyama K, Yamagiwa K, et al. Deep learning-based image quality improvement of (18) F-fluorodeoxyglucose positron emission tomography: a retrospective observational study. EJNMMI Phys 2021;8(1):31.

53. Liu CC, Qi J. Higher SNR PET image prediction using a deep learning model and MRI image. Phys Med Biol 2019;64(11):115004.

54. Sanaat A, Shiri I, Arabi H, et al. Deep learning-assisted ultra-fast/low-dose whole-body PET/CT imaging. Eur J Nucl Med Mol Imaging 2021;48(8):2405–15.

55. Chen KT, Toueg TN, Koran ME, et al. True ultra-low-dose amyloid PET/MRI enhanced with deep learning for clinical interpretation. Eur J Nucl Med Mol Imaging 2021;48(8):2416–25.

56. Katsari K, Penna D, Arena V, et al. Artificial intelligence for reduced dose 18F-FDG PET examinations: a real-world deployment through a standardized framework and business case assessment. EJNMMI Phys 2021;8(1):25.

57. Cui J, Gong K, Guo N, et al. PET image denoising using unsupervised deep learning. Eur J Nucl Med Mol Imaging 2019;46(13):2780–9.

58. Hashimoto F, Ohba H, Ote K, et al. Dynamic PET image denoising using deep convolutional neural networks without prior training datasets. IEEE Access 2019;7:96594–603.

59. Hashimoto F, Ohba H, Ote K, et al. 4D deep image prior: dynamic PET image denoising using an unsupervised four-dimensional branch convolutional neural network. Phys Med Biol 2021;66(1):015006.

60. Wu D, Gong K, Kim K, et al. Deep denoising of O-15 water dynamic PET images without training data. J Nucl Med 2020;61(supplement 1):433.

61. Yie SY, Kang SK, Hwang D, et al. Self-supervised PET denoising. Nucl Med Mol Imaging 2020;54(6):299–304.

62. Song TA, Chowdhury SR, Yang F, et al. Super-resolution PET imaging using convolutional neural networks. IEEE Trans Comput Imaging 2020;6:518–28.

63. Garehdaghi F, Meshgini S, Afrouzian R, et al. PET image super resolution using convolutional neural networks. In 2019 5th Iranian Conference on Signal Processing and Intelligent Systems (ICSPIS). Shahroud, Iran. December 18–19, 2019. pp. 1-5.

64. Chen WJ, McMillan A. Single subject deep learning-based partial volume correction for PET using simulated data and cycle consistent networks. J Nucl Med 2020;61(supplement 1):520.

65. Song TA, Chowdhury SR, Yang F, et al. PET image super-resolution using generative adversarial networks. Neural Netw 2020;125:83–91.

66. He K, Zhang X, Ren S, et al. Deep residual learning for image recognition. In 2016 IEEE conference on computer vision and pattern recognition (CVPR). Las Vegas, United States. June 27–30, 2016. pp.770-778.

67. Serrano-Sosa M, Spuhler K, DeLorenzo C, et al. PET image denoising using structural MRI with a novel dilated convolutional neural network. J Nucl Med 2020;61(supplement1):434.

68. Ronneberger O, Fischer P, Brox T. U-net: convolutional networks for biomedical image segmentation. In 2015 Medical image computing and computer assisted Intervention conference

(MICCAI). Cham,Switzerland. October 5–9, 2015. pp. 234-241. Springer Cham.

69. Goodfellow IJ, Pouget-Abadie J, Mirza M, et al. Generative adversarial nets. In: Proceedings of the 27th international Conference on neural information processing systems, vol. 2. Montreal, Canada: MIT Press; 2014. p.2672–2680.

70. Zhou B, Tsai YJ, Liu C. Simultaneous denoising and motion estimation for low-dose gated PET using a Siamese adversarial network with gate-to-gate consistency learning. In 2020 International conference on medical image computing and computer assisted Intervention conference (MICCAI). Lima, Peru, Virtual/Online. October 4–8, 2020. pp. 743-752. Springer Cham.

71. Zhu J-Y, Park T, Isola P, et al. Unpaired image-to-image translation using cycle-consistent adversarial networks. In 2017 IEEE conference on computer vision and pattern recognition (CVPR). Hawaii, United States. July 21-26, 2017. pp. 2223-2232.

72. Dong C, Loy CC, He K, et al. Image super-resolution using deep convolutional networks. IEEE Trans Pattern Anal Mach Intell 2015;38(2):295–307.

73. Kim J, Lee JK, Lee KM. Accurate image super-resolution using very deep convolutional networks. In 2016 IEEE conference on computer vision and pattern recognition (CVPR). Las Vegas, United States. June 27-30, 2016. pp. 1646-1654.

74. Lim B, Son S, Kim H, et al. Enhanced deep residual networks for single image super-resolution. In 2017 IEEE conference on computer vision and pattern recognition (CVPR). Hawaii, United States. July 21–26, 2017. pp. 136-144.

75. Ledig C, Theis L, Huszár F, et al. Photo-realistic single image super-resolution using a generative adversarial network. In 2017 IEEE conference on computer vision and pattern recognition (CVPR). Hawaii, United States. July 21–26, 2017. pp. 4681-4690.

76. Kim K, Wu D, Gong K, et al. Penalized PET reconstruction using deep learning prior and local linear fitting. IEEE Trans Med Imaging 2018;37(6): 1478–87.

77. Lehtinen J, Munkberg J, Hasselgren J, et al. Noise2Noise: learning image restoration without clean data. In Proceedings of the 35th International conference on machine learning (ICML). Stockholm,Sweden: PMLR; July 15–18, 2018. vol. 80. p. 2965–2974.

78. Chan C, Zhou J, Yang L, et al. Noise to noise ensemble learning for PET image denoising. In 2019 IEEE Nuclear Science Symposium and Medical Imaging Conference (NSS/MIC). Manchester, United Kingdom. October 26-November 2, 2019. pp. 1-3.

79. Moran N, et al. Noisier2Noise: learning to denoise from unpaired noisy data. In 2020 IEEE/CVF conference on computer vision and pattern recognition workshops (CVPRW). Seattle, United States, Virtual/Online. June 19, 2020. pp. 12064-12072.

80. Ulyanov D, Vedaldi A, Lempitsky V. Deep image prior. Int J Computer Vis 2020;128(7):1867–88.

81. Zhou W, Bovik AC, Sheikh HR, et al. Image quality assessment: from error visibility to structural similarity. IEEE Trans Image Process 2004;13(4): 600–12.

82. Liu H, Viswanath V, Karp J, et al. Investigation of lesion detectability using deep learning based denoising methods in oncology PET: a cross-center phantom study. J Nucl Med 2020;61(supplement 1):430.

83. Xu F, Pan B, Zhu X, et al. Evaluation of deep learning-based PET image enhancement method in diagnosis of lymphoma. J Nucl Med 2020; 61(supplement 1):431.

84. Nai YH, Schaefferkoetter J, Fakhry-Darian D, et al. Validation of low-dose lung cancer PET-CT protocol and PET image improvement using machine learning. Phys Med 2021;81:285–94.

85. Johnson J, Alahi A, Fei-Fei L. Perceptual losses for real-time style transfer and super-resolution. In 2016 European conference on computer vision (ECCV). Amsterdam, Netherlands. October 8–16, 2016. pp. 694-711. Springer science.

86. Simonyan K, Zisserman A. Very deep convolutional networks for large-scale image recognition. arXiv preprint arXiv: 2014, 1409.1556.

87. Zhuang F, Qi Z, Duan K, et al. A comprehensive survey on transfer learning. Proc IEEE 2021;109: 43–76.

88. Pan SJ, Yang Q. A survey on transfer learning. IEEE Trans Knowl Data Eng 2010;22(10):1345–59.

89. Chen KT, Schürer M, Ouyang J, et al. Generalization of deep learning models for ultra-low-count amyloid PET/MRI using transfer learning. Eur J Nucl Med Mol Imaging 2020;47(13):2998–3007.

90. ShellerMJ, Edwards B, Reina GA, et al. Federated learning in medicine: facilitating multi-institutional collaborations without sharing patient data. Sci Rep 2020;10(1):12598.

91. Li W, Milletarì F, Xu D, et al. Privacy-preserving federated brain tumor segmentation. In 2019 International workshop on machine learning in medical imaging (MLMI). Shenzhen, China, October 13, 2019. pp. 133-141. Springer, Cham.

92. Kumar R, Khan AA, Kumar J, et al. Blockchain-Federated-Learning and deep learning Models for COVID-19 detection using CT imaging. IEEE Sens J 2021;21(14):16301–14.

93. Dou Q, So TY, Jiang M, et al. Federated deep learning for detecting COVID-19 lung abnormalities

in CT: a privacy preserving multinational validation study. NPJ Digital Med 2021;4(1):60.

94. Qi J, Leahy RM. Resolution and noise properties of MAP reconstruction for fully 3-D PET. IEEE Trans Med Imaging 2000;19(5):493–506.

95. Stayman JW, Fessler JA. Regularization for uniform spatial resolution properties in penalized-likelihood image reconstruction. IEEE Trans Med Imaging 2000;19(6):601–15.

96. Smith RL, Ackerley IM, Wells K, et al. Reinforcement learning for object detection in PET imaging. In 2019 IEEE nuclear science symposium and medical imaging conference (NSS/MIC). Manchester,United Kingdom. October 26–November 2, 2019. pp. 1-4.

97. Furuta R, Inoue N, Yamasaki T. PixelRL: fully convolutional network with reinforcement learning for image processing. IEEE Trans Multimedia 2020; 22(7):1704–19.

98. Mo_zejko M, Latkowski T, Treszczotko L, et al. Super-kernel neural architecture search for image denoising. In 2020 IEEE/CVF conference on computer vision and pattern recognition workshops (CVPRW). Seattle, United States, Virtual/Online. June 19, 2020. pp. 484-485.

99. Yu K, Dong C, Lin L, et al. Crafting a toolchain for image restoration by deep reinforcement learning. In 2018 IEEE/CVF conference on computer vision and pattern recognition (CVPR). Salt Lake, United States, June 18-22, 2018. pp. 2443-2452.

100. Qiu S, Joshi PS, Miller MI, et al. Development and validation of an interpretable deep learning framework for Alzheimer's disease classification. Brain 2020;143(6):1920–33.

101. Lee E, Choi JS, Kim M, et al. Toward an interpretable Alzheimer's disease diagnostic model with regional abnormality representation via deep learning. Neuroimage 2019;202:116113.

102. Papanastasopoulos Z, Samala RK, Chan HP, et al. Explainable AI for medical imaging: deeplearning CNN ensemble for classification of estrogen receptor status from breast MRI. SPIE Medical Imaging, vol. 11314. SPIE; 2020.

103. Wu YH, Gao SH, Mei J, et al. JCS: an explainable COVID-19 diagnosis system by joint classification and segmentation. IEEE Trans Image Process 2021;30:3113–26.

104. Gunraj H, Wang L, Wong A. COVIDNet-CT: a tailored deep convolutional neural network design for detection of COVID-19 cases from chest CT images. Front Med (Lausanne) 2020;7:608525.

105. Monga V, Li Y, Eldar YC. Algorithm unrolling: interpretable, efficient deep learning for signal and image processing. IEEE Signal Process Mag 2021; 38(2):18–44.

106. Li Y, Tofighi M, Geng J, et al. Efficient and interpretable deep blind image deblurring via algorithm unrolling. IEEE Trans Comput Imaging 2020;6: 666–81.

107. Marivani I, Tsiligianni E, Cornelis B, et al. Multimodal deep unfolding for guided image superresolution. IEEE Trans Image Process 2020;29: 8443–56.

108. Huang Y, Li J, Gao X, et al. Interpretable detail-fidelity attention network for single image superresolution. IEEE Trans Image Process 2021;30: 2325–39.

109. Yokota T, Hontani H, Zhao Q, et al. Manifold modeling in embedded space: an interpretable alternative to deep image prior. IEEE Trans Neural Netw Learn Syst 2020;1–15. https://doi.org/10.1109/TNNLS.2020.3037923.

Toward High-Throughput Artificial Intelligence-Based Segmentation in Oncological PET Imaging

Fereshteh Yousefirizi, PhD[a],*, Abhinav K. Jha, PhD[b,c],
Julia Brosch-Lenz, PhD[a], Babak Saboury, MD, MPH, DABR, DABNM[d,e,f],
Arman Rahmim, PhD, DABSNM[g,h]

KEYWORDS

- Artificial intelligence • Nuclear medicine • PET • Convolutional neural network • Segmentation
- Metabolically active tumor volume

KEY POINTS

- The need for an automatic segmentation technique to support oncologic diagnosis as well as to assess the progression-free survival analysis by radiomics is vital.
- The lack of annotated data and publicly available data affect the generalizability of AI techniques that have been developed to this aim.
- Semisupervised or unsupervised AI techniques can be used to tackle the data scarcity and have the potential to improve consistency and quality of annotated data

INTRODUCTION

An array of artificial intelligence (AI) techniques in the field of medical imaging has emerged in the past decade for automated image segmentation.[1] Medical image segmentation seeks to extract regions with specific anatomic and/or functional features and to classify the pixels (voxels) in terms of gray level and spatial or textural features.[2,3] The pixels (voxels) may be segmented with varied amounts of uncertainty, given contextual information.

Accurate segmentation is also crucial for external beam therapy planning. In the last decade, the valuable role of radiomics[4,5] for image assessment and outcome prediction has been reported, for which segmentation is a vital step.[6–9] In clinical workflows, in the context of radiopharmaceutical therapies, segmentation of PET and/or single-photon emission computed tomographic (SPECT) images is also needed for image-based dosimetry as well as quantification of therapy response based on pretherapeutic and posttherapeutic images (see Julia Brosch-Lenz and

[a] Department of Integrative Oncology, BC Cancer Research Institute, 675 West 10th Avenue, Vancouver, British Columbia V5Z 1L3, Canada; [b] Department of Biomedical Engineering, Washington University in St. Louis, St Louis, MO 63130, USA; [c] Mallinckrodt Institute of Radiology, Washington University School of Medicine, St Louis, MO 63110, USA; [d] Department of Radiology and Imaging Sciences, Clinical Center, National Institutes of Health, 9000 Rockville Pike, Bethesda, MD 20892, USA; [e] Department of Computer Science and Electrical Engineering, University of Maryland Baltimore County, Baltimore, MD, USA; [f] Department of Radiology, Hospital of the University of Pennsylvania, 3400 Spruce Street, Philadelphia, PA 19104, USA; [g] Department of Radiology, University of British Columbia, BC Cancer, BC Cancer Research Institute, 675 West 10th Avenue, Office 6-112, Vancouver, British Columbia V5Z 1L3, Canada; [h] Department of Physics, University of British Columbia, Senior Scientist & Provincial Medical Imaging Physicist, BC Cancer, BC Cancer Research Institute, 675 West 10th Avenue, Office 6-112, Vancouver, British Columbia V5Z 1L3, Canada
* Corresponding author.
E-mail address: frizi@bccrc.ca

PET Clin 16 (2021) 577–596
https://doi.org/10.1016/j.cpet.2021.06.001

colleagues' article, "Role of AI in Theranostics: Towards Routine Personalized Radiopharmaceutical Therapies," in this issue). To streamline the tedious, prone-to-error, and subjective task of manual delineations (eg, leading to interobserver and intraobserver variabilities), there have been significant efforts toward automated tumor segmentation.[10–13]

Considering the quality of annotations, weak supervision can be categorized as follows: (1) incomplete supervision: when limited annotated data are provided in the training set, (2) inexact supervision: when bounding boxes and image-level annotations are provided, and (3) inaccurate supervision: where the provided labels are not always ground truth.[14]

In this review, we consider supervised, weakly supervised (as generalization of semisupervised techniques), and unsupervised AI techniques that have been used for tumor or normal organ segmentation in oncological PET and PET/computed tomographic (CT) imaging (more details in the following section). Translating AI techniques into routinely used clinical workflows requires collaboration between AI researchers, clinicians, and predefined frameworks for evaluating these techniques to be integrated into clinical applications.[15] We outline the needed steps for AI techniques to be applicable in clinical workflows in section titled Solutions to Tackle Limitations in Annotations. We conclude this article with a series of considerations for an AI technique to be applicable in the clinical workflow and future directions for automated segmentation.

ARTIFICIAL INTELLIGENCE TECHNIQUES FOR IMAGE SEGMENTATION IN ONCOLOGICAL PET IMAGING

Metabolic tumor volume (MTV) refers to the volume of the segmented tumor in fludeoxyglucose (FDG) PET images. MTV has also been referred to as metabolically active tumor volume.[16] There are significant studies on PET imaging using other tracers, for example, prostate-specific membrane antigen (PSMA) PET, in which case this is referred to as molecular tumor volume (MTV). MTV is an important metric for response assessment and outcome prediction.[17] MTV has also been referred to as metabolically active tumor volume (MTV), and total MTV (TMTV) if the metastatic regions and lymph nodes are taken into consideration. Most existing studies report techniques for primary tumor segmentation, whereas for TMTV, accurate segmentation of metastatic regions and/or lymph nodes is also needed. As an example, TMTV is a significant prognostic factor in a range

of lymphomas (diffuse large B cell lymphoma [DLBCL], primary mediastinal B cell lymphoma, and Hodgkin lymphoma). Owing to the small size of metastatic regions, their variant locations, and different tumor-to-background ratios, segmentation of metastatic regions and lymph nodes is a challenging task. **Fig. 1** depicts an AI application for the quantification of whole-body tumor volume: AI-based segmentation and differentiation between tumor lesions and physiologic tracer uptake in FDG PET and PSMA PET images are shown. Segmentation techniques range from 2D to volumetric segmentations to assess the entire tumor (bulk) and/or normal organs. Different levels of supervision can be used for training a segmentation model from pixel/voxel-level annotations in supervised learning, and image-level or inaccurate annotations in weakly supervised learning, to no annotations in unsupervised learning (**Fig. 2**).[18]

Supervised segmentation techniques are applicable if pixel-level annotations are available. In the case of limited annotated data (ie, limited in number), semisupervised techniques are helpful. If only bounding-box or image-level weak annotations (eg, annotations of objects and attributes without spatial localization or associations between them) are available, weakly supervised techniques can be applicable. When no labels are available, unsupervised techniques would be the solution. **Fig. 2** shows the different learning techniques for different levels of supervision. We note that it is possible to consider weakly supervised techniques to encompass data that are limited in quality (along x-axis) and semisupervised techniques for data that are limited in number (y-axis) (see Ref.[14]). As such, weakly supervised techniques can be thought as generalization of semisupervised techniques. Overall, it is worth noting that because large numbers of unannotated or weakly annotated images can be available, they can be potentially combined/cascaded with small yet well-annotated images.[19]

Deep learning (DL) techniques, especially convolutional neural networks (CNNs) have shown to be effective for medical image segmentation,[2,20] specifically for PET segmentation.[21] Furthermore, fully convolutional networks (FCNs)[22] have gained much attention for probability maps generation by extracting the high-level features of lesions and normal organs and producing coarse segmentation or bounding boxes to be used for tumor localization.[23]

Fig. 3 depicts a standard workflow for AI-based segmentation of PET and PET/CT images. These steps start with study design and data collection, and as we mentioned for supervised techniques, with manual delineations as the ground truth.

A B

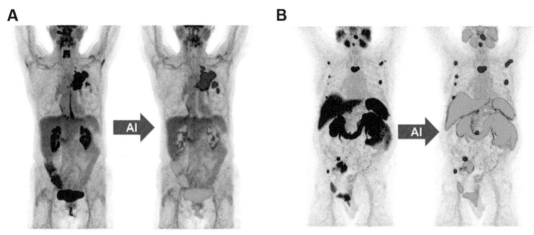

Fig. 1. AI framework assists nuclear medicine experts in the reading of whole-body scans. Example segmentations of tumor lesions and physiologic tracer uptake for FDG PET imaging of lung cancer (*A*) or PSMA PET imaging of prostate cancer (*B*). Physiologic uptake is shown in green, whereas pathologic uptake is in red. (*From* Seifert, R., et al., Artificial Intelligence and Machine Learning in Nuclear Medicine: Future Perspectives. Seminars in Nuclear Medicine, 2021. **51**(2): p. 170-177; with permission.)

PET/CT images need to be resampled to consistent sizes; considering a single or bimodal segmentation model, individual or multichannel data should be prepared as input to the model. Evaluation of the test results to check the reliability of the segmentation model should be optimally considered on data from independent centers that are captured under different conditions. The next step is data and model sharing along with the list of limitations and negative results of the proposed model.

We can consider fully automated segmentation as a 2-step process that includes separate detection and segmentation modules.[24,25] Lesion detection and segmentation can be performed simultaneously[25–27] or distinctly (back-to-back) as complementary tasks (using one model for detection[28] or 2 cascaded deep models for detection followed by segmentation[29]). Some existing segmentation techniques are designed based on the input from a detection step performed automatically[30] or manually[31] to localize the suspicious regions. In **Table 1**, a few studies that report detection performance, in addition to segmentation performance, are pointed out. Detection techniques are reviewed in another chapter.

Supervised Artificial Intelligence-Based Attempts for PET-Only Segmentation

Here we briefly describe some AI techniques used for PET segmentation. It is worth noting that

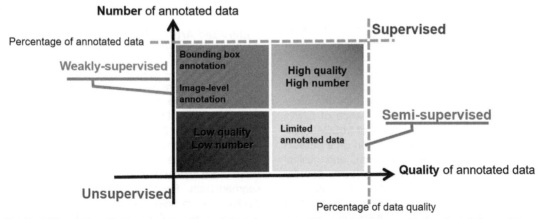

Fig. 2. Different levels of supervision for training a segmentation model. We emphasize that it is possible to consider weakly supervised techniques to encompass data that are limited in quality (along x-axis) and semisupervised techniques to encompass data that are limited in number (along y-axis), that is, weakly supervised techniques can be thought as generalization of semisupervised techniques. With high quality and high number of annotated data within the training data, one moves toward fully supervised AI techniques.

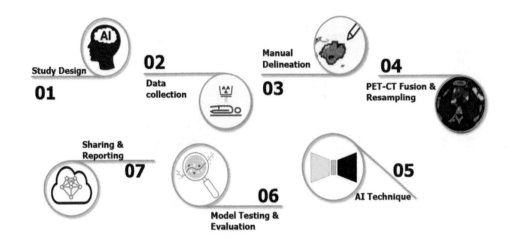

Fig. 3. Standard workflow for AI-based segmentation in PET and PET/CT images, consisting of the following steps: (1) study design such as the need for automated segmentation for TMTV calculation or radiomics analysis; (2) PET or PET/CT data collection from relevant study cohort; (3) manual delineations provided by physicians or by using semiautomatic thresholding techniques to be used for training the supervised technique; (4) data preparation including, cropping, resampling, and data fusion considering the application; (5) developing AI model (supervised/semisupervised); (6) model testing and evaluating the model to be applied on new data; (7) sharing the model for transfer learning.

performing accurate and reproducible tumor delineations on PET images is difficult due to partial-volume effects (PVEs), noise, motion artifacts, and varying shape, texture, and location of tumors.[11,13] Variations in image properties due to varying PET/CT scanners in real clinical practice is also a challenge. Most conventional and AI-based techniques for segmentation are based on classification of each voxel in the PET image to tumor (or a specific normal organ) versus background region, a task that is affected by these limitations. As an example, high repeatability of segmentation for smaller lesions in PET is hard to achieve because PVE affects the apparent tumor uptake.[32]

Czakon and colleagues[33] applied different AI techniques for PET-only segmentation, namely, 3D spatial distance-weighted fuzzy c-means,[34] dictionary-based model,[35] and CNN (eg, 3D U-net architecture) for PET segmentation, and CNN showed better performance than the other techniques. The superior performance of CNNs was also confirmed later by the first MICCAI challenge in 2018 on PET segmentation on a dataset composed of simulated, phantom, and clinical scans.[21] CNNs have nowadays become popular networks for PET segmentation; for instance, Blanc-Durand and colleagues[26] and Huang and colleagues[36] also used 3D U-net for automated tumor segmentation in gliomas and head and neck cases, respectively.

Most AI segmentation techniques in PET have been for FDG PET scans[26,33,36,37]; the other radiotracers have been rarely considered. As an example, Kostyszyn and colleagues[38] used a 3D U-net architecture to segment intraprostatic tumors in PSMA PET scans. Zhao and colleagues[39] developed a 2.5D U-Net architecture for segmentation of prostate lesions and local and secondary prostate tumors in lymph nodes and bones. Iantsen and colleagues [24] applied an SE U-net for tumor detection and segmentation in PET images of cervical cancer cases. Their proposed technique is capable of differentiating the pathologic and physiologic uptake in bladder successfully. In any case, most works have involved both PET and CT for segmentation, which we describe next.

Supervised Artificial Intelligence Techniques for Tumor Cosegmentation from PET/CT Images

Personalized therapy decision can be guided by PET/CT because the corresponding voxels in PET and CT contain complementary but distinct information.[40,41] **Table 1** summarizes the main studies on cosegmentation of tumors in bimodality PET and CT images. U-net,[42] 3D U-net,[43] and V-net[44] are widely used architectures for PET/CT segmentation. Recently, state-of-the-art frameworks such as skip connections,[45] dense-net,[46] recurrent residual CNN,[47] GAN[48] along with integrating squeeze and excitation modules,[49] Deepmedic,[50] and attention mechanism[51] have gained much attention for PET/CT segmentation. Details of such architectures are elucidated in the Tyler

Table 1
Supervised PET/computed tomographic segmentation studies

Investigators	Detection Performance Also Reported	Technique	Anatomic Interest/Dataset	Detection Performance	Segmentation Performance
Zhao et al,[58] 2018	✕	3D FCN	Lung, 84 PET/CT	-	Dice = 0.85
Zhong et al,[23] 2018	✕	3D U-Net + graph cut	Lung, 32 PET-CT	-	Dice (PET) = 0.76 Dice (CT) = 0.869
Zhong et al,[40] 2019	✕	FCN	NSCLC, 60 PET/CT	-	Dice (CT) = 0.861 ± 0.037 Dice (PET) = 0.828 ± 0.087
Li et al,[52] 2019	✕	FCN	NSCLC, 84 PET/CT	-	Dice = 0.86 ± 0.05 Sensitivity = 0.86 ± 0.07
Perk et al,[56] 2018	✕	VGG19	14 NaF PET/CT	-	Accuracy = 0.88 Sensitivity = 0.9 Specificity = 0.85
Moe et al,[142] 2019	✕	U-Net	197 H&N PET/CT	-	Dice (PET/CT) = 0.75 ± 0.12)
Zhao et al,[143] 2019	✕	FCN + auxiliary paths	30 H&N PET-CT	-	Dice = 0.8747
Kumar et al,[25] 2019	✔	CNN	50 NSCLC PET-CT	Precision: 64.6 ± 29.61 Sensitivity: 80.0 ± 28.3 Specificity: 99.89 ± 0.13 Accuracy: 99.85 ± 0.14	Dice = 0.6385
Andrearczyk et al,[119] 2020	✕	2D and 3D V-Net	202 H&N PET/CT	-	2D Dice (PET-CT) = 0.606 3D Dice = 0.597
Iantsen et al,[144] 2020	✕	U-Net with Squeeze & Excitation Normalization	254 H&N PET/CT	-	Dice = 0.759 Precision = 0.833 Recall = 0.74
Ma et al,[145] 2020	✕	CNN + hybrid active contours	254 H&N PET/CT	-	Dice = 0.752 Precision = 0.838 Recall = 0.717
Yousefirizi et al,[120] 2020	✕	GAN + Mumford-Shah loss + ACM	201 H&N PET/CT	-	Dice = 0.82 ± 0.06 Jaccard = 0.81 ± 0.07 HD = 1.72 ± 0.67
Weisman et al,[29] 2019	✔	Deepmedic	90 lymphoma PET/CT	Sensitivity = 87% (3 false positives per patient)	Dice = 0.64 (interquartile range:0.43–0.76)
Li et al,[19] 2019	✕	DenseX-Net	80 lymphoma PET/CT	-	Dice = 0.728
Jin et al,[53] 2019	✕	U-Net	110 esophageal PET/CT	-	Dice = 0.764 ± 0.134 HD = 47 ± 56 mm

Abbreviations: H&N, head and neck; NSCLC, non–small cell lung cancer.

J. Bradshawa and Alan B. McMillan's article, "Anatomy and Physiology of Artificial Intelligence in PET Imaging," in this issue.

Multimodality segmentation methods aim to use the functional information of PET images and anatomic localization of CT images simultaneously[25,39,52,53] or separately[25,54,55]; thus PET/CT fusion is needed for PET/CT segmentation. For tumor segmentation, because lesions can spread throughout the body, spatially variant fusion techniques can improve segmentation performance.[16] PET/CT fusion for segmentation can be varied from using a multichannel input (input-level fusion)[56] to the layer-level fusion of the modality-specific encoder branches.[23,40,54,57] In the modality-specific framework, multichannel input can consist of CT + PET or CT + maximum intensity projection PET images entered into the segmentation model.

CNN-based PET/CT segmentations are mainly carried out based on image patches around the tumor without considering tumor occurrence in different parts of the images.[23,52,58] To cope with this limitation, a spatially varied fusion map proposed by Kumar and colleagues[25] measures the relative significance of PET and CT features in the different parts of the images. Their suggested colearning scheme involves (1) a CNN that learns to extract the spatially varying fusion maps and a (2) fusion operation that prioritizes the features from each modality. **Fig. 4** shows the fusion technique proposed by Yuan and colleagues.[59] For DLBCL segmentation, they used 2 encoder branches for single-modality feature extraction and then used hybrid learning module in a supervised 3D CNN to create a prediction map of DLBCL lesions.

On the other hand, some existing multimodality PET-CT segmentation techniques are time consuming or require preprocessing steps including clipping, standardization, and resampling (isotropic or anisotropic) for one or both modalities and postprocessing steps.[58] Furthermore, the fact that these distinct modalities describe complementary but not identical characteristics of the same target is ignored in some studies.[60–62]

Artificial Intelligence Techniques for Unlabeled Data or Data with Scarce or Weak Annotations

The performance of AI-based techniques improves logarithmically with the size of training data.[63,64] At the same time, consistency of the labels is of primary importance. As an example, Weisman and colleagues[28] showed that the detection performance of the Deepmedic[50] model will not improve after training with 40 or more patients.

This finding can be explained as follows. Delineations by experts have in the past been mostly standard uptake value (SUV) based, impacting the reliability of supervised techniques. Limited number of annotations can be considered as the problem with "scarce annotations," that is, labeled data are rare, whereas "weak annotations" occur when the existing labels are noisy or roughly drawn or inaccurate. Data scarcity emerges from the class imbalance of medical images and time-consuming task of manual delineations. Meanwhile, limited consistency and reliability of annotations clearly affect AI task performance. These limitations motivate the use of advanced AI techniques that can be trained with limited supervision that is, semisupervised techniques[65–68] and unsupervised[69] methods.

Unsupervised techniques

A fully unsupervised and reliable segmentation framework for PET/CT remains to be demonstrated. Here, we briefly consider some existing studies to this end. Unsupervised techniques based on clustering have shown acceptable performance for tumor segmentation in PET images considering heterogeneous uptake patterns and vague edges. Addressing the inherent imprecision of PET, Lian and colleagues[70] suggested using Dempster-Shafer theory, to model the uncertainty along with an evidential clustering algorithm considering the intensity of the voxels and textural features of a patch surrounding the voxel. The same group also proposed a belief function to model uncertain image information and an adaptive distance metric to consider the spatial information.[62,71] Hu and colleagues[72] aggregated the voxels of 3D PET scans to supervoxels (a cluster of voxels) and subsequently used density-based spatial clustering with noise for segmentation.

Recently unsupervised AI techniques have been applied for anomaly detection in medical images based on normal images. The idea of using normal images (without anomalies) to train unsupervised anomaly detection and segmentation models has gained much attention mostly using encoder-decoder or CNNs.[73] For example, training a convolutional adversarial autoencoder on normal images can be used to learn a latent space that models the variant normal PET images. The residual map is then calculated to identify the PET images that are different from this manifold. Wu and colleagues[74] applied this technique on lung cancer images, and their method outperformed U-net. Klyuzhin and colleagues[75] used this idea for background removal to predict the physiologic PSMA-PET (18F-DCFPyL) uptake patterns from a pair of CT and low-resolution PET images.

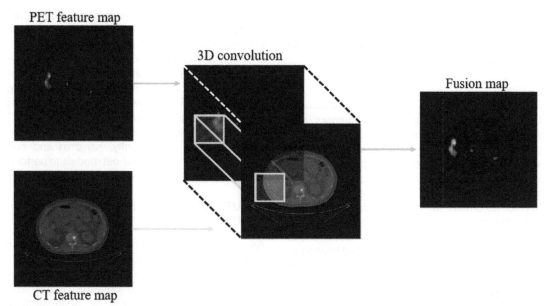

Fig. 4. Conceptual description of hybrid learning generating fusion maps by 3D CNNs. The encoder branches extract features form PET and CT images. This process (an example shown earlier) is repeated for different feature maps via different layers. The spatial fusion maps are generated by hybrid learning that quantifies the contribution of the complementary information from PET and CT images. The learned feature maps are then concatenated. (*From* Yuan, C., et al., Diffuse Large B-cell Lymphoma Segmentation in PET-CT Images via Hybrid Learning for Feature Fusion. Medical Physics, 2021; with permission.)

In a nutshell, as unsupervised learning techniques are less affected by the quality of labeled data which may be inadequate and biased with limited diversity. These approaches have the potential for flexible application to heterogeneous patient data, even for rare diseases, and can be combined with expert interpretations.

Weakly supervised and semisupervised techniques

Weakly supervised learning is a general term for training schemes under incomplete, inexact, and inaccurate supervision[14] as defined in the Introduction section. Afshari and colleagues[65] proposed a weakly supervised technique using FCN with modified Dice and Mumford-Shah loss functional for tumor segmentation in PET images of head and neck while only the bounding boxes around the tumors (weak annotations) were provided.

Semisupervised learning as a subcategory of weakly supervised learning techniques use unlabeled data along with a limited amount of labeled data for training. For instance, in the joint training strategy proposed by Li and colleagues,[19] the network parameters and the labels for unlabeled data were iteratively updated. During training, the optimal convolutional kernel is determined that improves the accuracy of the segmentation. The investigators used this parallel segmentation and

reconstruction flows for lesion segmentation in DLBCL PET/CT images.

Estimation-Based Approaches

PVEs in PET arise mainly due to 2 reasons: limited system resolution and finite voxel size.[76,77] The latter results in tissue-fraction effects (TFE), that is, a voxel containing more than a single tissue. Conventional segmentation methods (the term *conventional segmentation techniques* in this article refers to thresholding methods, region-growing methods, and statistical methods [ie, as opposed to AI techniques]; by contrast, *conventional segmentation techniques* in the literature sometimes refers to SUV-based thresholding techniques, which is only a subset of what we denote by this term), including DL-based approaches, classify each voxel as belonging to only one tissue type and thus have limited efficacy in addressing the TFE. To address this inherent limitation, recently, techniques have been proposed that estimate the volume that a tissue occupies within a voxel using an encoder-decoder network, which can then be used to define a segmentation.[60,78] The methods have shown improved accuracy compared with conventional methods, including U-net-based methods, on the task of segmenting tumors in patients with non–small cell lung cancer (NSCLC), as demonstrated in a study with the ACRIN 6668/

RTOG 0235 multicenter clinical trial data.[60] Furthermore, these approaches can also use training data derived from other modalities where the resolution may be higher[78] (**Fig. 5**).

Segmentation of Normal Organs

The occurrence of abnormalities (tumors and metastasis) can be very unpredictable and heterogeneous, whereas the spatial information of normal organs with physiologic uptakes are relatively stable; consequently, segmentation of normal organs from PET/CT can be a preliminary step for automatic tumor segmentation. Furthermore, the diverse size, variant shape, and unpredictable location of metastasis occurrences impose the need for diverse delineated images to achieve the generalizability and good performance of the segmentation model.[75]

Normal organ detection can be applied to determine reference level uptakes to help define the Deauville 5-point scale in lymphoma cases; that is, in reference to mediastinal blood pool and liver. Sadik and colleagues[79] trained an FCN to extract the liver and the mediastinal blood pool using CT images. Many normal organ segmentation approaches rely solely on CT, for example, using DL models[80,81] specifically there are publicly shared annotated CT images.[82] Yu and colleagues[83] segmented the normal organs based on CT images by applying a multiatlas method and removed them to obtain lymphoma lesions.[72,83] However, removing the organs that are considered as "normal" on CT images, may not take into account the possible abnormal uptakes that are observed in these organs. On the other hand, PET-based segmentation of normal organs can be challenging depending on the radiopharmaceutical with possible very low normal organ uptake. The existing studies are mostly based on PET/CT, and the corresponding CT images provide the anatomic reference.[75]

Seifert and colleagues[84] described a semiautomatic approach to distinguish normal organ uptake and tumor uptake in PSMA PET/CT imaging by applying a GAN following SUV thresholding to segment a range of normal organs on patient CT images and excluding the regions with physiologic PSMA uptake.[75,84] Recently, Klyuzhin and colleagues[85] applied a set of U-net models to perform segmentation of each normal organ.

SOLUTIONS TO TACKLE LIMITATIONS IN ANNOTATIONS

As we previously mentioned, the need for large and consistent labeled data,[86] in spite of the scarcity of labeled data in the field of medical imaging, should be addressed to develop reliable and generalizable AI techniques for segmentation. Based on the recommendations by the task group 211 of the AAPM (American Association of Physicists in Medicine), thorough, consistent, and sufficient evaluation of developed PET automatic segmentation method should be applied on (1) phantom images, (2) a combination of physical and numerically simulated phantom images, and (3) clinical images.[13] These recommendations arise from the fact that the volume of clinical images available for training and evaluation of segmentation models is often limited.[13]

Data Augmentation

Data augmentation (ie, flipping, shifting, rotating, and random cropping) is a preliminary solution to tackle the lack of labeled data. However, these augmentation techniques sometimes produce meaningless medical images; consequently,

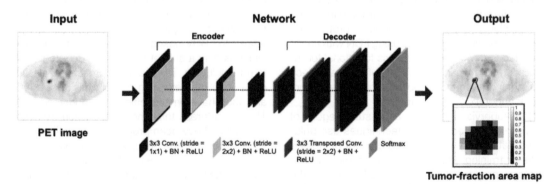

Fig. 5. The Bayesian approach proposed by Liu and colleagues[60] to tissue-fraction estimation for oncological PET segmentation. (*Adapted from* Liu Z, Mhlanga JC, Laforest R, Derenoncourt P-R, Siegel BA, Jha AK. "A Bayesian approach to tissue-fraction estimation for oncological PET segmentation" Phys Med Biol. 2021;66(12) Special Issue on Early Career Researchers. © Institute of Physics and Engineering in Medicine. Reproduced with permission. All rights reserved.)

realistically simulated or synthesized images can be used in this regard. GANs, for instance, can leverage data augmentation by synthesizing realistic-looking PET images based on existing PET or CT images. Studies on synthesizing PET images based on CT data have mostly used conditional GANs (cGANs)[87] and multichannel GANs.[88,89] Ben-Cohen and colleagues[90] used a cGAN to synthesize liver PET images based on CT images. cGANs can produce realistic PET images, but tumor regions are not very well reproduced.[91] On the other hand, FCNs have shown promising results for tumor synthesis, but the synthesized images are blurry. Consequently, using a combination of cGANs and FCNs showed improved performance.[90] Multichannel GANs (mGANs) was also applied to generate PET images based on CT and label images.[88]

Using Simulation Studies for Training

Using simulations to generate PET images with known tumor boundaries provides a way to address the challenge of limited accessibility of annotation. Briefly, an anthropomorphic digital phantom population, consisting of the tumors with known ground-truth boundaries, can be used to generate PET images using tools that model the PET imaging physics. There exist multiple mechanisms to generate such images. One approach is to use anthropomorphic phantoms, such as those based on XCAT[92,93] as inputs to software that models the PET physics. A second approach is synthetically generating tumors and inserting into clinical images. For example, Leung and colleagues[94] used a stochastic approach to simulate tumors with parameters such as shape/size/uptake similar to those in clinical images and used a projection-domain approach to insert these tumors into clinical images. **Fig. 6** depicts their proposed method. The investigators demonstrated that pretraining a network using these data led to improved segmentation accuracy and lower requirements of training data compared with a network that only used clinical data for training. Furthermore, the method was insensitive to PVEs and generalized across scanners. In using simulation-based strategies, it is important that the simulations be realistic, especially in terms of modeling the clinical characteristics. To evaluate this realism, observer-based strategies can be used.[95]

The consistency of ground truth
Annotations for standard training data have generally high cost and are laborious and time consuming for clinically experienced professionals. The delineations are made for different goals: for instance, masks generated for radiotherapy planning are generally larger than the original size of the tumors.[96,97] Depending on the interest in shell, surrounding tissue, and tumor region, delineations can vary. For instance, there has been increasing interest in peritumoral radiomics analyses, moving beyond typical delineated boundaries of tumors.[98,99] Besides, there are no actual hard edges between tumor and surrounding tissues even at the microscopic level. Furthermore, delineations based on fixed thresholding may be especially prone to error due to PVEs. Semiautomated algorithms can help obtain more consistent and accurate ground truths, such as fuzzy locally adaptive Bayesian (FLAB).[100]

Majority voting between manual segmentation by different experts has been used to enhance consistency. Web-based or freely available tools for crowdsourcing can also be used based on labels made by untrained or nonexpert trainees as a cost-effective alternative especially for organ segmentations.[64,101] Mehta and colleagues[101] showed that the performance of their 3D U-net model for kidney segmentation trained on crowdsourcing labels was not significantly different compared with the segmentation model trained on expert-labeled data. Heim and colleagues[102] used majority voting on labels for liver segmentation; they showed that crowd segmentation matched expert segmentation. There are strong observations that a large collection of naïve but independent analyses can outperform individual performance even by experts.[103] Furthermore, techniques have been developed to underemphasize the delineations made by lower expertise.[65]

EVALUATION OF ARTIFICIAL INTELLIGENCE TECHNIQUES

Conventionally, segmentation methods are evaluated by comparing the estimated segmentation with the gold-standard (ground-truth) segmented masks and quantifying performance by some measure of distance. For evaluating segmentation techniques, the use of at least 3 metrics is recommended because some of them are correlated (ie, Dice score [DSC], Jaccard score [JSC], Hausdorff distance [HD], average distance, and the Mahalanobis distance are highly correlated)[104]; for instance, DSC, true-positive rate, and false-negative rate can be used.[105] Based on the recommendations by AAPM TG 211, positive predictive value (PPV) and sensitivity should also be considered. For radiotherapy planning applications, sensitivity evaluation should be preferred, whereas for radiomics/quantification purposes, PPV is more informative (several frequently invoked metrics are listed in **Table 2**).

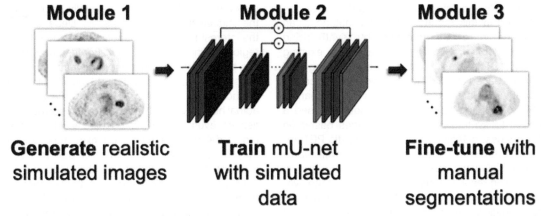

Fig. 6. Simulation-based segmentation framework proposed by Leung and colleagues. (*From* Leung, K.H., et al., A physics-guided modular deep-learning-based automated framework for tumor segmentation in PET.Physics in Medicine & Biology, 2020. 65(24):p. 245032.; with permission. © Institute of Physics and Engineering in Medicine. Reproduced with permission. All rights reserved.)

Clearly, this evaluation metrics can be affected by the ground-truth accuracy being not defined based on the ultimate task that segmentation is performed for; in this section we consider the no-gold-standard evaluation (NGSE)[106] that has been proposed to tackle this problem.

State-of-the-art DL segmentation models remain to be broadly translated to routine clinical workflow.[107] Such a high bar requires tacking of significant challenges with generalizability, repeatability, reproducibility, and trustworthiness of AI-based segmentation techniques, which we describe next.

No-Gold-Standard Evaluation

Conventionally, segmentation methods are evaluated by comparing the estimated segmentation with the ground-truth segmentation and quantifying performance by some measure of distance, such as DSC and JSC that quantify spatial overlap or HD that quantifies shape similarity. However, this strategy suffers from 2 issues. The first issue is the lack of such ground-truth segmentations. Although manually defined segmentations serve as surrogate ground truth, they can be erroneous, suffer from interreader and intrareader variability and can be difficult to obtain (time, expense). A second issue is that medical images, including PET images, are segmented for tasks such as quantification. Evaluation methodologies that quantify the distance between the measured and surrogate ground-truth segmentations may not correlate with that task.[108]

A segmentation method is developed to measure a certain quantitative feature from an image, so it should be evaluated based on how well the method performs on the task of reliably measuring that feature. However, this evaluation requires knowledge of the true quantitative parameter, or some gold-standard measurement. However, that is often unavailable or difficult to obtain. To address this issue, NGSE techniques have been proposed,[106,109–112] including in the context of evaluating PET segmentation methods on the task of estimating MTV[113,114] and, most recently, on evaluating PET partial volume compensation methods on the task of measuring activity uptake.[115]

Given measurements from multiple quantitative imaging methods, the NGSE techniques assume a linear relationship between the true quantitative values and the quantitative values obtained with

Table 2
Evaluation criteria for segmentation

Evaluation Measure	Definition
DSC	$\dfrac{2TP}{2TP+FP+FN}$
JSC	$\dfrac{TP}{TP+FP+FN}$
HD	$max\,\{sup_{x\in X}d(x,Y),\\ sup_{y\in Y}d(X,y)\}$
Sensitivity	$\dfrac{TP}{TP+FN}$
Specificity	$\dfrac{TN}{TN+FP}$
PPV or precision	$\dfrac{TP}{TP+FP}$

Abbreviations: FN, false-negative; FP, false-positive; PPV, positive predictive value; TN, true-negative; TP, true-positive.

each imaging method. This relationship is parameterized by a slope, bias, and a Gaussian distributed noise term described by a standard deviation. As we would expect, estimating these terms can yield a measure of how reliably the quantitative values are estimated (**Fig. 1** in Ref.[113]). Next, assuming that the true values are sampled from a certain parametric distribution, the NGSE technique derives a statistical model of the measurements obtained with the different imaging methods. The technique then estimates the parameters of the linear relationship that maximize the probability of occurrence of these measurements. The ratios of the noise standard deviation and slope terms (noise-to-slope ratio) for each method are then used to rank the methods based on how precisely they measure the true quantitative value. As has been shown in multiple studies,[106,109–112] this technique is able to accurately rank different quantitative imaging methods based on how precisely these methods measure the true value. For example, in **Fig. 7**, we show the performance of the NGSE technique in ranking 3 different quantitative SPECT methods. We observe that the NGSE technique, even in the absence of ground truth, yielded the same ranking as when the ground truth was known.

This NGSE technique promises to address a major barrier with clinical evaluation of segmentation methods for PET, but several challenges need to be addressed. As an example, existing NGSE techniques assume that the noise between the different methods is correlated. However, Liu and colleagues[114] recently proposed a strategy to model correlated noise. Another challenge is that NGSE techniques may require large amounts of patient images (N >200). A Bayesian approach to reduce the number of patient studies needed by the NGSE technique has demonstrated promise to address this issue.[116] Overall, these ongoing studies provide promise that NGSE techniques are well poised to provide a mechanism for clinical evaluation of PET segmentation methods on quantitative tasks.

Generalizability

Most AI techniques for medical imaging suffer from (1) the bias in the training population, (2) data leakage (the test data are not actually "unseen" in these studies), or (3) overfitting that results in the lack of generalizability of the AI models.[117] AI techniques should be evaluated on data from different scanners, centers, and patient populations with different clinical characteristics and demographics.[94,118] The cross-center generalizability of the model can be considered in 2 ways: (1) training the segmentation model on the data from one center (scanner) and testing on data from another center and (2) training the model on data from one center (scanner) and testing on data from other centers (scanners).[94] The leave-one-center-out cross-validation can also help the generalizability[119,120] in which one

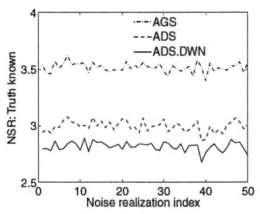
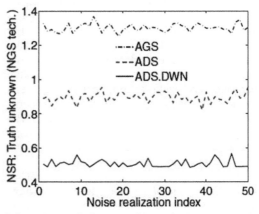

Fig. 7. Results from a study showing the performance of the NGSE technique. In this study, 3 reconstruction methods for quantitative SPECT (AGS, ADS, and ADS.DWN) were evaluated on the task of measuring regional uptake values. The figure on the left shows the rankings of the methods on the task of precisely measuring the true values, as quantified by the noise-to-slope ratio (NSR), that were obtained when the true uptake values were known. The figure on the right shows the results using the NGSE technique that did not use the knowledge of the true uptake values. The experiment was repeated for 50 noise realizations. We observe that even in the absence of the ground truth, the NGSE technique yielded the same ranking as the rankings obtained when the ground-truth values were known. (*Adapted from Jha, A.K., B. Caffo, and E.C. Frey, A no-gold-standard technique for objective assessment of quantitative nuclear-medicine imaging methods. Physics in Medicine & Biology, 2016. **61**(7): p. 2780.*)

center can be taken as the test set and the remaining centers as the training set. AI techniques for automatic segmentation have been mainly tested on limited dataset (in terms of the number of data and heterogeneity). Consequently semiautomatic thresholding methods remain as the main segmentation method in practice.[32]

Repeatability and Reproducibility

Repeatability measures the amount of variable results in repeated evaluations with same data, scanner type, reconstruction algorithm, and image noise levels. On the other hand, reproducibility considers the variability of the results when one or more of the above-mentioned conditions are variable. There are limited studies that consider the repeatability of AI segmentation techniques, whereas many more studies have reported the reproducibility of them. A repeatable segmentation technique produces comparable results on test-retest images (PET or PET/CT) of the same patient with similar physiologic conditions[121]; Pfaehler and colleagues[32] considered the repeatability of 2 segmentation techniques, that is, U-net framework and textural feature + random forest classifier. The investigators used a fully independent test-retest dataset of 10 PET/CT NSCLC recorded on 2 consecutive days. The investigators concluded that AI-based segmentation approaches have shown better repeatability compared with segmentation methods.[122]

Reproducibility analysis can be performed by intraclass correlation that helps to compare intra-individual and interindividual variabilities. For repeatability analysis, to assess within-subject variability under identical conditions,[123] percent test-retest differences in PET imaging are often quantified. For visual assessment of the mean versus differences of test-retest observations, Bland-Altman plots are also very helpful.[124] The reader is especially referred to the review article by Lodge[125] to understand the links between different metrics to quantify repeatability.

Furthermore, we note that there are a variety of evaluation metrics for segmentation, and multiple metrics may need to be used for more thorough assessment. For instance, a metric (eg, DSC, JSC) can consider the intersection of the predicted mask and ground truth, although it is not able to consider the edge details of the predicted mask achieved by other metrics (eg, HD).[104]

In manual or semiautomatic delineations, interobserver variability for delineations refers to the different segmentations obtained by different physicians, whereas intraobserver variability is for segmentations made by a physician at different instances. For automated AI methods, for example, DL methods, variabilities for segmentation originate from (1) the inherent variability of dataset, (2) random initialization of network parameters, (3) the stochastic optimization process, (4) variable selection of hyperparameters, and (5) variability of the infrastructure. These variabilities challenge high reproducibility.[105] To tackle this, several recommendations have been made. As shown in **Fig. 8**, these include providing (1) adequate descriptions for the DL frameworks as well as (2) analysis of variability due to different factors, arriving at (3) overall analysis for the sources of variability, toward efficient evaluation of segmentation results.[105] There are also several checklists to this aim (CLAIM [Checklist for Artificial Intelligence in Medical Imaging][126]).

Trustworthiness

AI techniques should be designed to allow physicians make better decisions, fostering their autonomy and minimizing automation bias ("human agency") and preserving the security and privacy of patients. Transparency is a crucial component of trustworthiness for an AI technique, which is challenged by "black box" models. More discussion on this topic appears in the Amirhosein Toosi and colleagus' article, "A Brief History of AI : How to Prevent Another Winter (A Critical Review)," in this issue.

The performance of AI techniques and the demand to use them in clinics can be improved if AI systems are able to represent uncertainties in given tasks. Two main categories of uncertainty are (1) epistemic uncertainty that refers to the uncertainty in the model and (2) aleatoric uncertainty that addresses the noise or randomness[127] and the spatial transformation of the input images.[128] These uncertainties can be considered by AI techniques such as Bayesian dilated CNN to predict the segmentation and generate corresponding spatial uncertainty map. Deep ensembles was also suggested to estimate the uncertainty as the variance of predictions by multiple models.[129]

The segmented regions with high uncertainty can be referred to radiologists; this helps to improve the quality of decision systems based on AI techniques. Consequently, radiologists can evaluate this uncertainty as a "human-in-the-loop" setting to improve the segmentation performance. This setting also helps to suppress implausible segmentations that are impossible to be produced by a radiologist.[107,130]

The performance monitoring of AI techniques when applied on real data in clinics should also

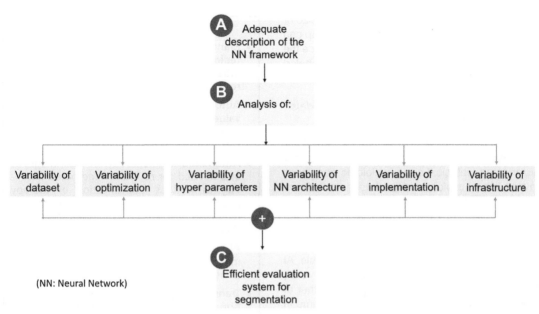

Fig. 8. Three main recommendations (*A, B, C*) to address the potential issues with reproducibility of DL frameworks for medical image segmentation. (*From* Renard, F., et al., Variability and reproducibility in deep learning for medical image segmentation. Scientific Reports, 2020. **10**(1): p. 1-16; with permission. This article is licensed under a Creative Commons Attribution 4.0 International License: http://creativecommons.org/licenses/by/4.0/.)

be iteratively evaluated for continual improvement. It is also recommended that safety and robustness of AI techniques be evaluated based on the updated methodology.[131]

FURTHER ADVANCEMENTS

Scarce annotations, as previously mentioned, result in supervised segmentation models with limited generalizability. To tackle these, several newer methods, beyond the above-mentioned efforts, are also being developed and explored, which we briefly discuss next.

Federated Learning

AI techniques for segmentation have faced challenges with generalizability due to limited volumes of data, having heterogeneity and variability in size, shape, texture, and site of the pathologies.[105] Federated learning (FL) enables training a centralized AI model across institutions instead of transferring the deidentified data from different centers to the centralized data storage. Parallel and sequential approaches have been proposed. In parallel training, the data are divided and different models are trained on each part, and the weights are transferred to the central model.[132,133] In sequential approach, the model is trained on the data from each institution and cyclic weight transfer is applied.[134]

FL faces several limitations and challenges. Data from different institutions with different infrastructure, imaging workflows, and different standards for delineations are heterogeneous with limited scalability. There may also exist ambiguity in preprocessing steps that are done differently in each institution. Finally, although only weights are supposed to be shared in FL, leakage of sensitive information is still possible, which needs to be tackled.[64,135]

Self-Training Techniques

As we discussed earlier, semisupervised learning techniques use the information of unlabeled data to train the model when limited and/or weakly annotated data are available.[136] Self-training is a semisupervised technique increasingly explored to estimate labels for unlabeled data during training. The predicted "pseudolabels" are weighted based on their confidence and then concatenated with labeled data to retrain the network by augmented training data. Self-training techniques remain to be thoroughly explored toward PET segmentation. As a limitation, incorrect early predictions can be propagated back to the network during the training process,[137] although this issue can be suppressed by techniques such as curriculum learning.[138] Curriculum learning that uses regression networks to predict the target region can overcome this limitation by enforcing the predictions of the unlabeled images to be close to the inferred label (in terms of target size or global label distributions). The regression step can regularize the segmentation model and reduce the errors of predicted pseudolabels for the unlabeled data.

Neurosymbolic Artificial Intelligence Models for PET Segmentation

Clinicians refer to a set of conditions, different imaging modalities, patient treatment and surgery history, and biological and physiologic conditions to evaluate a suspicious lesion based on their experiences.[139] By incorporating data, images, as well as "rules" into the AI models for detection and segmentation, more accurate and reliable AI-based tasks are expected. As such, use of neurosymbolic neural networks and explainable AI techniques[140] may add significant value. Overall, the future of AI may lie in the bringing together of 2 historically distinct and divergent paradigms in AI (symbolic vs connectionist) as discussed Amirhosein Toosi and colleagus' article, "A Brief History of AI : How to Prevent Another Winter (A Critical Review)," in this issue. Recently, use of hypertexts[141] and interactive reporting[64] have been considered to extract rules, toward generation of more generalizable models from limited data.

SUMMARY

Segmentation is a vital task for MTV calculation, radiotherapy planning, and radiomics analysis. Although AI techniques have significant potential for automated segmentation of oncology PET and PET/CT images, major challenges remain in terms of lack of consensus for manual delineations, and interobserver/intraobserver variabilities, to build consistent training sets for supervised techniques. It has indeed been shown that for supervised AI techniques, consistency in the training data is of higher importance compared with access to large amounts of data.[29] Meanwhile, to tackle issues with limited (annotated) data, several approaches such as semisupervised, self-training framework, FL, and neurosymbolic AI are being actively explored. For an AI-based segmentation technique to translate to routine clinical workflow, significant efforts are needed for improved generalizability and trustworthiness. Overall, AI-based segmentation methods applied to oncological PET images hold significantly promise and potential to help enable personalization of therapy for patients with cancer.

CLINICS CARE POINTS

- Manual delineation approaches are mostly tedious, subjective and prone to inter- and intra-observer variabilities, hampering routine deployment.
- Automated segmentation has significant value for external beam therapy planning, radiomics analysis and outcome prediction, towards personalized medicine.
- Automated segmentation of PET images is also needed for routine image-based dosimetry as well as quantification of therapy response based on pre- and post-therapeutic images in the context of radiopharmaceutical therapies.
- AI techniques enable reliable, robust, automated tumor and/or normal organ segmentations in oncological PET and PET/CT imaging.
- Translational AI techniques require collaboration between AI researchers and clinicians, and standardized frameworks to evaluate these techniques for integration into routine clinical workflows.

ACKNOWLEDGMENTS

This project was in part supported by the Natural Sciences and Engineering Research Council of Canada (NSERC) Discovery Grant RGPIN-2019-06467 and the Canadian Institutes of Health Research (CIHR) Project Grant PJT-173231. The authors would also like to acknowledge Dr Ghassan Hamarneh and Kumar Abhishek from Simon Fraser University for very valuable discussions.

DISCLOSURE

The authors do not have anything to disclose regarding conflict of interest with respect to this article.

REFERENCES

1. Langlotz CP, Allen B, Erickson BJ, et al. A roadmap for foundational research on artificial intelligence in medical imaging: from the 2018 nih/rsna/acr/the academy workshop. Radiology 2019;291(3):781–91.
2. Litjens G, Kooi T, Bejnordi BE, et al. A survey on deep learning in medical image analysis. Med Image Anal 2017;42:60–88.
3. Vial A, Stirling D, Field M, et al. The role of deep learning and radiomic feature extraction in cancer-specific predictive modelling: a review. Transl Cancer Res 2018;7(3):803–16.

4. Zwanenburg A, Vallières M, Abdalah MA, et al. The image Biomarker standardization Initiative: standardized Quantitative radiomics for High-Throughput image-based Phenotyping. Radiology 2020;295(2):328–38.

5. Starmans MP, Van Der Voort SR, Tovar JMC, et al. Radiomics: data mining using Quantitative medical image features. In: Handbook of medical image Computing and Computer Assisted Intervention. Elsevier; 2020. p. 429–56.

6. Klyuzhin IS, Gonzalez M, Shahinfard E, et al. Exploring the Use of shape and texture descriptors of Positron Emission Tomography Tracer distribution in imaging studies of neurodegenerative disease. J Cereb Blood Flow Metab 2016;36(6):1122–34.

7. Van Velden FH, Kramer GM, Frings V, et al. Repeatability of radiomic features in non-small-cell lung cancer [18 F] fdg-Pet/ct studies: Impact of reconstruction and delineation. Mol Imaging And Biol 2016;18(5):788–95.

8. Guezennec C, Bourhis D, Orlhac F, et al. Inter-observer and segmentation method variability of textural analysis in pre-therapeutic fdg Pet/ct in Head and neck cancer. PLoS One 2019;14(3):E0214299.

9. Yang F, Simpson G, Young L, et al. Impact of contouring variability on oncological Pet radiomics features in the lung. Sci Rep 2020;10(1):1–10.

10. Caldwell CB, Mah K, Ung YC, et al. Observer Variation in contouring Gross tumor Volume in Patients with Poorly defined non-small-cell lung tumors on ct: the Impact of 18fdg-Hybrid Pet fusion. Int J Radiat Oncol Biol Phys 2001;51(4):923–31.

11. Foster B, Bagci U, Mansoor A, et al. A review on segmentation of Positron Emission Tomography images. Comput In Biol And Med 2014;50:76–96.

12. Hansen S, Kuttner S, Kampffmeyer M, et al. Unsupervised supervoxel-based lung tumor segmentation across Patient scans in Hybrid Pet/mri. Expert Syst Appl 2021;167:114244.

13. Hatt M, Lee JA, Schmidtlein CR, et al. Classification and evaluation strategies of auto-segmentation approaches for Pet: report of aapm task Group No. 211. Med Phys 2017;44(6):E1–42.

14. Zhou Z-H. A Brief introduction to weakly supervised learning. Natl Sci Rev 2018;5(1):44–53.

15. Cheung H, Rubin D. Challenges and Opportunities for artificial intelligence in oncological imaging. Clin Radiol 2021. https://doi.org/10.1016/j.crad.2021.03.009.

16. Hatt M, Cheze-Le Rest C, Van Baardwijk A, et al. Impact of tumor size and Tracer Uptake Heterogeneity in 18f-fdg Pet and ct non–small cell lung cancer tumor delineation. J Nucl Med 2011;52(11):1690–7.

17. Im H-J, Bradshaw T, Solaiyappan M, et al. Current methods to define metabolic tumor Volume in Positron Emission Tomography: which One is Better? Nucl Med And Mol Imaging 2018;52(1):5–15.

18. Taghanaki SA, Abhishek K, Cohen JP, et al. Deep semantic segmentation of natural and medical images: a review. Artif Intelligence Rev 2021;54(1):137–78.

19. Li H, Jiang H, Li S, et al. Densex-net: an End-to-End model for lymphoma segmentation in whole-Body Pet/ct images. Ieee Access 2019;8:8004–18.

20. Zhou T, Ruan S, Canu S. A review: deep learning for medical image segmentation using multi-modality fusion. Array 2019;3:100004.

21. Hatt M, Laurent B, Ouahabi A, et al. The first miccai challenge on Pet tumor segmentation. Med Image Anal 2018;44:177–95.

22. Long J, Shelhamer, E, Darrell T. Fully Convolutional Networks For Semantic Segmentation. In Proceedings Of The Ieee Conference On Computer Vision And Pattern Recognition. 2015. Boston, Ma, Usa.

23. Zhong Z, Kim Y, Zhou L, et al. 3d Fully Convolutional Networks For Co-Segmentation Of Tumors On Pet-Ct Images. In 2018 Ieee 15th International Symposium On Biomedical Imaging (Isbi 2018). 2018. Washington, Dc, Usa: Ieee.

24. Iantsen A, Ferreira M, Lucia F, et al. Convolutional neural networks for Pet functional Volume fully automatic segmentation: development and Validation in A multi-center setting. Eur J Nucl Med Mol Imaging 2021;1–13.

25. Kumar A, Fulham M, Feng D, et al. Co-learning feature fusion maps from Pet-ct images of lung cancer. IEEE Trans Med Imaging 2019;39(1):204–17.

26. Blanc-Durand P, Van Der Gucht A, Schaefer N, et al. Automatic lesion detection and segmentation of 18f-fet Pet in Gliomas: a full 3d U-net convolutional neural network study. PLoS One 2018;13(4):E0195798.

27. Zhu Z, Jin D, Yan K, et al. Lymph Node Gross Tumor Volume Detection And Segmentation Via Distance-Based Gating Using 3d Ct/Pet Imaging In Radiotherapy. In International Conference On Medical Image Computing And Computer-Assisted Intervention. 2020. Lima, Peru: Springer.

28. Weisman AJ, Kieler MW, Perlman SB, et al. Convolutional neural networks for automated Pet/ct detection of diseased lymph node Burden in Patients with lymphoma. Radiol Artif Intelligence 2020;2(5):E200016.

29. Weisman A, Kieler M, Perlman S, et al. Automated quantification of lymphoma on fdg Pet/ct images using cascaded convolutional neural networks. In: Medical Physics. Hoboken (NJ): Wiley; 2019.

30. Andrearczyk V, Oreiller V, Depeursinge A. Oropharynx detection in Pet-ct for tumor segmentation. In: Irish Machine Vision and image Processing. Ireland: Sligo; 2020. p. 109–12.

31. Weisman AJ, Kieler MW, Perlman S, et al. Comparison of 11 automated Pet segmentation methods in lymphoma. Phys Med Biol 2020;65(23):235019.

32. Pfaehler E, Mesotten L, Kramer G, et al. Repeatability of Two semi-automatic artificial intelligence approaches for tumor segmentation in Pet. Ejnmmi Res 2021;11(1):1–11.

33. Czakon J, Drapejkowski F, Zurek G, et al. Machine learning methods for accurate delineation of tumors in Pet images. Arxiv 2016.

34. Guo Y, Liu K, Wu Q, et al. A new spatial fuzzy C-means for spatial clustering. Wseas Trans Computer 2015;14:369–81.

35. Dahl AL, Larsen R. Learning Dictionaries of Discriminative image Patches. Scotland, Uk: Bmvc; 2011.

36. Huang B, Chen Z, Wu P-M, et al. Fully automated delineation of Gross tumor Volume for Head and neck cancer on Pet-ct using deep learning: a dual-center study. Contrast Media Mol Imaging 2018;2018:8923028.

37. Smith RL, Paisey SJ, Evans N, et al. Deep Learning Pre-Clinical Medical Image Segmentation For Automated Organ-Wise Delineation Of Pet, In Annual Congress Of The European Association Of Nuclear Medicine. 2018: Barcelona, Spain.2018.Barcelona, Spain.

38. Kostyszyn D, Fechter T, Bartl N, et al. Intraprostatic Tumour segmentation on Psma-Pet images in Patients with Primary Prostate cancer with A convolutional neural network. J Nucl Med 2020;120: 254623.

39. Zhao Y, Gafita A, Vollnberg B, et al. Deep neural network for automatic characterization of lesions on 68 Ga-Psma-11 Pet/ct. Eur J Nucl Med Mol Imaging 2020;47(3):603–13.

40. Zhong Z, Kim Y, Plichta K, et al. Simultaneous co-segmentation of tumors in Pet-ct images using deep fully convolutional networks. Med Phys 2019;46(2):619–33.

41. Pantel AR, Mankoff DA. Molecular imaging to Guide systemic cancer therapy: Illustrative Examples of Pet imaging cancer Biomarkers. Cancer Lett 2017;387:25–31.

42. Ronneberger O, Fischer P, Brox T. U-Net: Convolutional Networks For Biomedical Image Segmentation. In International Conference On Medical Image Computing And Computer-Assisted Intervention. 2015. Munich, Germany: Springer.

43. Çiçek Ö, Abdulkadir A, Lienkamp SS, et al. 3d U-Net: Learning Dense Volumetric Segmentation From Sparse Annotation. In International Conference On Medical Image Computing And Computer-Assisted Intervention. 2016. Athens, Greece: Springer.

44. Milletari F, Navab N, Ahmadi S-A. V-Net: Fully Convolutional Neural Networks For Volumetric Medical Image Segmentation. In 2016 Fourth International Conference On 3d Vision (3dv). 2016. Stanford, Ca, Usa: Ieee.

45. Zhou Z, Sodha V, Siddiquee MMR, et al. Models Genesis: Generic Autodidactic Models For 3d Medical Image Analysis. In International Conference On Medical Image Computing And Computer-Assisted Intervention. 2019. Shenzhen, China: Springer.

46. Li X, Chen H, Qi X, et al. H-denseunet: Hybrid densely connected Unet for liver and tumor segmentation from ct Volumes. IEEE Trans Med Imaging 2018;37(12):2663–74.

47. Alom MZ, Hasan M, Yakopcic C, et al. Recurrent residual convolutional neural network based on U-net (R2u-Net) for medical image segmentation. Arxiv 2018.

48. Goodfellow I, Pouget-Abadie J, Mirza M, et al. Generative Adversarial Nets. In Advances In Neural Information Processing Systems 2014.

49. Roy AG, Navab N, Wachinger C. Concurrent Spatial And Channel 'Squeeze & Excitation'in Fully Convolutional Networks. In International Conference On Medical Image Computing And Computer-Assisted Intervention. 2018. Springer.

50. Kamnitsas K, Ledig C, Newcombe VF, et al. Efficient multi-scale 3d cnn with fully connected crf for accurate Brain lesion segmentation. Med Image Anal 2017;36:61–78.

51. Oktay O, Schlemper J, Folgoc LL, et al. Attention U-net: learning where to look for the Pancreas. Arxiv 2018.

52. Li L, Zhao X, Lu W, et al. Deep Learning for Variational Multimodality tumor segmentation in Pet/Ct. Neurocomputing; 2019.

53. Jin D, Guo D, Ho T-Y, et al. Accurate Esophageal Gross Tumor Volume Segmentation In Pet/Ct Using Two-Stream Chained 3d Deep Network Fusion. In International Conference On Medical Image Computing And Computer-Assisted Intervention. 2019. Springer.

54. Teramoto A, Fujita H, Yamamuro O, et al. Automated detection of Pulmonary nodules in Pet/ct images: Ensemble false-Positive reduction using A convolutional neural network technique. Med Phys 2016;43(6part1):2821–7.

55. Bi L, Kim J, Kumar A, et al. Automatic detection and classification of regions of fdg Uptake in whole-Body Pet-ct lymphoma studies. Comput Med Imaging Graph 2017;60:3–10.

56. Bradshaw T, Perk T, Chen S, et al. Deep learning for classification of Benign and malignant Bone

lesions in [F-18] naf Pet/ct images. J Nucl Med 2018;59(Supplement 1):327.

57. Van Tulder G, De Bruijne M. Representation learning for cross-modality classification. In: Medical Computer Vision and Bayesian and Graphical Models for Biomedical imaging. Athens (Greece): Springer; 2016. p. 126–36.

58. Zhao X, Li L, Lu W, et al. Tumor Co-segmentation in Pet/ct using multi-modality fully convolutional neural network. Phys Med Biol 2018;64(1):015011.

59. Yuan C, Zhang M, Huang X, et al. Diffuse large B-cell lymphoma segmentation in Pet-ct images via Hybrid learning for feature fusion. Med Phys 2021;48(7):3665–78.

60. Liu Z, Mhlanga J, Laforest R, et al. A Bayesian Approach To Tissue-Fraction Estimationfor Oncological Pet Segmentation. Physics In Medicine & Biology, 2021(Special Issue On Early Career Researchers).

61. Lian C, Ruan S, Denoeux T, et al. Accurate Tumor Segmentation In Fdg-Pet Images With Guidance Of Complementary Ct Images. In 2017 Ieee International Conference On Image Processing (Icip). 2017. Beijing, China: Ieee.

62. Lian C, Li H, Vera P, et al. Unsupervised Co-Segmentation Of Tumor In Pet-Ct Images Using Belief Functions Based Fusion. In 2018 Ieee 15th International Symposium On Biomedical Imaging (Isbi 2018). 2018. Washington, Dc, Usa: Ieee.

63. Sun C, Shrivastava A, Singh S, et al. Revisiting Unreasonable Effectiveness Of Data In Deep Learning Era. In Proceedings Of The Ieee International Conference On Computer Vision. 2017. Venice, Italy.

64. Willemink MJ, Koszek WA, Hardell C, et al. Preparing medical imaging data for machine learning. Radiology 2020;295(1):4–15.

65. Afshari S, Bentaieb A, Mirikharaji Z, et al. Weakly supervised fully convolutional network for Pet lesion segmentation. In: Medical imaging 2019: image Processing. International Society For Optics And Photonics; 2019.

66. Hu Y, Modat M, Gibson E, et al. Weakly-supervised convolutional neural networks for multimodal image registration. Med Image Anal 2018;49:1–13.

67. Zhou Y, Wang Y, Tang P, et al. Semi-Supervised 3d Abdominal Multi-Organ Segmentation Via Deep Multi-Planar Co-Training. In 2019 Ieee Winter Conference On Applications Of Computer Vision (Wacv). 2019. Waikoloa, Hi, Usa: Ieee.

68. Cheplygina V, De Bruijne M, Pluim JP. Not-so-supervised: a survey of semi-supervised, multi-Instance, and Transfer learning in medical image analysis. Med Image Anal 2019;54:280–96.

69. Kamnitsas K, Baumgartner C, Ledig C, et al. Unsupervised Domain Adaptation In Brain Lesion Segmentation With Adversarial Networks. In International Conference On Information Processing In Medical Imaging. 2017. Boone, Nc, Usa: Springer.

70. Lian C, Ruan S, Denœux T, et al. Spatial Evidential clustering with adaptive distance metric for tumor segmentation in fdg-Pet images. Ieee Trans Biomed Eng 2017;65(1):21–30.

71. Lian C, Ruan S, Denœux T, et al. Joint tumor segmentation in Pet-ct images using Co-clustering and fusion based on Belief functions. IEEE Trans Image Process 2018;28(2):755–66.

72. Hu H, Decazes P, Vera P, et al. Detection and segmentation of lymphomas in 3d Pet images via clustering with Entropy-based Optimization strategy. Int J Comput Assist Radiol Surg 2019;14(10):1715–24.

73. Baur C, Wiestler B, Albarqouni S, et al. Deep Autoencoding Models For Unsupervised Anomaly Segmentation In Brain Mr Images. In International Miccai Brainlesion Workshop. 2018. Granada, Spain: Springer.

74. Wu X, Bi L, Fulham M, et al. Unsupervised Positron Emission Tomography Tumor Segmentation Via Gan Based Adversarial Auto-Encoder. In 2020 16th International Conference On Control, Automation, Robotics And Vision (Icarcv). 2020. Shenzhen, China: Ieee.

75. Klyuzhin I, Xu Y, Harsini S, et al, Unsupervised Background Removal By Dual-Modality Pet/Ct Guidance: Application To Psma Imaging Of Metastases, In 2021 Snmmi Annual Meeting. 2021: Washington Dc.2021.Washington Dc.

76. Soret M, Bacharach SL, Buvat I. Partial-volume Effect in Pet tumor imaging. J Nucl Med 2007;48(6): 932–45.

77. Rousset O, Rahmim A, Alavi A, et al. Partial Volume correction strategies in Pet. Pet Clin 2007;2(2): 235–49.

78. Liu Z, Moon HS, Laforest R, et al. Fully automated 3d segmentation of dopamine Transporter spect images using an Estimation-based approach. Arxiv 2021.

79. Sadik M, Lind E, Polymeri E, et al. Automated quantification of reference levels in liver and mediastinal Blood Pool for the deauville therapy response classification using fdg-Pet/ct in Hodgkin and non-Hodgkin lymphomas. Clin Physiol Funct Imaging 2019;39(1):78–84.

80. Wang H, Zhang N, Huo L, et al. Dual-modality multi-atlas segmentation of Torso organs from [18 F] fdg-Pet/ct images. Int J Comput Assist Radiol Surg 2019;14(3):473–82.

81. Rister B, Yi D, Shivakumar K, et al. Ct organ segmentation using Gpu data augmentation, unsupervised labels and Iou loss. Arxiv 2018.

82. Rister B, Yi D, Shivakumar K, et al. Ct-org, A new dataset for multiple organ segmentation in computed Tomography. Scientific Data 2020;7(1): 1–9.

83. Yu Y, Decazes P, Gardin I, et al. 3d lymphoma segmentation in Pet/ct images based on fully connected crfs. In: Molecular imaging, Reconstruction and analysis of Moving Body organs, and Stroke imaging and Treatment. Springer; 2017. p. 3–12.

84. Seifert R, Weber M, Kocakavuk E, et al. Artificial intelligence and machine learning in nuclear medicine: future Perspectives. Semin Nucl Med 2021; 51(2):170–7.

85. Klyuzhin I, Chausse G, Bloise I, et al. Automated Deep Segmentation Of Healthy Organs In Psma Pet/Ct Images, In 2021 Snmmi Annual Meeting. 2021: Washington Dc.2021.Washington Dc.

86. Zhang P, Zhong Y, Deng Y, et al. A Survey On Deep Learning Of Small Sample In Biomedical Image Analysis. Arxiv Preprint Arxiv:1908.00473, 2019.

87. Isola P, Zhu J-Y, Zhou T, et al. Image-To-Image Translation With Conditional Adversarial Networks. In Proceedings Of The Ieee Conference On Computer Vision And Pattern Recognition. 2017. Honolulu, Hi, Usa.

88. Bi L, Kim J, Kumar A, et al. Synthesis of Positron Emission Tomography (Pet) images via multi-channel Generative adversarial networks (Gans). In: Molecular imaging, Reconstruction and analysis of Moving Body organs, and Stroke imaging and Treatment. Springer; 2017. p. 43–51.

89. Ben-Cohen A, Klang E, Raskin SP, et al. Virtual Pet Images From Ct Data Using Deep Convolutional Networks: Initial Results. In International Workshop On Simulation And Synthesis In Medical Imaging. 2017. Québec City, Qc, Canada: Springer.

90. Ben-Cohen A, Klang E, Raskin SP, et al. Cross-modality synthesis from ct to Pet using fcn and Gan networks for improved automated lesion detection. Eng Appl Artif Intell 2019;78:186–94.

91. Kazeminia S, Baur C, Kuijper A, et al. Gans for medical image analysis. Artif Intelligence In Med 2020;109:101938.

92. Segars WP, Sturgeon G, Mendonca S, et al. 4d Xcat Phantom for multimodality imaging research. Med Phys 2010;37(9):4902–15.

93. Leung K, Marashdeh W, Wray R, et al. A deep-learning-based fully automated segmentation approach to delineate tumors in fdg-Pet images of Patients with lung cancer. J Nucl Med 2018; 59(Supplement 1):323.

94. Leung KH, Marashdeh W, Wray R, et al. A Physics-Guided modular deep-learning based automated framework for tumor segmentation in Pet. Phys Med Biol 2020;65(24):245032.

95. Liu Z, Laforest R, Mhlanga J, et al. Observer study-based evaluation of A stochastic and Physics-based method to generate oncological Pet images. In: Medical imaging 2021: image Perception, observer Performance, and Technology assessment. International Society For Optics And Photonics; 2021.

96. Andrearczyk V, Oreiller V, Jreige M, et al. Overview of the Hecktor challenge at miccai 2020: automatic Head and neck tumor segmentation in Pet/ct. In: 3d Head and Neck tumor segmentation in Pet/Ct Challenge. Springer; 2020.

97. Vallieres M, Kay-Rivest E, Perrin LJ, et al. Radiomics strategies for risk assessment of Tumour failure in Head-and-neck cancer. Sci Rep 2017;7(1): 1–14.

98. Kadota K, Nitadori J-I, Sima CS, et al. Tumor spread through air spaces is an Important Pattern of Invasion and Impacts the frequency and location of recurrences after limited resection for small stage I lung adenocarcinomas. J Thorac Oncol 2015;10(5):806–14.

99. Dou TH, Coroller TP, Van Griethuysen JJ, et al. Peritumoral radiomics features Predict distant metastasis in locally advanced nsclc. PLoS One 2018; 13(11):E0206108.

100. Hatt M, Le Rest CC, Turzo A, et al. A fuzzy locally adaptive Bayesian segmentation approach for Volume determination in Pet. IEEE Trans Med Imaging 2009;28(6):881–93.

101. Mehta P, Sandfort V, Gheysens D, et al. Segmenting The Kidney On Ct Scans Via Crowdsourcing. In 2019 Ieee 16th International Symposium On Biomedical Imaging (Isbi 2019). 2019. Venice, Italy: Ieee.

102. Heim E, Roß T, Seitel A, et al. Large-scale medical image annotation with crowd-Powered algorithms. J Med Imaging 2018;5(3):034002.

103. Surowiecki J. The Wisdom of Crowds. New York: Doubleday; 2005. Anchor.Newyork.

104. Taha AA, Hanbury A. Metrics for evaluating 3d medical image segmentation: analysis, selection, and Tool. Bmc Med Imaging 2015;15(1):1–28.

105. Renard F, Guedria S, De Palma N, et al. Variability and reproducibility in deep learning for medical image segmentation. Sci Rep 2020;10(1):1–16.

106. Jha AK, Caffo B, Frey EC. A No-Gold-Standard technique for Objective assessment of Quantitative nuclear-medicine imaging methods. Phys Med Biol 2016;61(7):2780.

107. Sander J, De Vos BD, Wolterink JM, et al. Towards Increased Trustworthiness of deep learning segmentation methods on cardiac mri. In: Medical imaging 2019: image Processing. International Society For Optics And Photonics; 2019.

108. Zhu Y, Yousefirizi F, Liu Z, et al. Comparing clinical evaluation of Pet segmentation methods with reference-based metrics and No-Gold-Standard evaluation technique. In: Snmmi 2021. 2021. Washington Dc: Soc Nuclear Med; 2021.

109. Jha AK, Kupinski MA, Rodríguez JJ, et al. Evaluating segmentation algorithms for diffusion-weighted mr images: a task-based approach. In:

Medical imaging 2010: image Perception, observer Performance, and Technology assessment. International Society For Optics And Photonics; 2010.

110. Jha AK, Kupinski MA, Rodriguez JJ, et al. Task-based evaluation of segmentation algorithms for diffusion-weighted mri without using A Gold standard. Phys Med Biol 2012;57(13):4425.

111. Lebenberg J, Buvat I, Lalande A, et al. Nonsupervised ranking of different segmentation approaches: application to the Estimation of the left Ventricular Ejection fraction from cardiac cine mri sequences. IEEE Trans Med Imaging 2012;31(8):1651–60.

112. Jha AK, Song N, Caffo B, et al. Objective evaluation of reconstruction methods for Quantitative spect imaging in the absence of Ground Truth. In: Medical imaging 2015: image Perception, observer Performance, and Technology assessment. International Society For Optics And Photonics; 2015.

113. Jha AK, Mena E, Caffo BS, et al. Practical No-Gold-Standard evaluation framework for Quantitative imaging methods: application to lesion segmentation in Positron Emission Tomography. J Med Imaging 2017;4(1):011011.

114. Liu J, Liu Z, Moon HS, et al. A No-Gold-Standard technique for Objective evaluation of Quantitative nuclear-medicine imaging methods in the Presence of correlated noise. J Nucl Med 2020;61(Supplement 1):523.

115. Zhu Y, Liu Z, Bilgel M, et al. No-Gold-Standard evaluation of partial Volume compensation methods for Brain Pet. In: Snmmi 2021. 2021,. Washington, DC: Soc Nuclear Med; 2021.

116. Jha, A. And E. Frey. Incorporating Prior Information In A No-Gold-Standard Technique To Assess Quantitative Spect Reconstruction Methods. In International Meeting On Fully 3d Reconstruction In Radiology And Nuclear Medicine. 2015. Newport, Rhode Island, Usa.

117. Buvat I, Orlhac F. The True checklist for Identifying Impactful ai-based findings in nuclear medicine: is it True? Is it reproducible? Is it useful? Is it Explainable? J Nucl Med 2021;62(7).

118. Chang K, Balachandar N, Lam C, et al. Distributed deep learning networks among Institutions for medical imaging. J Am Med Inform Assoc 2018;25(8):945–54.

119. Andrearczyk V, Oreiller V, Vallieres M, et al. Automatic segmentation of Head and neck tumors and nodal metastases in Pet-ct scans, In Medical imaging with Deep Learning Midl. 2020: Montreal.2020.Montreal.

120. Yousefirizi F, Rahmim A. Gan-based Bi-modal segmentation using mumford-shah loss: application to Head and neck tumors in Pet-ct images. In: First Challenge, Hecktor 2020, Held in Conjunction with Miccai 2020. Lima, Peru: Springer; 2020.

121. National Academies of Sciences, Engineering, and Medicine. Reproducibility and Replicability in Science. Washington, DC: National Academies Press; 2019.

122. Bi WL, Hosny A, Schabath MB, et al. Artificial intelligence in cancer imaging: clinical challenges and applications. CA Cancer J Clin 2019;69(2):127–57.

123. Baumgartner R, Joshi A, Feng D, et al. Statistical evaluation of Test-retest studies in Pet Brain imaging. Ejnmmi Res 2018;8(1):1–9.

124. Bland JM, Altman DG. Measuring agreement in method comparison studies. Stat Methods Med Res 1999;8(2):135–60.

125. Lodge MA. Repeatability of suv in oncologic 18f-fdg Pet. J Nucl Med 2017;58(4):523–32.

126. Mongan J, Moy L, Kahn JCE. Checklist for artificial intelligence in medical imaging (claim): a Guide for authors and reviewers. Radiol Artif Intelligence 2020;2(2):E200029.

127. Kendall A, Gal Y. What Uncertainties Do We Need In Bayesian Deep Learning For Computer Vision? Arxiv Preprint Arxiv:1703.04977, 2017.

128. Wang G, Li W, Aertsen M, et al. Aleatoric uncertainty Estimation with Test-Time augmentation for medical image segmentation with convolutional neural networks. Neurocomputing 2019;338:34–45.

129. Lakshminarayanan B, Pritzel A, Blundell C. Simple and scalable predictive uncertainty Estimation using deep Ensembles. Adv In Neural Inf Process Syst 2017;30.

130. Kwon Y, Won J-H, Kim BJ, et al. Uncertainty quantification using Bayesian neural networks in classification: application to Ischemic stroke lesion segmentation. Comput Stat Data Anal 2018;142.

131. Stephens K. Fda releases artificial intelligence/machine learning action Plan. Axis Imaging News 2021.

132. Dean J, Corrado GS, Monga R, et al. Large Scale Distributed Deep Networks, In Proceedings Of Nips. 2012. P. 1232–1240.2012.

133. Su H, Chen H. Experiments On Parallel Training Of Deep Neural Network Using Model Averaging. Arxiv Preprint Arxiv:1507.01239, 2015.

134. Kairouz P, Mcmahan HB, Avent B, et al. Advances And Open Problems In Federated Learning. Arxiv Preprint Arxiv:1912.04977, 2019.

135. Zerka F, Barakat S, Walsh S, et al. Systematic review of Privacy-Preserving distributed machine learning from federated databases in Health care. JCO Clin Cancer Inform 2020;4:184–200.

136. Iglesias JE, Liu C-Y, Thompson P, et al. Agreement-Based Semi-Supervised Learning For Skull Stripping. In International Conference On Medical Image Computing And Computer-Assisted Intervention. 2010. Beijing, China: Springer.

137. Li X, Yu L, Chen H, et al. Semi-Supervised Skin Lesion Segmentation Via Transformation

Consistent Self-Ensembling Model. Arxiv Preprint Arxiv:1808.03887, 2018.

138. Kervadec H, Dolz J, Granger É, et al. Curriculum Semi-Supervised Segmentation. In International Conference On Medical Image Computing And Computer-Assisted Intervention. 2019. Shenzhen, China: Springer.

139. Manhaeve R, Dumancic S, Kimmig A, et al. Deep-problog: neural Probabilistic logic Programming. Adv In Neural Inf Process Syst 2018;31:3749–59.

140. Došilović FK, Brčić M, Hlupić N. Explainable Artificial Intelligence: A Survey. In 2018 41st International Convention On Information And Communication Technology, Electronics And Microelectronics (Mipro). 2018. Opatija, Croatia: Ieee.

141. Folio LR, Machado LB, Dwyer AJ. Multimedia-enhanced radiology reports: concept, components, and challenges. Radiographics 2018;38(2):462–82.

142. Moe YM, Groendahl AR, Tomic O, et al. Deep learning-based auto-delineation of Gross Tumour Volumes and Involved nodes in Pet/ct images of Head and neck cancer Patients. Eur J Nucl Med Mol Imaging 2021;1–11.

143. Zhao L, Lu Z, Jiang J, et al. Automatic nasopharyngeal carcinoma segmentation using fully convolutional networks with auxiliary Paths on dual-modality Pet-ct images. J Digit Imaging 2019; 32(3):462–70.

144. Iantsen A, Visvikis D, Hatt M. Squeeze-and-excitation normalization for automated delineation of Head and neck Primary tumors in combined Pet and ct images. In: 3d Head and Neck tumor segmentation in Pet/Ct Challenge. Lima, Peru: Springer; 2020.

145. Ma J, Yang X. Combining cnn and Hybrid active contours for Head and neck tumor segmentation in ct and Pet images. In: 3d Head and Neck tumor segmentation in Pet/Ct Challenge. Lima, Peru: Springer; 2020.

Radiomics in PET Imaging:
A Practical Guide for Newcomers

Fanny Orlhac, PhD[a],*, Christophe Nioche, PhD[a], Ivan Klyuzhin, PhD[b,c],
Arman Rahmim, PhD, DABSNM[b,c], Irène Buvat, PhD[a]

KEYWORDS

• Radiomics • PET • Texture • Heterogeneity • Harmonization

KEY POINTS

- In the literature, promising results report links between the radiomic feature values measured on PET images and the biological characteristics of lesions, patient prognosis, and response to treatments.
- Each step in the radiomic analysis pipeline influences the feature values and should be carefully reported to allow other teams to reproduce the findings.
- Harmonization methods will play a key role in the development of radiomic models using heterogeneous data and in their deployment for multicenter validation.
- Deep-learning methods can be used to extract new features and could bring a new and complementary perspective to current engineered features.

INTRODUCTION

The term "radiomics" was first introduced in 2010 by Gillies and colleagues[1] and was later defined as *"the conversion of digital images into mineable high-dimensional data."*[2] The analysis of these high-dimensional data is intended to provide information on the biological characteristics of tumors, patient prognosis, or the response to treatments. These data can reflect the signal intensity distribution, texture, or shape of the signal in a given volume of interest (VOI) in the image. Although the term "radiomics" is relatively new, many studies have reported on advanced image analysis in the past and investigated the relationship between sophisticated measurements and biological characteristics. For instance, even before the 2000s, investigators were studying the relationship between fractal analysis and striatal dopamine uptake[3] and the use of a cooccurrence matrix to classify

lung nodules.[4] Since 2007, the Quantitative Imaging Biomarkers Alliance working groups have also published recommendations "*to advance quantitative imaging and the use of imaging biomarkers in clinical trials and clinical practice.*"[5] Among the 2970 articles associated with the keyword "*radiomics*" on PubMed (between january 2012 and december 2020), 424 mention PET imaging (**Fig. 1**). These articles mainly concern oncologic applications regarding the lungs (30%), the head and neck (16%), the esophagus (7%), breast cancer (6%), and lymphoma (6%). In these articles, the authors investigated the relationship between radiomic feature values and the biological characteristics of the lesions (39%), patient prognosis (27%), or the response to treatments (24%). Features were mainly extracted from PET images obtained after injection of 18F-fluorodeoxyglucose (18F-FDG, 87%) but also using other radiotracers such as 18F-fluoroethyl-L-tyrosine (18F-FET, 2%),

[a] Institut Curie Centre de Recherche, Centre Universitaire, Bat 101B, Rue Henri Becquerel, CS 90030, 91401 Orsay Cedex, France; [b] Department of Integrative Oncology, BC Cancer Research Institute, 675 West 10th Avenue, Vancouver, BC V5Z 1L3, Canada; [c] Department of Radiology, University of British Columbia, 675 West 10th Avenue, Vancouver, BC V5Z 1L3, Canada
* Corresponding author. Institut Curie, Université PSL, Inserm, U1288, Institut Curie Centre de Recherche, Centre Universitaire, Bat 101B, Rue Henri Becquerel, CS 90030, 91401 Orsay Cedex, France.
E-mail address: orlhacf@gmail.com

PET Clin 16 (2021) 597–612
https://doi.org/10.1016/j.cpet.2021.06.007
1556-8598/21/© 2021 Elsevier Inc. All rights reserved.

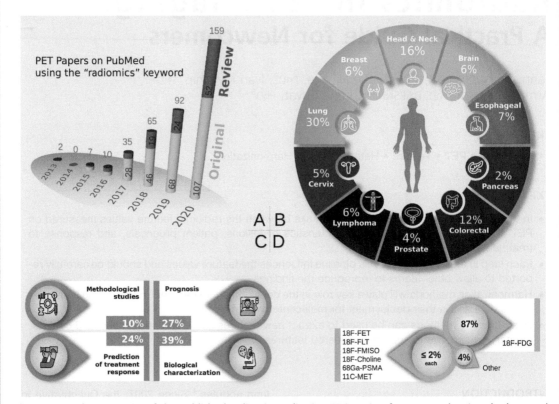

Fig. 1. Main characteristics of the published radiomic studies in PET imaging from a search using the keywords "radiomics AND PET" on PubMed (between january 2012 and december 2020). (*A*) Number of original articles and reviews per year. (*B*) Percentage of articles according to the organ studied in cancerology. (*C*) Question of interest studied in the articles. (*D*) Distribution of articles according to the tracer used.

11C-methionine (11C-MET, 2%) and 68Ga-prostate-specific membrane antigen (68Ga-PSMA, 2%). A small proportion of articles (10%) report methodological contributions regarding the impact of acquisition and reconstruction parameters of PET images and of the different steps of the radiomic analysis pipeline on feature values based on phantom and/or clinical data.

Many reviews published in recent years (30% of the articles published in the radiomics field) have explained the potential of radiomics in medical imaging and the current limitations, and interested readers might want to refer to those.[6–8] However, when starting a radiomic study, many practical questions arise.

First, it is important to realize that radiomics includes 2 approaches. The first approach consists of extracting "handcrafted" features from the images, where handcrafted features refer to features obeying a precise mathematical definition, such as maximum standardized uptake value (SUVmax), metabolic volume, sphericity, or entropy. The resulting radiomic feature values are then used to perform statistical tests relevant to the task of interest or as an input for a multivariate classifier, most often designed using a machine-learning approach, such as the logistic regression, support vector machine, or random forest.

A second approach consists of using images or image VOIs directly as input to a neural network, such as a convolutional neural network (CNN), to obtain a classification or a prediction. This approach can be called deep radiomics, as it still treats the images as high-dimensional mineable data (each voxel is an input variable); however, the radiomic features are no longer predefined as when using handcrafted features but are learned by the CNN itself as a function of the input images and of the task.

Deep radiomics can also consist of extracting "deep" features using a CNN and then providing these features to a classifier.[9,10] Alternatively, deep radiomics can first involve the calculation of radiomic parametric images using the definition of handcrafted features and then inputs these maps into a deep neural network. In short, deep radiomics will be used thereafter anytime a deep neural network is used in a certain step of the radiomic pipeline.

The difficulty for physicians to precisely quantify heterogeneity, the lack of intraobserver and interobserver reproducibility, and the challenge of coanalyzing many pieces of information at the same time are all arguments in favor of radiomics. Several studies have proven that radiomic indices can quantify the heterogeneity perceived by physicians[11,12] and that the macroscopic phenotypes measured from images are related to the density and spatial organization of cells at the microscopic scale.[13–15] Despite the indisputable potential of radiomics in PET, no model has yet proven its superiority over existing methods based on common features (eg, SUVmax or metabolic volume) in multicenter and multicohort settings and by different independent investigators. To produce sound radiomic models amenable to clinical translation, a thorough understanding of the impact of the choices made in each step of a radiomic study is absolutely necessary.

Therefore, the main objective of this article is to offer a practical guide to help interested readers establish a radiomic study involving PET images and "handcrafted" features. In addition, the authors discuss key aspects to consider when analyzing the literature in this field. Finally, they explain how deep radiomics can complement handcrafted radiomics.

CHECKLIST TO DESIGN A RELIABLE RADIOMIC STUDY

Before initiating a radiomic study, several questions should be considered to determine if the study is relevant and feasible. The major points to be examined are listed in **Fig. 2**.

Identify a Relevant Question

As with any scientific study, the question of interest will determine the impact of the investigation. From a clinical point of view, the question of interest may relate to patient management (for instance, the prediction of patient response or survival) or to a better understanding of a disease (for instance, the distinction between different molecular subtypes from phenotypic data). The level of performance that would make the radiomic approach appealing compared with state-of-the-art approaches should be indicated or, alternatively, the reason a radiomic approach would be desirable. From a physics point of view, the goal might be to better understand radiomics or the factors that can influence feature values and/or to propose corrections or improvements for enhanced radiomic models. The relevance of the question and previous contributions addressing it should be carefully inspected based on a bibliographic search.

Review the State-of-the-Art

In radiomics, there is at least as much value in confirming a previously published result as in establishing a new model.[16] As obvious as this may seem, the first instinct should be to review the existing literature on the subject of interest to determine whether the question has already been addressed by others and how. In particular, it is useful to know if a clinical question has already been investigated using conventional features (for instance, SUVmax, metabolic volume, and total lesion glycolysis) and which added value is expected from the use of more sophisticated radiomic features. If a clinical question has already been dealt with using radiomics, the first step could be to try to reproduce the findings. Indeed, at the moment, although hundreds of radiomic models are published, publications that independently validate radiomic models published by others are scarce, if they even exist.[16] This lack of reproducible results is certainly the greatest bottleneck for advancing the field, and it is an essential prerequisite for clinical translation.

Collect Data

Once the question of interest has been identified and well defined, the availability of the data needed to conduct the study with the expected statistical power should be checked. Of course, the data should comply with the legislation regarding data privacy (for instance, it should be GDPR-compliant in Europe). When collecting the data, the inclusion/exclusion criteria should be precisely defined and later clearly reported in any publication. In most cases, images alone are insufficient; additional data, such as that on age, sex, cancer subtype, comedication, and treatment, must be accessible and collected, as these factors can influence the measurements made from the images. For example, the age of patients can influence the radiomic feature values measured in breast cancer lesions[17] and thus be a confounding factor. For supervised learning, a ground truth or surrogate ground truth must be available and can be based on histologic analysis (eg, subtype and the presence of mutations), radiological evaluation (eg, response to treatment evaluated via RECIST), or follow-up (eg, recurrence, progression-free survival, and overall survival). In practice, this ground truth might be imperfect, especially when it is derived from a physician's diagnosis, and this might influence the performance of the model and its generalization.

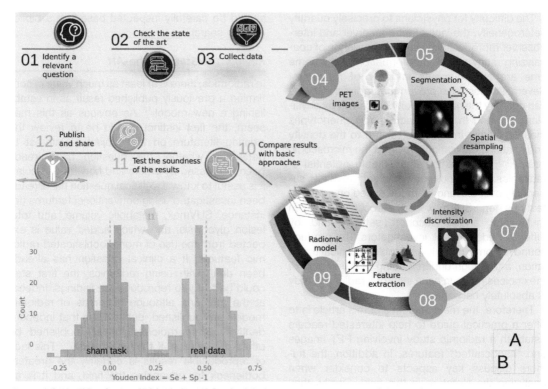

Fig. 2. (*A*) Checklist for a reliable radiomic study. (*B*) Sham test: comparison of the performances using real labels and randomly assigned labels to test the significance of findings.

The quantity of images needed for a specific investigation does not obey a simple rule. It depends on the difficulty of the task, the complexity of the mathematical model, and the approaches used (handcrafted or deep radiomics). If the biological signal is weak or the data have high heterogeneity, several hundred or even thousand patients may be needed. If the biological signal is well reflected by the radiomic features, fewer than 100 patients might be sufficient to build and validate a handcrafted radiomic model using cross-validation.[18] Moreover, the required number of images may grow when several hundred radiomic features are investigated to account for an increased false discovery rate. A downsampling strategy can be used to obtain some insights into how the performance evolves as a function of the number of patients and the number of patients needed to achieve a given performance.[19] Overall, as the definition of handcrafted features is fixed, a smaller number of patients is typically needed in handcrafted radiomics compared with when designing models based on deep features. In deep learning, a recent meta-analysis[20] for detecting disease from medical images reported that all sound and well-validated models were built using cohorts involving at least 800 patients.

Include a Comparison with Basic Approaches

Even when the question of interest has not been addressed or reported previously, a good practice is to always compare and report the performance of a radiomic model with that obtained using current approaches that may involve visual analysis (for instance, the visual 4-point "Lizarraga" scale for brain tumors[21]) or when building a model based on usual PET features, such as SUVs and/or metabolic volume only.

Test the Soundness of the Results

To ensure the stability of the results, the investigators should check if the findings remain similar when using slightly different statistical methods. Indeed, if information relevant to the task is captured by some radiomic features, it is unlikely that it can only be found using a single model or a single set of features.[22] Using a cross-validation design when building a model is a good approach to select the model and test the stability of the results as a function of the validation fold and makes it possible to compare the consistency of the models identified based on the different training sets. This procedure can be repeated several times (eg, using so-called nested cross-validation) in order not to be biased by the drawing of the folds. When using cross-validation, once the average performance and their variability have been characterized based on the different folds, the final model should be retrained using all the patients of the training set to be later deployed. The practice of "cherry picking," which consists of carrying forward only the best results obtained with a single approach while omitting contradictory results obtained with a slightly different approach, is strongly discouraged. The reliability of a set of results or of a model should ideally be tested by evaluating the model on an independent data set, that is, on data that have neither contributed to the model design nor been kept aside from the original data set. It is recommended that these data be external data, that is, acquired on a different device or from a different center to validate the performance in slightly different conditions, to better demonstrate the validity of the findings. Another useful evaluation approach is to test the extensive model building or data analysis pipeline using sham data.[19] Using sham data involves randomly assigning the real labels to the actual data and comparing the performance with that obtained when the labels are correctly assigned. For this approach to be informative, the complete analysis process should be applied to the sham data (including the feature selection process, if any), and several sham data sets (corresponding to several random drawings) should be used so that the statistical distribution of the relevant figures of merit can be determined in sham conditions. The figures of merit measured on the real data can then be compared with those statistical distributions to establish the significance of the results (see **Fig. 2**). Other approaches, such as image simulations,[11,23] can be used to check the robustness of the results and/or the interpretation of features.

The use of a hypothesis-driven approach can help to minimize false discovery. For example, this is the case when a new feature is designed to quantify a characteristic perceived by physicians as predictive or prognostic (for instance, the quantification of the presence of a necrosis in a tumor). The investigation of the biological plausibility of a radiomic model by deciphering the information reflected by the different features and the associated weights improves the confidence in the results. The use of unsupervised feature selection methods, test-retests, or studies investigating the influence of segmentation methods can eliminate irrelevant or insufficiently robust variables and thus reduce false discoveries.

Publish and Share

A scientific study should be replicable, and its impact will actually depend on the ability of independent researchers to confirm the findings. To make that possible, the steps used to produce the results should be precisely described (see later discussion), and the images (or extracted radiomic feature values) and/or the algorithm could be shared whenever possible. If the source code does not have to be shared, an executable file or information regarding how to access a prototype implementing the model can be sufficient. This allows colleagues to challenge, and confirm the results on the same data or test the classification or prediction model independently on other data. The huge importance of data sharing was recently well illustrated by Welch and colleagues,[23] who were able to demonstrate the spurious interpretation of a previously published prognostic signature through an independent reanalysis of the data provided by the investigators.

Sharing the data and methods should prompt the investigators to clearly define the limitations of their findings, including the description of the situations in which they expect their model to fail or conclusions not to be true. Reporting negative results is essential to avoid the misuse of algorithms or excessive generalization of results.[16]

HOW TO READ AN ARTICLE REPORTING A RADIOMICS STUDY

As in any scientific discipline, reading an article in the radiomics field calls for the reader's critical sense. The Materials and Methods section is as important as if not more important than the results, and scrutinization of the supplemental data is often needed to avoid misinterpretation. The reader should in particular pay attention to whether the data are homogeneous (well-defined patient cohort, same acquisition protocol for all patients, same treatment, or such) and, if not, to the strategy implemented to rule out or account for possible confounding factors caused by that heterogeneity. The validation approach used in the article should be examined carefully to determine whether the corresponding results support the claim. The positioning of the results with respect to clinical practice or previous work addressing the same topic should be reported so that the findings are put into perspective. Last, whether the conclusion can be checked by others will actually determine the impact of the findings.

Recently, a Radiomic Quality Score has been proposed to assess the quality of radiomic studies.[24] This score, including 16 criteria related to the acquisition protocol up to data sharing, is provided in order to *"both reward and penalize the methodology and analyses of a study, consequently encouraging the best scientific practice"*[24] according to the investigators. However, this score does not necessarily reflect the reliability of the results and of their interpretation. Indeed, the study by Aerts and colleagues[25] had a score of 55.6%, according to Sanduleanu and colleagues,[26] which is higher than all other articles mentioned in this article (range: 0%–50%). However, it was still highly biased, including a spurious interpretation of the findings.[23] Other checklists not specifically dedicated to radiomic studies, such as transparent reporting of a multivariable prediction model for individual prognosis or diagnosis (TRIPOD)[27] and Checklist for Artificial Intelligence in Medical Imaging (CLAIM),[28] for example, can also be considered when conducting radiomic studies, as they include good practice rules that are very relevant to radiomic studies.

Therefore, the best way to judge the quality of a radiomic study is to become familiar with the various steps of the pipeline and to understand their influences on the results. These different steps are thus explained in later discussion.

HANDCRAFTED RADIOMICS

A handcrafted radiomics pipeline can be described using 5 steps. The investigator builds a database of medical images, and VOIs are defined. This is followed by a spatial resampling step and an intensity discretization step (except for shape features) before the calculation of radiomic features (see **Fig. 2**). As many different practices have been reported in the literature,[29] an international consortium named the Image Biomarker Standardization Initiative (IBSI) involving 25 teams[30] has been established to precisely define the different options for each step and provide benchmark data to check that different radiomic software programs provide the same value for specific well-defined features. This standardization step remains a fundamental prerequisite to ensure that the calculated radiomic values follow a reference standard that others can replicate. The IBSI has produced a reference guide[31] with definitions of features and has listed most options for the preprocessing steps. Reference to this guide is then extremely useful to explain how a specific step (eg, interpolation) in the radiomic feature calculation process is performed. However, based on this guide, it may be difficult to choose the optimal setting among all the available options because it depends on the type of medical images that are analyzed, the

device used, the imaging protocol, the type of cancer, and the question of interest. Many methodological choices remain the responsibility of the investigator. Based on the authors' experience and the data from the literature, some guidelines are presented to perform radiomic analysis in PET.

Segmentation

There is no consensus regarding how the structure of interest should be segmented before subsequent radiomic analysis.[32,33] However, it has been widely demonstrated that radiomic features are sensitive to the segmentation method used,[34–38] with an intraclass correlation coefficient that can vary from 0.0 to 1 depending on the segmentation methods and the radiomic features. For the sake of reproducibility, it therefore seems preferable to use an automatic or semiautomatic method rather than manual segmentation. In addition, the impact that the segmentation method has on the radiomic model performance should be systematically analyzed, unless the radiomic features involved in the models have already been demonstrated not to be sensitive to the region delineation (eg, SUVmax).

In tumor imaging, the primary tumor is usually segmented, and radiomic analysis is performed using this single VOI. However, extending the radiomic analysis to the peritumoral area (sometimes called ring) at the interface between the lesion and the surrounding healthy tissue[39] to possibly capture relevant information related to the tumor environment has been proposed. When multiple tumor sites are present, there are no rules as to how to combine the radiomic features measured in different lesions, and specific features reflecting the distribution of lesions can also be extracted.[40,41]

In patients with cancer, there is an increasing interest in studying metabolism and its heterogeneity in "healthy" organs, especially lymphoid organs, to determine whether such features might provide valuable information to prognostic or predictive models. This is often performed by locating a small volume of a fixed size (on the order of a few milliliters) in the organ of interest, such as the liver, spleen, bone marrow, or adipose tissue, to derive radiomic features.[42]

To reduce the variability in radiomic feature values because of the VOI definition, the rule is to use the same strategy for all patients in the cohort (eg, the same threshold corresponding to 40% of SUVmax or the anatomic contour based on computed tomographic [CT] or MR images). When this is not possible, the influence of the difference in VOI delineation should be considered in the analysis of the results. For biological characterization (eg, to distinguish between tumor subtypes), focusing on the tumor VOI may be sufficient. Conversely, if the objective is to predict the response to treatments (especially in the case of immunotherapy) or the survival of the patients, considering radiomic features measured in organs other than the tumors might be useful.[43]

Spatial Resampling

When the radiomic algorithm uses neighboring voxel values to compute a texture feature, it is implicitly assumed that the voxels are isotropic, that is, that all the neighbors of a voxel are located at the same distance in the 3 directions. Spatial resampling is thus needed when this is not the case. This makes the extraction of textural features rotationally invariant. In addition, the size of the voxels strongly influences the values of some features.[44,45] Therefore, feature values should be compared only if they are calculated from images with the same voxel size. Spatial resampling involves interpolation, such as nearest neighbor, trilinear, tricubic convolution, and tricubic spline interpolation, and the choice of the method influences the feature values.[46] For this resampling step, there is no single best option. For instance, if the voxel size in the original image is $1 \times 1 \times 3$ mm^3, it is possible to resample them to $1 \times 1 \times 1$ mm^3, $2 \times 2 \times 2$ mm^3, or $3 \times 3 \times 3$ mm^3, but it would not make sense to resample to 0.1 or 10 mm. The rule is to choose the same isotropic voxel size with the same interpolation method for all patients in the cohort. After a resampling strategy is used and a successful model is validated, it is always recommended that whether the model performance is highly dependent on the resampling settings be checked.

Intensity Discretization

Intensity discretization is a mandatory step to calculate some radiomic features in order to group close gray levels together to reduce the impact of noise. In the literature, 2 techniques are mostly used: relative discretization, corresponding to setting the number of gray levels or bins; and absolute discretization, corresponding to setting the bin size. This step greatly influences the values of the features,[47,48] and it is important to understand what each approach implies. The relative discretization consists of grouping the gray levels in a fixed number of bins between the minimum (SUVmin) and maximum intensity (SUVmax) of each lesion:

$$R(x) = floor\left(NBin \times \frac{I(x) - SUV_{min}}{SUV_{max} - SUV_{min}} \right) + 1$$

where $R(x)$ is the resampled value in voxel x, $I(x)$ is the value in voxel x in the original image, and $NBin$ corresponds to the number of bins.

For example, consider 2 lesions with uptakes between 3 and 7 SUV for lesion 1 and between 2 and 12 SUV for lesion 2 (Fig. 3). Setting the number of bins to 4, after discretization with the relative method, lesion 1 has 4 bins of size 1, and lesion 2 has 4 bins of size 2.5. The first bin corresponds to uptake between 3 and 4 SUV for lesion 1 and uptake between 2 and 4.5 for lesion 2, so a bin number does not encompass the same SUV range for all lesions.

The absolute discretization consists of grouping the gray levels in bins of a fixed size between 2 fixed bounds (Bound$_{min}$ and Bound$_{max}$):

$$R(x) = floor\left(NBin \times \frac{I(x) - Bound_{min}}{Bound_{max} - Bound_{min}} \right) + 1$$

The number of bins and the bin size are related by the following equation:

$$Bin\ size = \frac{Bound_{max} - Bound_{min}}{NBin}$$

Using the previous example, if the bin size is set to 1 between 0 and 13 SUV, lesion 1 has 4 bins of size 1, and lesion 2 has 10 bins of size 1 (see Fig. 3). Therefore, a bin number corresponds to the same SUV range for all lesions. For instance, bin 4 corresponds to an uptake between 3 and 4 SUV for all lesions.

These 2 methods lead to different correlations of the radiomic feature values with the metabolic volume or SUV. In Orlhac and colleagues,[48] VOIs were segmented in a homogenous phantom, lung lesions, and healthy liver tissue. With relative discretization, the entropy values are highly correlated with metabolic volume and are not different between the 3 regions (phantom, lung lesion, and liver region), whereas visually, the heterogeneity is quite different. With absolute discretization, the entropy values are different between the 3 regions (with higher values for the tumor than for the liver tissue and higher values in the liver compared with the phantom), and the features are much less dependent on the volume but are more correlated with SUVs. As seen from this example, in PET, features calculated using absolute discretization thus better reflect visual impression. The choice of the bin size influences the results.[44] A tradeoff must be found between the quantification of the heterogeneity and the influence of noise. For instance, in PET images, a difference in 0.01 SUV

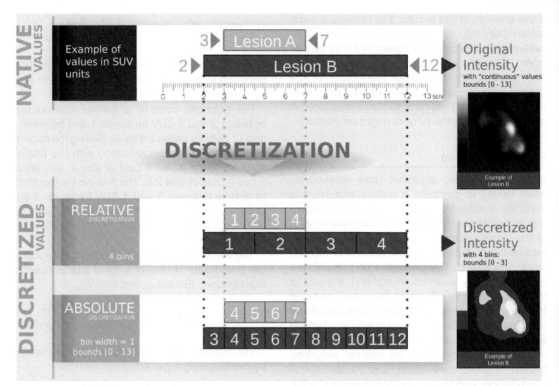

Fig. 3. Intensity discretization consists of converting continuous values into discretized levels. Two approaches are commonly used: relative discretization, which sets the number of bins (for instance, number of bins = 4), and absolute discretization, which sets the width of the bin (for instance, bin width = 1). Here, the authors illustrate the discretization step for 2 lesions (A and B), the intensities of which vary between 3 and 7 SUV and 2 and 12 SUV, respectively, before discretization.

unit is meaningless, so using a bin size of 0.01 SUV unit does not make sense. The authors therefore recommend, for example, setting the bin size to 0.3 SUV unit between 0 and 20 SUV units (representing 64 bins) or between 0 and 40 SUV (ie, 128 bins) if some lesions have a SUVmax greater than 20. The rule is to use the same range and bin size for all patients.

Handcrafted Features

The calculation of the radiomic features is performed in the segmented region after spatial resampling and intensity discretization, except for "native" features that do not need any binning to be calculated, such as the SUVmax, SUVmean, SUVpeak intensity features, or the metabolic volume or total lesion glycolysis. The goal is to quantitatively characterize the intensity distribution of voxel values, the shape of the VOI, and the spatial relationship between voxel values within the VOI. To do this, 3 types of features can be used.

So-called shape features include the volume, the surface of a region of interest, and its sphericity or compactness. In the case of the segmentation of several tumor volumes, it is possible to characterize the spatial distribution of tumor foci using dedicated features, by measuring, for example, the distance between the 2 most distant foci[41,49] or the volume of the bounding box, including all segmented tumors.[40] These features are much less dependent on the acquisition and reconstruction parameters than first- or second-order features. However, some of them are highly dependent on the segmentation method.

The first-order or histogram features describe the distribution of values of individual voxels without accounting for spatial relationships. The histogram features are therefore not textural features. From the histogram, the minimum, maximum (different from the SUVmax, obtained before intensity discretization), mean (respectively SUVmean), median, first quartile, third quartile, standard deviation, skewness, kurtosis, energy, and entropy can be calculated, among other values.

The third category corresponds to textural features. They describe spatial interrelationships between voxels with similar (or dissimilar) values. In the literature, 4 matrices are often used: the gray-level cooccurrence matrix, gray-level run length matrix, gray-level zone length matrix, and neighborhood gray-level difference matrix. All these matrices were initially designed to be computed for 2-dimensional (2D) images. To extend their use to 3-dimensional (3D) volumes of interest, several options are possible, as listed in the IBSI guide; the most common option consists of calculating 13 matrices in 13 directions (to cover all space without redundancy), extracting the features from each of the matrices and then taking the average of the 13 values. As texture analysis consists of studying the relationships between voxels, small lesions composed of only a few voxels can be a challenge. Some investigators recommend not performing texture analysis below a certain volume (5, 10, or even 45 mL)[50–52] because below this cutoff volume, the features would mostly depend on the volume and would not reflect the texture. Other investigators do not set limits. What matters is the number of voxels and not the volume in milliliters because the algorithm does not consider the size of the voxels and only considers the number of voxels. If the VOI is $3 \times 3 \times 3$ voxels, only the voxel at the center has 26 neighbors in 3 dimensions; therefore, it is the only voxel contributing to the computation of texture matrices in all directions. It might not be robust to calculate a texture based on 1 voxel only. Thus, the authors recommend calculating textural features in regions that contain at least 64 voxels, which correspond to $4 \times 4 \times 4$ voxels for cubic regions. When several VOIs are segmented for the same patient, the textural features can be calculated for each VOI independently or by merging the contributions of each VOI within the same texture matrices. The use of several VOIs in texture analysis is still marginal and does require special attention, as there is currently no best way to aggregate values measured in each VOI.

Finally, histogram and textural features can be calculated from the original images or after initial image filtering, such as using wavelets or Gabor filters. Given the number of possible wavelet and Gabor filters, such prefiltering considerably increases the number of calculable features. Few results using such filters on PET imaging are currently available,[53] and the definition of these filters is the subject of ongoing effort by the IBSI consortium.

Radiomic Models

Radiomic feature extraction is usually followed by designing a model to solve a classification, prognostic, or predictive task. Given the initially high number of features, a preliminary step of variable selection is often used to reduce overfitting and build more parsimonious models that might be easier to interpret in a clinical context and that also might be better generalizable to other data. Feature selection can be based on one or more of the following criteria:

- The redundancy: a single feature from a group of highly correlated radiomic features is selected or dimensionality reduction techniques, such as principal component analysis, can be used;
- The robustness of the features: by preselecting only radiomic features that have been previously shown to be robust with respect to different segmentation methods or based on test-retest studies, for instance;
- The importance of the features for the task of interest: for instance, for a 2-group classification task, only radiomic features that are significantly different between the 2 groups (eg, P value of the Wilcoxon test lower than 5%) can be retained (so-called univariate feature selection).

Feature selection can also be integrated into the training of the model, for instance, using recursive feature elimination[54] or the least absolute shrinkage and selection operator (LASSO).[55]

A radiomic model can then be trained using different machine-learning approaches, such as logistic regression, support vector machine, random forest, or neural networks, to mention just a few. The performance of the model often depends on the variable selection method and machine-learning approach. For example, when designing a prognostic model using radiomic features extracted from CT images of patients with head and neck cancer, Parmar and colleagues[56] observed an area under the receiver operating characteristic curve (AUC) ranging from 0.50 (uninformative model) to 0.79 (fair performance) when combining 13 feature selection methods with 11 classification methods. To compare several models and select the best performing, investigators can use different performance metrics, such as the Akaike Information Criterion (AIC), the Bayesian Information Criterion (BIC), the accuracy (or balanced accuracy in case of class imbalance data set) or AUC measured on the test set. Each of these metrics has advantages and limitations, and there is no single one that should always be preferred. Different cross-validation techniques[57] can be used to assess the performances: leave-one out, k-fold, or bootstrap, for example. As mentioned above, the cross-validation procedures must be repeated several times in order not to be biased by the selection of folds. Finally, at a similar or near-similar level of performance, a more parsimonious model may be considered preferable, as it might be easier to interpret and possibly more generalizable on new data. For this purpose, it is possible to apply the "one-standard-error-rule,"[58] consisting of selecting the most parsimonious model (ie, the model with the lowest complexity), the performance of which is no more than 1 standard error below that of the best performing model.

Given the different steps involved in radiomic feature calculation and the development of a radiomic model, it is necessary to report how radiomic features were calculated and combined (**Box 1**) so that other teams can evaluate published radiomic models while ensuring they process the data as reported in the original studies.

Even when radiomic features are calculated in exactly the same way as described in a publication and using the same feature selection and classification method, the evaluation of a radiomic model on a different cohort of data often leads to different, often not as good, results. One possible reason might be differences in the image properties (spatial resolution, contrast, and signal-to-noise ratio) that affect the feature values. This calls for addressing the issue of heterogeneous data.

HOW TO MANAGE HETEROGENEOUS DATA

To increase the number of patients and hence the statistical power, pooling data from different centers or imaging protocols can be an option. However, feature values are sensitive to the acquisition and reconstruction parameters,[59–63] such as the reconstruction algorithm, the number of iterations, or postreconstruction smoothing, if

---

Box 1
Checklist of information to be reported in radiomic articles

Minimum information to be provided:

- Name of the software, version number, and IBSI compliance (yes/no)

- Segmentation method used

- Interpolation method and voxel size (before and after resampling)

- Discretization method (absolute or relative) and parameters (bin size and bounds)

- Feature selection and classification method used, including metrics on test set and cross-validation scheme

---

any. The consequence is that a radiomic model developed on data from 1 PET scanner applied to data acquired with another device of a different generation might not perform well,[64] especially when the model involves some features that are very sensitive to the center effect, such as the entropy. It is thus always useful to assess the impact of the center effect on the features involved in the model. This can be achieved easily using unsupervised analysis, such as principal component analysis, or by observing the statistical distribution of each feature in a reference region (eg, cerebellum and healthy liver) where it is assumed to be the same for all patients wherever they have been scanned.

The way the center effect can be handled depends on whether the study is retrospective or prospective. In prospective studies, imaging protocols can be harmonized before data acquisition by following, for example, the resEARch 4 Life accreditation program (EARL) recommendations.[65,66] In retrospective studies, this is not always possible, as this would require access to the scanners to perform phantom acquisitions. It is sometimes even complicated to access the images directly.

When the data cannot be harmonized before acquisition, the center effect should be accounted for in the statistical analysis, for example, by introducing a covariate. A method initially described in Genomics,[67] called ComBat, can also reduce the center effect. ComBat was designed to correct for the batch effect, which is a technical source of variations caused by the handling of samples by different laboratories, by different technicians, and on different days. ComBat harmonization has then been used to normalize cortical thickness measurements from MR images.[68] In the radiomics field,[69] ComBat assumes that the values of one feature are the sum of an average value, an additive scanner effect, and a multiplicative scanner effect. ComBat estimates the model parameters using a maximum likelihood approach based on the set of available observations. ComBat thus determines one transformation for each feature separately and for each type of tissue (for instance, different transformations for tumors and healthy liver tissue). Schematically, ComBat consists of adjusting and translating a distribution so as to make the distributions overlap (**Fig. 4**). ComBat has many advantages. The method is easily available and fast. The transformations are estimated based on the observed feature values without the need to return to images or to perform phantom experiments, and no learning set is needed. If the patient groups have different characteristics (for instance, different proportions of

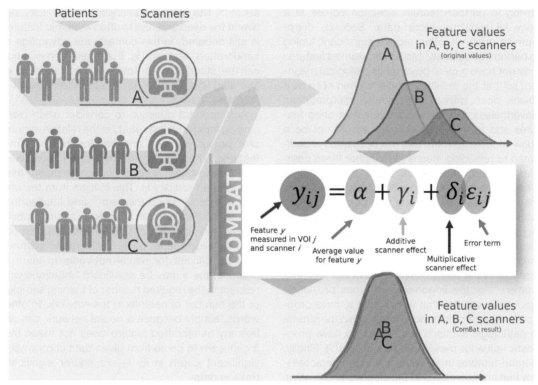

Fig. 4. Harmonization using the ComBat method that realigns the distributions of feature values obtained in different centers considering additive and multiplicative scanner effects.

healthy subjects and diseased patients), the covariates of interest may be used in the ComBat method to account for this difference. A limitation of the method is that it is necessary to have at least 20 patients per batch or per imaging protocol to correctly estimate the transformations. Other harmonization approaches using generative adversarial networks in particular are currently under development.[70] These techniques that process the images (unlike ComBat, which only needs the feature values) aim to convert an image measured using a scanner into the same image but with image properties (noise, contrast, and spatial resolution) similar to those of images acquired using a different scanner (or protocol).

Even with careful feature extraction, the signal captured by handcrafted features may not be sufficient to answer the clinical question of interest. Deep features might be able to capture other types of information, as now discussed.

HANDCRAFTED VERSUS DEEP FEATURES

The training of deep neural networks consists of iterative optimization of tunable network parameters. In this process, deep features that help recognize salient and persistent patterns become encoded within the network. The type of features that the network learns is determined by the training data, neural network architecture, optimization algorithm and task.

This ability to learn disease-relevant deep features from the data is what gives deep learning its power. In contrast to handcrafted features, automatic feature learning eliminates the need to perform feature engineering or selection for a particular task. Feature selection is replaced by the selection of a deep architecture. In addition, feature learning and predictive modeling can be performed in one step (referred to as "end-to-end" training). Another possible advantage of deep-learning approaches is that neural networks might automatically identify the parts of the image that are most relevant for the task of interest; in more advanced architectures, this is achieved using the so-called attention modules.[71] Thus, there is no need to perform image segmentation before analysis, in contrast to handcrafted features where a VOI needs to be specified for feature extraction. The associated drawback is the need for added training data given the large collection of voxels being considered, as discussed later.

The limitations of deep-learning features are closely related to their advantages. First, not having to perform feature selection comes at a price of requiring more data. Second, deep-learning methods often require significant tuning to perform adequately. Moreover, learned features may not have a clear physical or biological meaning, so that the resulting model is often seen as a "black box" without any simple interpretation. Nevertheless, the black-box aspect of deep features and associated networks should not be a show-stopper as more and more research is dedicated to providing means to decipher these complex models. In addition, these models might ultimately provide evidence of sophisticated information "hidden" in the data that could be turned into new hypotheses later amenable to testing using dedicated experiments. In fields other than nuclear medicine, model-agnostic interpretation methods have led to new discoveries, such as differences in the retina observed between men and women,[72] or the importance of areas previously ignored by experts that were found to have prognostic values (for instance, areas within the stroma in pathologic sections were found to have prognostic value for mesothelioma patients[73]). Finally, learned features may capture image characteristics that are not related to the diagnostic objective. For example, they may capture image properties related to a particular scanner or imaging protocol.[74,75] Methods are more and more frequently used to identify the regions of the image that contributed the most to the decision made by a neural network. Such methods facilitate the understanding of the models, although their results should sometimes be interpreted with caution.[76]

Because deep features are determined in large part for a particular data set, they are subject to population biases and may show poor descriptive performance when applied to a different data set.[77,78] The relative generalization capacity between the deep and handcrafted radiomic features is still debated. In this context, the advantage of handcrafted features is that their computation can be standardized; however, no standards or standard libraries currently exist for deep radiomic features.

An important question to consider when planning an image analysis study is the relative expressive power of deep and handcrafted radiomic features. Theory suggests that deep neural networks have much greater expressive power than handcrafted radiomics. This follows from the universal approximation theorem[79] and implies that all handcrafted features are merely a small subset of deep radiomic features. However, despite theoretic considerations, some handcrafted features may be difficult for neural networks to learn in practice: there may be significant limitations with respect to the required number of training samples or the number of neurons in the network. In other words, simply because a neural network can act like any handcrafted feature does not mean that it can learn to do so from given data (it may need significant depth in its layers and/or significant training data).

Because data sets are limited in practice and neural networks have finite sizes, there may be biases to the types of deep radiomic features that can be learned from a given set of images. In a recent work, the authors trained CNNs to function like common handcrafted features of the tumor intensity, texture, and shape.[80,81] In other words, the authors tested how well the deep networks can learn these features. They found that CNNs were negatively biased in capturing shape information (Fig. 5). This finding may have significant implications for CNN-based quantitative

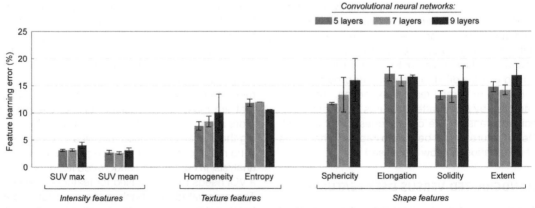

Fig. 5. Feature learning errors for CNNs with 5, 7, and 9 convolutional layers, expressed in percent of the ground truth values of handcrafted features. The names of the tested handcrafted features are given on the x-axis. The CNNs were trained on 4000 synthetic 2D PET images containing realistic lesions and tested on a separate set of 500 images.

medical image analysis because shape features represent an important subset of handcrafted radiomics.[30] Thus, deep features may not be as effective as handcrafted features at capturing and leveraging certain lesion properties that have previously been associated with clinical outcomes. Therefore, handcrafted radiomic features appear to be complementary to deep radiomic features rather than redundant, although additional studies in this area are needed.

Ultimately, the choice between handcrafted and deep radiomic features depends on the study objectives and data availability. Handcrafted features can be recommended for inference studies, where the objective is to establish a link between biologically meaningful features and a particular clinical metric. These studies can be performed with a relatively low number of samples, which can be determined based on the required power of the study. If a very large number of samples is available, deep radiomics might achieve higher performance than models based on handcrafted features.

SUMMARY

Radiomic analysis of PET images is a promising approach to extract subtler information and continuously evolves with advances in artificial intelligence. Using deep-learning methods, new disease-specific deep features can also be learned directly from data and appear to complement conventional handcrafted features. However, in order to create models that can be clinically translated and benefit patients, investigators should be aware of the ins and outs of each step of the radiomic pipeline. Particular attention must be paid to the comparison of the results obtained with state-of-the-art approaches and to the findings previously reported in the literature in order to advance knowledge in the field.

CLINICS CARE POINTS

- Radiomic models require thorough external validation before clinical translation.
- Previously published spurious model interpretations call for extra caution before the deployment of radiomic models in a clinical setting.

DISCLOSURE

The authors have nothing to disclose.

REFERENCES

1. Gillies RJ, Anderson AR, Gatenby RA, et al. The biology underlying molecular imaging in oncology: from genome to anatome and back again. Clin Radiol 2010;65(7):517–21.
2. Gillies RJ, Kinahan PE, Hricak H. Radiomics: images are more than pictures, they are data. Radiology 2016;278(2):563–77.
3. Kuikka JT, Tiihonen J, Karhu J, et al. Fractal analysis of striatal dopamine re-uptake sites. Eur J Nucl Med 1997;24(9):1085–90.
4. McNitt-Gray MF, Wyckoff N, Sayre JW, et al. The effects of co-occurrence matrix based texture parameters on the classification of solitary pulmonary nodules imaged on computed tomography. Comput Med Imaging Graphics 1999;23(6):339–48.
5. Quantitative Imaging Biomarkers Alliance. Available at: https://www.rsna.org/research/quantitative-imaging-biomarkers-alliance. Accessed May 18, 2021.
6. Reuzé S, Schernberg A, Orlhac F, et al. Radiomics in nuclear medicine applied to radiation therapy: methods, pitfalls, and challenges. Int J Radiat Oncol Biol Phys 2018;102(4):1117–42.
7. Zwanenburg A. Radiomics in nuclear medicine: robustness, reproducibility, standardization, and how to avoid data analysis traps and replication crisis. Eur J Nucl Med Mol Imaging 2019;46(13):2638–55.
8. Mayerhoefer ME, Materka A, Langs G, et al. Introduction to radiomics. J Nucl Med 2020;61(4):488–95.
9. Bizzego A, Bussola N, Salvalai D, et al. Integrating deep and radiomics features in cancer bioimaging. Siena, Italy; IEEE Conference on Computational Intelligence in Bioinformatics and Computational Biology (CIBCB). 9-11 july 2019; 18936077. https://doi.org/10.1101/568170.
10. Peng H, Dong D, Fang M-J, et al. Prognostic value of deep learning PET/CT-based radiomics: potential role for future individual induction chemotherapy in advanced nasopharyngeal carcinoma. Clin Cancer Res 2019;25(14):4271–9.
11. Orlhac F, Nioche C, Soussan M, et al. Understanding changes in tumor texture indices in PET: a comparison between visual assessment and index values in simulated and patient data. J Nucl Med 2017;58(3):387–92.
12. Martin-Gonzalez P, de Mariscal EG, Martino ME, et al. Association of visual and quantitative heterogeneity of 18F-FDG PET images with treatment response in locally advanced rectal cancer: a feasibility study. PLoS One 2020;15(11):e0242597.
13. Orlhac F, Thézé B, Soussan M, et al. Multiscale texture analysis: from 18F-FDG PET images to histologic images. J Nucl Med 2016;57(11):1823–8.

14. Hoeben BAW, Starmans MHW, Leijenaar RTH, et al. Systematic analysis of 18F-FDG PET and metabolism, proliferation and hypoxia markers for classification of head and neck tumors. BMC Cancer 2014;14:130.

15. Bashir U, Weeks A, Goda JS, et al. Measurement of 18F-FDG PET tumor heterogeneity improves early assessment of response to bevacizumab compared with the standard size and uptake metrics in a colorectal cancer model. Nucl Med Commun 2019; 40(6):611–7.

16. Buvat I, Orlhac F. The dark side of radiomics: on the paramount importance of publishing negative results. J Nucl Med 2019;60(11):1543–4.

17. Boughdad S, Nioche C, Orlhac F, et al. Influence of age on radiomic features in 18F-FDG PET in normal breast tissue and in breast cancer tumors. Oncotarget 2018;9(56):30855–68.

18. Papp L, Pötsch N, Grahovac M, et al. Glioma survival prediction with combined analysis of in vivo 11C-MET PET features, ex vivo features, and patient features by supervised machine learning. J Nucl Med 2018;59(6):892–9.

19. Dirand A-S, Frouin F, Buvat I. A downsampling strategy to assess the predictive value of radiomic features. Sci Rep 2019;9(1):1–13.

20. Liu X, Faes L, Kale AU, et al. A comparison of deep learning performance against health-care professionals in detecting diseases from medical imaging: a systematic review and meta-analysis. Lancet Digit Health 2019;1(6):e271–97.

21. Lizarraga KJ, Allen-Auerbach M, Czernin J, et al. 18) F-FDOPA PET for differentiating recurrent or progressive brain metastatic tumors from late or delayed radiation injury after radiation treatment. J Nucl Med 2014;55(1):30–6.

22. Parmar C, Leijenaar RTH, Grossmann P, et al. Radiomic feature clusters and prognostic signatures specific for lung and head & neck cancer. Sci Rep 2015; 5:11044.

23. Welch ML, McIntosh C, Haibe-Kains B, et al. Vulnerabilities of radiomic signature development: the need for safeguards. Radiother Oncol 2019;130: 2–9.

24. Lambin P, Leijenaar RTH, Deist TM, et al. Radiomics: the bridge between medical imaging and personalized medicine. Nat Rev Clin Oncol 2017;14(12): 749–62.

25. Aerts HJWL, Velazquez ER, Leijenaar RTH, et al. Decoding tumour phenotype by noninvasive imaging using a quantitative radiomics approach. Nat Commun 2014;5:4006.

26. Sanduleanu S, Woodruff HC, de Jong EEC, et al. Tracking tumor biology with radiomics: a systematic review utilizing a radiomics quality score. Radiother Oncol 2018;127(3):349–60.

27. Collins GS, Reitsma JB, Altman DG, et al. Transparent reporting of a multivariable prediction model for individual prognosis or diagnosis (TRIPOD): the TRIPOD statement. Br J Cancer 2015;112(2):251–9.

28. Mongan J, Moy L, Kahn CE. Checklist for artificial intelligence in medical imaging (CLAIM): a guide for authors and reviewers. Radiol Artif Intelligence 2020;2(2):e200029.

29. Buvat I, Orlhac F, Soussan M. Tumor texture analysis in PET: where do we stand? J Nucl Med 2015;56(11): 1642–4.

30. Zwanenburg A, Vallières M, Abdalah MA, et al. The Image Biomarker Standardization Initiative: standardized quantitative radiomics for high throughput image-based phenotyping. Radiology 2020;295(2): 328–38.

31. Zwanenburg A, Leger S, Vallières M, et al. Image biomarker standardisation initiative. arXiv 2016. https://doi.org/10.1148/radiol.2020191145.

32. Foster B, Bagci U, Mansoor A, et al. A review on segmentation of positron emission tomography images. Comput Biol Med 2014;50:76–96.

33. Hatt M, Lee JA, Schmidtlein CR, et al. Classification and evaluation strategies of auto-segmentation approaches for PET: report of AAPM task group No. 211. Med Phys 2017;44(6):e1–42.

34. Klyuzhin IS, Gonzalez M, Shahinfard E, et al. Exploring the use of shape and texture descriptors of positron emission tomography tracer distribution in imaging studies of neurodegenerative disease. J Cereb Blood Flow Metab 2016;36(6):1122–34.

35. van Velden FHP, Kramer GM, Frings V, et al. Repeatability of radiomic features in non-small-cell lung cancer [(18)F]FDG-PET/CT studies: impact of reconstruction and delineation. Mol Imaging Biol 2016; 18(5):788–95.

36. Guezennec C, Bourhis D, Orlhac F, et al. Inter-observer and segmentation method variability of textural analysis in pre-therapeutic FDG PET/CT in head and neck cancer. PLoS One 2019;14(3):e0214299.

37. Yang F, Simpson G, Young L, et al. Impact of contouring variability on oncological PET radiomics features in the lung. Sci Rep 2020;10(1):369.

38. Klyuzhin IS, Fu JF, Shenkov N, et al. Use of generative disease models for analysis and selection of radiomic features in PET. IEEE Trans Radiat Plasma Med Sci 2019;3(2):178–91.

39. Beichel RR, Ulrich EJ, Smith BJ, et al. FDG PET based prediction of response in head and neck cancer treatment: assessment of new quantitative imaging features. PLoS One 2019;14(4):e0215465.

40. Decazes P, Camus V, Bohers E, et al. Correlations between baseline 18F-FDG PET tumour parameters and circulating DNA in diffuse large B cell lymphoma and Hodgkin lymphoma. EJNMMI Res 2020;10(1):120.

41. Cottereau A-S, Nioche C, Dirand A-S, et al. 18F-FDG PET dissemination features in diffuse large B-cell lymphoma are predictive of outcome. J Nucl Med 2020;61(1):40–5.

42. Seban R-D, Moya-Plana A, Antonios L, et al. Prognostic 18F-FDG PET biomarkers in metastatic mucosal and cutaneous melanoma treated with immune checkpoint inhibitors targeting PD-1 and CTLA-4. Eur J Nucl Med Mol Imaging 2020;47(10):2301–12.

43. Seban R-D, Nemer JS, Marabelle A, et al. Prognostic and theranostic 18F-FDG PET biomarkers for anti-PD1 immunotherapy in metastatic melanoma: association with outcome and transcriptomics. Eur J Nucl Med Mol Imaging 2019;46(11):2298–310.

44. Papp L, Rausch I, Grahovac M, et al. Optimized feature extraction for radiomics analysis of 18F-FDG PET imaging. J Nucl Med 2019;60(6):864–72.

45. Crandall JP, Fraum TJ, Lee M, et al. Repeatability of 18F-FDG PET radiomic features in cervical cancer. J Nucl Med 2021;62(5):707–15.

46. Whybra P, Parkinson C, Foley K, et al. Assessing radiomic feature robustness to interpolation in 18F-FDG PET imaging. Sci Rep 2019;9(1):9649.

47. Leijenaar RTH, Nalbantov G, Carvalho S, et al. The effect of SUV discretization in quantitative FDG-PET radiomics: the need for standardized methodology in tumor texture analysis. Sci Rep 2015;5:11075.

48. Orlhac F, Soussan M, Chouahnia K, et al. 18F-FDG PET-derived textural indices reflect tissue-specific uptake pattern in non-small cell lung cancer. PLoS One 2015;10(12):e0145063.

49. Cottereau A-S, Meignan M, Nioche C, et al. Risk stratification in diffuse large B-cell lymphoma using lesion dissemination and metabolic tumor burden calculated from baseline PET/CT. Ann Oncol 2021; 32(3):404–11.

50. Brooks FJ, Grigsby PW. The effect of small tumor volumes on studies of intratumoral heterogeneity of tracer uptake. J Nucl Med 2014;55(1):37–42.

51. Orlhac F, Soussan M, Maisonobe J-A, et al. Tumor texture analysis in 18F-FDG PET: relationships between texture parameters, histogram indices, standardized uptake values, metabolic volumes, and total lesion glycolysis. J Nucl Med 2014;55(3): 414–22.

52. Pfaehler E, Mesotten L, Zhovannik I, et al. Plausibility and redundancy analysis to select FDG-PET textural features in non-small cell lung cancer. Med Phys 2021;48(3):1226–38.

53. Shiri I, Maleki H, Hajianfar G, et al. Next-generation radiogenomics sequencing for prediction of EGFR and KRAS mutation status in NSCLC patients using multimodal imaging and machine learning algorithms. Mol Imaging Biol 2020;22(4):1132–48.

54. Guyon I, Weston J, Barnhill S. Gene selection for cancer classification using support vector machines. Machine Learn 2002;46:389–422.

55. Tibshirani R. Regression shrinkage and selection via the Lasso. J R Stat Soc Ser B (Methodological) 1996;58(1):267–88.

56. Parmar C, Grossmann P, Rietveld D, et al. Radiomic machine-learning classifiers for prognostic biomarkers of head and neck cancer. Front Oncol 2015;5:272.

57. Papp L, Spielvogel CP, Rausch I, et al. Personalizing medicine through hybrid imaging and medical big data analysis. Front Phys 2018;6.

58. Hastie T, Tibshirani R, Friedman J. The elements of statistical learning - data mining, inference, and prediction, Second Edition. Springer. Available at: https://www.springer.com/gp/book/9780387848570. Accessed June 18, 2021.

59. Blinder SAL, Klyuzhin I, Gonzalez ME, et al. Texture and shape analysis on high and low spatial resolution emission images. In: 2014 Seattle, WA, USA; IEEE Nuclear Science Symposium and Medical Imaging Conference (NSS/MIC). 8-15 november 2014:1-6. https://doi.org/10.1109/NSSMIC.2014. 7430910.

60. Yan J, Chu-Shern JL, Loi HY, et al. Impact of image reconstruction settings on texture features in 18F-FDG PET. J Nucl Med 2015;56(11):1667–73.

61. Shiri I, Rahmim A, Ghaffarian P, et al. The impact of image reconstruction settings on 18F-FDG PET radiomic features: multi-scanner phantom and patient studies. Eur Radiol 2017;27(11):4498–509.

62. Ketabi A, Ghafarian P, Mosleh-Shirazi MA, et al. Impact of image reconstruction methods on quantitative accuracy and variability of FDG-PET volumetric and textural measures in solid tumors. Eur Radiol 2019;29(4):2146–56.

63. Pfaehler E, van Sluis J, Merema BBJ, et al. Experimental multicenter and multivendor evaluation of the performance of PET radiomic features using 3-dimensionally printed phantom inserts. J Nucl Med 2020;61(3):469–76.

64. Reuzé S, Orlhac F, Chargari C, et al. Prediction of cervical cancer recurrence using textural features extracted from 18F-FDG PET images acquired with different scanners. Oncotarget 2017;8(26): 43169–79.

65. Boellaard R, Delgado-Bolton R, Oyen WJG, et al. FDG PET/CT: EANM procedure guidelines for tumour imaging: version 2.0. Eur J Nucl Med Mol Imaging 2015;42(2):328–54.

66. Kaalep A, Sera T, Rijnsdorp S, et al. Feasibility of state of the art PET/CT systems performance harmonisation. Eur J Nucl Med Mol Imaging 2018;45(8): 1344–61.

67. Johnson WE, Li C, Rabinovic A. Adjusting batch effects in microarray expression data using empirical Bayes methods. Biostatistics 2007;8(1):118–27.

68. Fortin J-P, Cullen N, Sheline YI, et al. Harmonization of cortical thickness measurements across scanners and sites. Neuroimage 2018;167:104–20.

69. Orlhac F, Boughdad S, Philippe C, et al. A postreconstruction harmonization method for multicenter radiomic studies in PET. J Nucl Med 2018;59(8):1321–8.

70. Xie Z, Baikejiang R, Li T, et al. Generative adversarial network based regularized image reconstruction for PET. Phys Med Biol 2020;65(12):125016.

71. Oktay O, Schlemper J, Folgoc LL, et al. Attention U-net: learning where to look for the pancreas. arXiv: 180403999 [cs]. Published online May 20, 2018. Available at: http://arxiv.org/abs/1804.03999. Accessed March 16, 2021.

72. Holm EA. In defense of the black box. Science 2019; 364(6435):26–7.

73. Courtiol P, Maussion C, Moarii M, et al. Deep learning-based classification of mesothelioma improves prediction of patient outcome. Nat Med 2019;25(10):1519–25.

74. Zech JR, Badgeley MA, Liu M, et al. Variable generalization performance of a deep learning model to detect pneumonia in chest radiographs: a cross-sectional study. PLOS Med 2018;15(11):e1002683.

75. Badgeley MA, Zech JR, Oakden-Rayner L, et al. Deep learning predicts hip fracture using confounding patient and healthcare variables. Npj Digit Med 2019;2(1):1–10.

76. Hooker S, Erhan D, Kindermans P-J, et al. A benchmark for interpretability methods in deep neural networks. arXiv:180610758 [cs, stat]. Published online November 4, 2019. Available at: http://arxiv.org/abs/1806.10758. Accessed March 16, 2021.

77. Chen IY, Szolovits P, Ghassemi M. Can AI help reduce disparities in general medical and mental health care? AMA J Ethics 2019;21(2):167–79.

78. Mårtensson G, Ferreira D, Granberg T, et al. The reliability of a deep learning model in clinical out-of-distribution MRI data: a multicohort study. Med Image Anal 2020;66:101714.

79. Hornik K, Stinchcombe M, White H. Multilayer feedforward networks are universal approximators. Neural Networks 1989;2(5):359–66.

80. Klyuzhin I, Rahmim R. Shape analysis in PET images using convolutional neural nets: limitations of standard architectures. Available at: https://virtual.aapm. org/aapm/2020/eposters/301769/ivan.klyuzhin. shape.analysis.in.pet.images.using.convolutional. neural.nets.html?f=menu%3D17%2Abrowseby% 3D8%2Asortby%3D2%2Amedia%3D2%2Atopic% 3D23585. Accessed March 16, 2021.

81. Klyuzhin IS, Xu Y, Ortiz A, et al. Testing the ability of convolutional neural networks to learn radiomic features. medRxiv 2020. https://doi.org/10.1101/2020. 09.19.20198077.

Total-Body PET Kinetic Modeling and Potential Opportunities Using Deep Learning

Yiran Wang[a,b], Elizabeth Li[a], Simon R. Cherry, PhD[a,b], Guobao Wang, PhD[b,*]

KEYWORDS

• Total-body PET • Dynamic imaging • Kinetic modeling • Parametric imaging • Deep learning

KEY POINTS

• Total-body PET kinetic modeling on the uEXPLORER PET/CT system addresses several factors that serve as barriers to implementation of dynamic whole-body PET imaging on conventional PET scanners.
• Total-body kinetic modeling with increased detection sensitivity supports multiparametric imaging which has clinical potential, but also brings several technical challenges.
• Deep learning provides multiple opportunities in total-body kinetic modeling, including noninvasive input function estimation, kinetic model selection, and kinetic parameter estimation. Applications of deep learning can help with further improvement of accuracy, robustness, and efficiency.

INTRODUCTION

PET is a sensitive molecular imaging method that uses radiolabeled tracers to monitor the biological and physiologic function of the scanned subject *in vivo*.[1] PET is commonly used in the clinic to acquire static images of radioactivity distribution at a specific time interval (eg, 60 minutes) after radiotracer injection. The standardized uptake value (SUV) is provided as a semiquantitative measure of tracer uptake, which, however, is affected by many factors, including body habitus, dietary preparation, and scan timing. Dynamic PET imaging can also be performed by taking multiple consecutive frames, typically starting at the time of injection. The acquired four-dimensional (4D: 3D space and 1D time) data from dynamic PET may reflect a broad spectrum of physiologic and metabolic information, including blood flow, tracer delivery, transport, and metabolism. Dynamic PET data are commonly analyzed using compartmental modeling to quantify physiologic parameters in a region of interest (ROI) or at the image voxel level (ie, parametric imaging).[2,3]

Although dynamic PET with tracer kinetic modeling has many potential advantages over static PET imaging, its widespread use and clinical implementation have been hampered by several factors such as high noise, the need of blood input function, long scan time, and so forth.[4] Dynamic PET also has been largely restricted to single-organ imaging, for example, for brain and heart, due to the short axial field-of-view (AFOV) of conventional PET scanners (usually ~20 cm).[5] Implementation of whole-body dynamic imaging has become feasible on conventional PET scanners,[6–8] but it is challenging to achieve high temporal resolution, and the data are sparse in the temporal domain due to the need to move the subject relative to the scanner to image different parts of the body.

---

[a] Department of Biomedical Engineering, University of California, 451 E. Health Sciences Drive, Davis, CA 95616, USA; [b] Department of Radiology, University of California Davis Medical Center, Ambulatory Care Center, Building Suite 3100, 4860 Y Street, Sacramento, CA 95817, USA
* Corresponding author.
E-mail address: gbwang@ucdavis.edu

PET Clin 16 (2021) 613–625
https://doi.org/10.1016/j.cpet.2021.06.009

The recent advent of the uEXPLORER total-body PET system (and other long AFOV scanners that cover all or most of the vital organs[9,10]) provides unprecedented levels of detection sensitivity and simultaneous coverage of the entire body for dynamic imaging.[5,11,12] The total-body kinetic modeling and parametric imaging enabled by this system may have potential in both molecular imaging research and clinical applications.[13–16] Meanwhile, challenging technical problems coexist with the opportunities given the large scale of total-body dynamic data sizes and the need for consideration of physiologic heterogeneities in different organs and of the presence of motion that occurs throughout the dynamic series of images. This article provides a brief introduction of total-body dynamic PET imaging and kinetic modeling, describes its potential benefits and limitations, and discusses potential directions to address the challenging problems using deep learning. Image examples shown in this article are mainly from the widely used tracer ^{18}F-fluoro-deoxyglucose (FDG), but the concept is also applicable to most other radiotracers.

TOTAL-BODY DYNAMIC PET AND ITS POTENTIAL FOR KINETIC MODELING
Basis of Dynamic PET and Kinetic Modeling

Fig. 1 shows the flowchart for dynamic PET imaging and kinetic modeling. An example of tracer kinetic modeling with compartmental models[17] for metabolic imaging is given in **Fig. 2** for ^{18}F-FDG. The FDG net influx rate $K_i = \frac{K_1 k_3}{k_2 + k_3}$ is directly proportional to the metabolic rate of glucose and is a macro parameter of interest.[2,3] Compartmental modeling usually needs nonlinear curve fitting to estimate the kinetic parameters, which is computationally expensive and also sensitive to noise. As an alternative to compartmental modeling, the Patlak model[18] is a linear graphical method that can approximate K_i using the slope of a graphical plot of the blood input function and tissue time-activity curve (TAC). It has the advantages of computational efficiency and noise robustness for parametric imaging. Examples of compartmental models and graphical methods for modeling ligand-receptor kinetics are reviewed by Watabe and colleagues[19] The potential of kinetic modeling and parametric imaging has been demonstrated in both research studies and clinical diagnosis.[20,21]

One challenge of kinetic modeling is to obtain the input function $C_p(t)$. Conventionally, it would be obtained using arterial blood sampling, which, however, is invasive. To reduce invasiveness, population-based input functions can be used in combination with one or two blood samples.[22] As the spatial resolution of PET scanners has improved over time, it has become feasible to noninvasively derive a blood input function from dynamic PET images if a large blood region (eg, left ventricle or aorta) is available in the scanner FOV. This type of input function is usually referred to as the image-derived input function (IDIF).

Limitations of Dynamic Whole-Body Imaging on Conventional PET Scanners

Conventional PET scanners have a short AFOV, typically 15 to 30 cm, as shown in **Fig. 3**A. To acquire a set of whole-body dynamic images in sequence, the scanner must use multiple bed positions and multiple passes,[8,23] as shown in **Fig. 3**B. As a result, early-phase data that have unique information linked to blood flow and blood volume are only available for the organs imaged in the first bed position for conventional scanners but is missing for most of the body. There are also large temporal gaps in dynamic frames at any given scanned location. Furthermore, owing to the isotropic nature of the annihilation photon emission, the detection sensitivity within the short AFOV is low,[11] leading to a high noise level in dynamic images.

The acquisition of an input function $C_p(t)$ for whole-body kinetic modeling with short AFOV PET scanners is another challenge. If measuring of the IDIF is desired, the location of the first bed position may need to be shifted from the main organ of interest (eg, the brain) to a location covering the aorta, losing valuable early information in the organ of interest. This means some (complex) kinetic models (eg, two-tissue compartment model) can no longer be used for analyzing the tissue of interest.

Total-Body Dynamic Imaging on uEXPLORER

The development of the uEXPLORER total-body PET/CT system,[12] with a 194 cm AFOV, is an important step in addressing some limitations of conventional PET scanners, as shown in **Fig. 4**. It allows simultaneous dynamic imaging of the entire body. This eliminates the large temporal gaps in conventional dynamic whole-body imaging. The total-body axial coverage also increases the scanner detection sensitivity by 20 to 40 fold and the image signal-to-noise ratio by 5 to 6 fold[5] for imaging the entire body. In addition, the high sensitivity allows dynamic imaging with much higher temporal resolution (HTR), such as 1 s per time frame[13] or even 0.1 s per frame[24] compared to 10 to 40 s per frame in traditional protocols, which may be used to explore novel clinical applications.

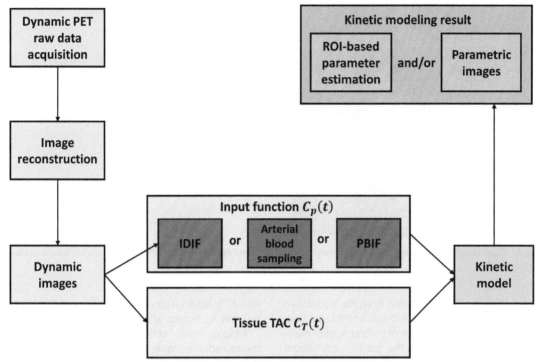

Fig. 1. Flowchart of PET kinetic modeling and parametric imaging. Raw PET projection data in the format of sinogram or list-mode are acquired and reconstructed into dynamic images. For each image voxel or a ROI, a time-activity curve (TAC) $C_T(t)$ is extracted from the dynamic sequence and fitted using a kinetic model and a blood input function to estimate kinetic parameters. The input function can be either noninvasively derived from the dynamic images or invasively measured by arterial blood sampling or is a population-based input function (PBIF). Kinetic modeling can be ROI-based or voxel-based (ie, parametric imaging).

Potential Benefits of Total-Body Dynamic PET for Kinetic Modeling: Examples

Noninvasive Image-Derived Input Function

Total-body dynamic images acquired from the uEXPLORER system bring several potential benefits for noninvasive IDIF determination. As compared to dynamic whole-body imaging on conventional PET scanners, the total-body coverage of uEXPLORER allows an IDIF to be

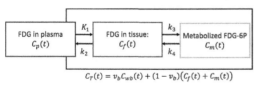

$$C_T(t) = v_b C_{wb}(t) + (1 - v_b)(C_f(t) + C_m(t))$$

Fig. 2. Two-tissue compartment model for ^{18}F-FDG. FDG is transported from plasma to tissue cells with the delivery rate K_1 and from tissue to plasma with the rate k_2. FDG is phosphorylated in cells into FDG 6-phosphate with the rate k_3 and the process can be reversed at the rate k_4. The total activity measured by PET is $C_T(t)$ that is, a sum of different compartments. v_b denoting the fractional blood volume and $C_{wb}(t)$ is FDG activity in the whole blood.

extracted from major blood pools in the body without compromising the temporal resolution of imaging any other organs. This is advantageous even for single-organ dynamic PET imaging. For example, for dynamic brain imaging with conventional PET, the carotid arteries are the largest available blood pool present in the FOV from which to derive an IDIF; with a diameter of 5 to 6 mm, the carotids have little signal and suffer from severe partial volume effects. Total-body dynamic PET overcomes this problem by providing a low-noise IDIF from the large blood pool present in the FOV such as the left ventricle or ascending/descending aorta. **Fig. 5** shows an example of brain parametric imaging from a healthy subject scan on the uEXPLORER, where carotid partial volume effects result in increased K_i estimates.

The ability to acquire low-noise input functions, noninvasively, and measured using the same device as the tissue TACs, aids in unbiased kinetic parameter estimation.

Although most organs are supplied by a single blood input from the arterial system, some organs have dual blood supplies. The liver, for example, is supplied by both the hepatic artery and the portal

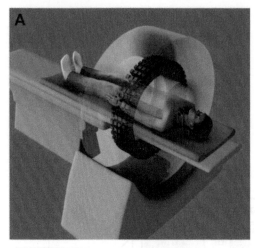

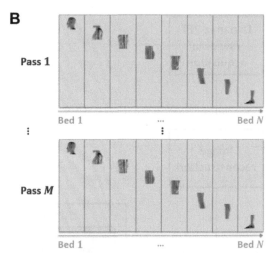

Pass 1

Bed 1   ...   Bed N

Pass M

Bed 1   ...   Bed N

Fig. 3. Illustration of dynamic whole-body imaging on a conventional PET scanner[11] (A) with a multibed multipass strategy (B).

vein. However, IDIF extraction from the portal vein is difficult with conventional dynamic PET imaging, due to the combined effect of limited spatial resolution, the small size of the portal vein (about 10 mm), and high noise levels present in a small ROI. This challenge can be reduced by total-body dynamic PET imaging on uEXPLORER which with much higher sensitivity and higher spatial resolution will allow better estimation of the IDIF from such vessels.

Multiparametric imaging

Limited by the short AFOV, conventional PET scanners cannot simultaneously capture total-body kinetic signals, especially in the early phase of radiotracer bolus distribution. Thus, parametric imaging has usually been limited to the linear Patlak plot method in dynamic whole-body PET studies with conventional scanners. This method provides a slope image for the macro kinetic parameter K_i and an intercept image related to a combination of fractional blood volume v_b and volume of distribution. However, the full potential of compartmental modeling that allows quantification of micro kinetic parameters (eg, the tracer delivery rate K_1 and fractional blood volume v_b) are difficult to explore with such systems. For example, a whole-body K_i image can be obtained with conventional scanners, whereas a whole-body K_1 image cannot.

Total-body dynamic imaging with the uEXPLORER system has the potential to address this shortcoming and enable high-quality total-body kinetic modeling and parametric imaging of micro kinetic parameters. **Fig. 6** shows an example for parametric imaging of FDG uptake

rate K_i, fractional blood volume v_b, and FDG delivery rate K_1 from a uEXPLORER scan.[16]

Among the different kinetic parameters measured, the tracer delivery rate K_1 is of particular clinical interest because of its connection to blood flow.[25] This parameter is different from the influx rate K_i and hence can provide complementary information, for example, potentially for simultaneous evaluation of perfusion-metabolism mismatch using FDG for myocardial viability.[26] Parametric imaging of the relative delivery rate R_1 (ratio of K_1 between a tissue region and a reference region) of tau tracers and beta amyloid tracers is also being explored as a surrogate of cerebral blood flow to simultaneously assess both blood flow and misfolded protein changes in neurodegenerative disease using a single tracer. Readers are referred to section III.D of a recent review article on parametric imaging for more details.[4]

Total-body parametric imaging of the fractional blood volume v_b may also add useful physiologic and pathologic information. For example, chronic obstructive pulmonary disease changes lung blood volume.[27] v_b may also reveal the local blood supply and microenvironment of a tumor, thus may be helpful to improve tumor diagnosis and characterization.[28]

High-temporal resolution kinetic modeling

The ability of uEXPLORER for HTR imaging (eg, 1 s per frame) allows not only better temporal sampling of the blood input function but also more accurate modeling of fast tracer kinetics. For example, after bolus injection, radiotracer signal in the lungs is supplied by the pulmonary artery and bronchial artery. However, differentiation of

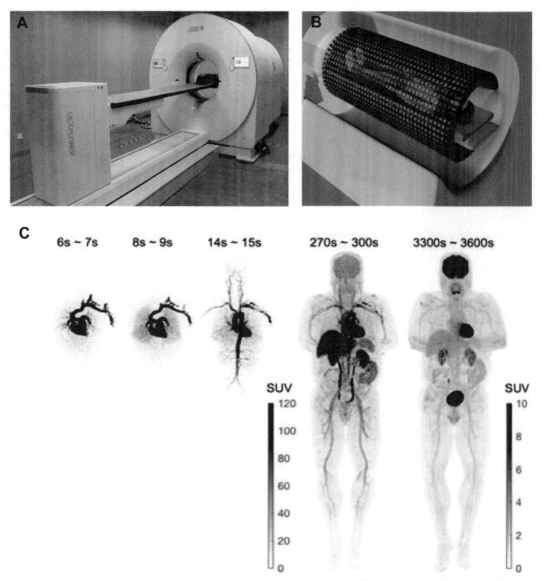

Fig. 4. Total-body dynamic PET imaging using uEXPLORER. (*A*) The uEXPLORER total-body PET system.[13] (*B*) Total-body imaging.[11] (*C*) Total-body dynamic ^{18}F-FDG images of a healthy subject. The images were reconstructed with no point spread function modeling and no postreconstruction smoothing.

the contributions from the two blood supplies is challenging if the temporal resolution of dynamic imaging is insufficient. With total-body dynamic PET, it becomes feasible to measure lung TACs with high temporal resolution and derive the bronchial arterial input function and pulmonary arterial input function from the left ventricle and right ventricle, respectively. Our preliminary results have demonstrated that HTR imaging has a significant effect on the quantification of ^{18}F-FDG K_1 and v_b in the lungs.[29]

The second example is the multiphase Patlak plot. Patlak plots derived with standard temporal

resolution commonly show a single late-time linear phase. With HTR imaging, preliminary results from Zuo and colleagues[30] demonstrated two additional approximately linear phases: one at around 20 to 30 s (first-pass) and the other at around 1 to 2 minutes (early-time) (**Fig. 7**). Total-body parametric images of the slopes of the first-pass, early-time, and standard late-time linear phases also demonstrate different spatial patterns. It is worth noting that the Patlak plot has been used with high temporal resolution in dynamic contrast-enhanced MR imaging for assessing blood-brain barrier permeability.[31] Thus, we postulated that

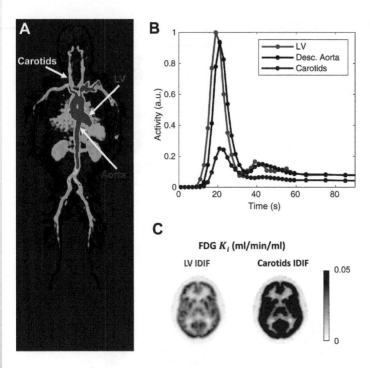

Fig. 5. Total-body IDIF extraction. (*A*) Maximum intensity projection (MIP) image of the dynamic, uEXPLORER data set of a healthy volunteer. (*B*) Example IDIFs derived from different blood pool ROIs. (*C*) Parametric images of FDG net influx rate K_i using different ROIs for IDIF extraction. The carotid-extracted IDIF results in much higher K_i estimates than the LV-extracted IDIF.

the first-pass and early-time Patlak slopes may be related to blood flow and tracer permeability, though the precise meaning and physiologic basis for these earlier linear phases remain to be determined.

Another example of HTR kinetic modeling is for the separation of blood flow and tracer-specific transport from the overall tracer delivery rate K_1, for example, through time-varying kinetic

modeling that is currently under development.[32,33] For ^{18}F-FDG, HTR kinetic modeling may make it possible to derive blood flow, glucose transport, and glucose metabolism simultaneously from a single dynamic scan.

Dual-tracer dynamic PET imaging

Single-scan dual-tracer (or multi-tracer) PET imaging has attracted a lot of interest over the past decades (see the review paper from Kadrmas and

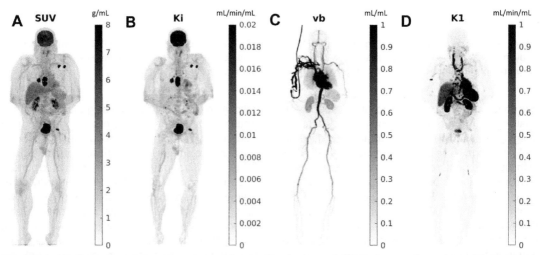

Fig. 6. Total-body parametric images estimated from a 60-min dynamic ^{18}F-FDG scan of a patient with metastatic cancer on the uEXPLORER: (*A*) SUV, (*B*) FDG net influx rate K_i, (*C*) fractional blood volume v_b, and (*D*) FDG delivery rate K_1.

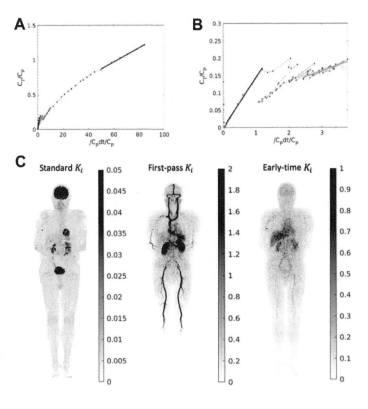

Fig. 7. High temporal resolution Patlak plot and parametric imaging.[30] (*A*) Patlak plot of 1-hour dynamic FDG data; (*B*) zoom-in of the first 2-min data; (*C*) parametric images of the slope at 3 different phases—standard K_i (30–60 minutes), first-pass K_i (20–30 s), and early-time K_i (1–2 minutes). Shown are the MIP images. The unit of K_i is mL/min/mL.

Hoffman[34]). To recover separate images of each tracer from the same scan, dynamic imaging and kinetic modeling can be used to separate the two tracer signals from each other. The robustness of single-scan dual-tracer methods has typically been limited by data noise. The increased sensitivity of total-body PET scanners is offering new opportunities to make this framework more robust and feasible for clinical investigation. The total-body coverage will also allow simultaneous dual-tracer dynamic imaging of the entire body.

Potential Clinical Impact

Compared to the semiquantitative SUV used routinely in the clinic today, total-body kinetic modeling on the uEXPLORER opens up the window for studying systemic diseases quantitatively and in a multiparametric fashion using a single radiotracer.

One obvious example is studying the heterogeneity of metastatic tumor characteristics, both before and after treatment. Total-body PET allows for kinetic data to be acquired simultaneously for all metastatic lesions in the body, and multiparametric imaging may provide a sensitive assay for assessing the response or likely response of each lesion to treatment. For example,

dysregulated cellular metabolism and angiogenesis are both hallmarks of cancer.[35] High-quality multiparametric imaging of FDG K_i (reflecting metabolism) and K_1 (reflecting perfusion and glucose transport) has the potential to provide complementary information of tumor metabolism and angiogenesis for more accurate tumor characterization for response assessment.

Similar approaches could be used to quantify inflammatory or infection burden across the entire body with appropriate radiotracers. For example, in arthritis, total-body dynamic imaging allows all the joints of the body to be assessed simultaneously with kinetic modeling approaches. Finally, absolute quantification of perfusion and blood volume across the entire body would likely have a broad clinical impact, especially if scans can be performed quickly and at relatively low radiation dose. Clinical applications would include a range of cardiovascular diseases (for example, peripheral arterial disease) where the vascular health of the entire body can be assessed and quantified. Whole-body parametric imaging of rapid physiologic processes and tracer distributions is particularly challenging on conventional short axial field of scanners as there simply is insufficient time to move the bed and collect data across the entire body.

Limitations of Total-Body Dynamic PET

Although total-body dynamic PET brings several potential benefits, some limitations of conventional dynamic PET imaging still remain. For example, parametric imaging of FDG K_i usually requires a 1-hour long scan, which is one of the main hurdles that limit the widespread adoption of dynamic FDG-PET in clinics. This hurdle remains with total-body dynamic PET imaging. Many radiotracers have the issue of being metabolized during the imaging time. Metabolite correction is needed for determining the true parent plasma input function,[36] which remains a challenge for total-body kinetic modeling, though new noninvasive methods are being explored. Another limitation of total-body dynamic PET imaging is the limited availability of total-body PET systems. At the time of writing, there are approximately 10 installations of total-body or long (>1 m) AFOV scanner worldwide. This implies that initially total-body dynamic PET studies will be only conducted in a small number of institutions, although the number of these scanners is expected to increase quite quickly in the coming years.

Total-body kinetic modeling also brings new significant challenges, including the large scale of total-body dynamic data sets and wide physiologic heterogeneity in different organs that should be accounted for using organ and tissue appropriate models. Total-body parametric imaging is further complicated by nonrigid subject motion that occurs throughout the dynamic acquisition. Kinetic parameter estimation with compartmental modeling is also highly nonlinear, suffers from local minima, and is sensitive to noise, resulting in a challenging task for conventional ROI-based modeling that is exacerbated when performing parametric imaging where models are applied on a voxel-by-voxel basis. In addition, the computational efficiency of nonlinear parametric imaging needs to be further improved for practical use because up to 10 million image voxels per acquisition are typically processed in total-body parametric imaging.

OPPORTUNITIES USING DEEP LEARNING FOR TOTAL-BODY KINETIC MODELING

Deep learning has attracted broad attention for its huge potential in almost every field, including PET.[37,38] One major advantage of deep learning is its ability for end-to-end training of a mapping from problem inputs to answers. Once the model is trained, the prediction is fast. In this section, we discuss a few examples of potential deep learning-based solutions to address the specific challenges in total-body kinetic modeling.

Voxel-wise Corrections for Blood Input Function

In total-body dynamic PET, the IDIF is usually extracted from an ROI selected within a large central blood pool. For a peripheral tissue region that is far from the blood ROI, the arrival time of the radiotracer is delayed compared with the start time of the extracted blood input function. Thus, this time delay of the input function needs to be corrected to achieve accurate kinetic quantification. Time delay correction has been considered impactful only for high-temporal resolution imaging in conventional dynamic PET but is also essential in total-body imaging because the time delay can be 30 to 40 s in peripheral tissues. In addition, a dispersion correction to account for the mixing of the injected radiotracer in the blood may also be critical to model the input function for a specific organ.[14,39]

Corrections for these factors can be pursued by joint estimation, which estimates the parameters simultaneously with other kinetic parameters during the fitting of TACs. A recent example is given by Feng and colleagues[14] in total-body imaging of early FDG kinetics. However, the joint estimation method can be computationally expensive. Alternatively, time delay can be corrected voxel-wise before parametric imaging.[40] Such a precorrection method has the advantage of reducing the computational burden. Although analytical approaches such as the leading-edge method may not achieve the best accuracy, one of our ongoing efforts is to explore deep learning for regression to train a model that can predict the time delay and/or dispersion of the blood input from the tissue TAC data in combination with the blood input function. The labeling data for training can be built from patient data using the joint estimation method.

Learning-Based Input Function

For tracer kinetic modeling, a plasma input function is what is actually needed, while an IDIF represents the tracer activity in the whole blood. The tracer fraction in plasma may be predetermined based on population data, but it is challenging to adapt this to individual patients.[41] In addition, an IDIF may suffer from partial volume and spill-over effects, which leads to a potential discrepancy between the IDIF and true blood input function.

Machine learning has the potential to provide a robust and fast prediction of the input function from tissue TACs. For example, Kuttner and colleagues estimated the IDIF from multiple blood pool TACs or multiple tissue TACs using a Gaussian process model and a long short-term memory network.[42] Instead of requiring manual

ROI placements, machine learning can also estimate the IDIF directly from dynamic images.[43]

Metabolite correction is needed for some radiotracers[36] and can be done by arterial blood sampling (or if the metabolism is slow and the arterial-venous difference is small, venous blood sampling may be sufficient) followed by high-performance liquid chromatography analysis, which is complex and invasive, and therefore is often mainly used to derive a population-based model. Mathematical metabolite correction[44–46] is an alternative solution that jointly estimates the parent plasma input function during TAC fitting.[47] However, this method requires a complex optimization because of the high nonlinearity of the model and can easily get stuck at a local minimum and has a high computational cost. One possible solution is to use deep learning to learn an end-to-end solution from the TAC data using the global optimization or arterial sampling result as the training labels. Once trained in this manner, the model can be efficient to use.

Voxel-wise Kinetic Model Selection

In conventional parametric imaging with short AFOV scanners, one kinetic model is commonly used for the kinetic parameter estimation for all image voxels. However, the physiology varies among organs in the body and is beyond the descriptive ability of a single kinetic model. An oversimplified model causes biased quantification, while a too complex model leads to unstable parameter estimation. This issue can be addressed by voxel-wise model selection, which chooses the best of two or more candidate models **Fig. 8**A. As shown in **Fig. 8**B, the parametric image generated by a standard two-tissue irreversible compartment model produces artifacts in the ventricular blood pool and blood vessels (pointed out by arrows). These artifacts can be suppressed by the appropriate model selection, as shown in **Fig. 8**C.

Conventional methods for model selection use statistical metrics to balance the trade-off between the curve-fitting error and the model complexity. Golla and colleagues compared several model selection metrics, including Akaike Information Criterion, Model Selection Criterion, and Schwartz Criterion, and found strong agreement across them.[48] These methods can be implemented in a voxel-wise manner but are time-consuming for total-body imaging.

Deep learning may bring an efficient solution to kinetic model selection by formulating model selection as a binary or multiclass classification problem. The spatial correlation of neighboring voxels can also be incorporated into the learning

model. Such an approach has been recently explored by Klyuzhin and colleagues[49] and Fuller and colleagues[50] for detecting transient responses in neurotransmitter PET.

Fast and Robust Prediction of Kinetic Parameters

Machine learning has also been applied for directly predicting kinetic parameters from the TAC data. A trained model has the potential to generate parametric images very efficiently and be robust to noise. Early attempts were demonstrated in 2001 using a shallow neural network for ^{13}N-ammonia perfusion parametric imaging by Golish and colleagues,[51] in 2011, using a support vector machine for kinetic prediction with a shortened dynamic FDG-PET protocol,[52,53] and recently using a deep convolutional neural network for predicting the parametric images of macro parameters.[54]

Although learning a direct mapping from the TAC space to kinetic parameter space remains a big challenge, it is more feasible to predict high-quality parametric images from low-quality parametric images generated by conventional kinetic modeling. For example, parametric imaging commonly uses an indirect approach that reconstructs the dynamic images first and then performs kinetic modeling voxel by voxel to generate parametric images, as discussed in the previous sections. In comparison, the "direct method" combines the kinetic model into the forward projection model of PET image reconstruction and estimates the parametric images directly from the projection data. Direct parametric image reconstruction has been demonstrated to outperform the indirect method.[55] However, direct parametric image reconstruction requires a more complex optimization and is time-consuming. Feng and colleagues[56] and Xie and colleagues[57] used convolutional neural network learning to recover high-quality Patlak parametric images (estimated by the direct method) from the Patlak images estimated by the indirect method.

Single-Subject Deep Learning

One general challenge with deep learning is the requirement of collecting a large number of patient scans for building the training data set. This is particularly challenging for deep learning for kinetic modeling because each patient has only one blood input function, although many tissue TACs are available for building a database. With a limited number of blood input functions, the generalization capability of a trained model remains a concern.

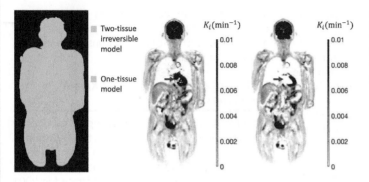

Fig. 8. Total-body kinetic model selection. (*A*) The model selection map. (*B*) Total-body K_i image using the 2-tissue irreversible model without model selection. (*C*) Total-body K_i image with model selection.

Single-subject deep learning may be a feasible alternative solution and is being pursued in our group. In this method, a deep learning model is trained on the fly with a low computational cost using a small fraction of voxels labeled with conventional kinetic modeling. The remaining voxels are unlabeled but will be predicted efficiently using the trained model. One advantage of this learning method is all the training and testing samples share the same blood input function. The labeled and unlabeled data can be further combined through a semisupervised learning framework.[58]

Voxel-wise Motion Correction

As the image data size and FOV increase with total-body PET, various types of subject motion, involuntary (eg, respiratory, cardiac, bladder filling) and voluntary (eg, head tilting) are always present in the FOV. For the purposes of total-body parametric imaging, positioning changes in the tissue will be reflected in the individual voxel TACs, which in turn may affect kinetic parameter estimation. Motion tracking hardware[59,60] and data-driven methods[61] such as the centroid of distribution method[62–64] can be applied to total-body dynamic imaging. Note that total-body motion is generally nonrigid and requires time-consuming algorithms for motion correction. Deep-learning–based solutions may have the advantage to efficiently and nonrigidly register respiratory-gated PET images,[65] and may provide improved results with high-quality images generated from total-body PET.

SUMMARY

Total-body kinetic modeling on the uEXPLORER system enables quantitative multiparametric imaging of the entire body simultaneously. With recent developments in deep learning, the remaining challenges of total-body kinetic modeling and parametric imaging may be addressed. Many opportunities are emerging for exploiting total-body kinetic modeling in various research and clinical applications.

CLINICS CARE POINTS

- Total-body 18F-FDG PET parametric imaging provides simultaneous imaging of glucose delivery rate and glucose metabolism, which may allow multiparametric multiorgan characterization for phenotying of systemic diseases.

TECHNICAL TERMS

Total-body PET, dynamic imaging, kinetic modeling, parametric imaging, image-derived input function, high temporal resolution, dual-tracer, time-delay correction, model selection, deep learning, convolutional neural network.

ACKNOWLEDGMENTS

The authors acknowledge the contribution of all EXPLORER team members. They also thank the two anonymous reviewers for helpful comments that led to the improvement of this article.

DISCLOSURE

The authors have a research agreement with United Imaging Healthcare. UC Davis also has a revenue-sharing agreement with United Imaging Healthcare. This work was funded in part by NIH grant R01 CA206187.

REFERENCES

1. Jones T, Townsend D. History and future technical innovation in positron emission tomography. J Med Imag 2017;4(1):011013.

2. Morris ED, Endres CJ, Schmidt KC, et al. Kinetic modeling in positron emission tomography. In Miles N. Wernick and John N. Aarsvold eds. Emission Tomography: The Fundamentals of PET and SPECT (pp. 499-540). Elsevier Inc.. https://doi.org/10.1016/B978-012744482-6.50026-0.

3. Carson RE. Tracer kinetic modeling in PET. In: Bailey D, Townsend D, Valk P, Maisey M, editors. Positron emission tomography. London, UK: Springer-Verlag; 2005. p. 127–59.

4. Wang G, Rahmim A, Gunn RN. PET parametric imaging: past, present, and future. IEEE Trans Radiat Plasma Med Sci 2020;4(6):663–75.

5. Cherry SR, Jones T, Karp JS, et al. Total-body PET: Maximizing sensitivity to Create new opportunities for clinical research and patient Care. J Nucl Med 2018;59(1):3–12.

6. Karakatsanis NA, Lodge MA, Tahari AK, et al. Dynamic whole-body PET parametric imaging: I. Concept, acquisition protocol optimization and clinical application. Phys Med Biol 2013;58(20):7391–418.

7. Hu J, Panin V, Smith AM, et al. Design and implementation of Automated clinical whole body parametric PET with Continuous bed motion. IEEE Trans Radiat Plasma Med Sci 2020;4(6):696–707.

8. Rahmim A, Lodge MA, Karakatsanis NA, et al. Dynamic whole-body PET imaging: principles, potentials and applications. Eur J Nucl Med Mol Imaging 2019;46(2):501–18.

9. Karp JS, Viswanath V, Geagan MJ, et al. PennPET explorer: design and preliminary performance of a whole-body imager. J Nucl Med 2020;61(1):136–43.

10. Alberts I, Hünermund J-N, Prenosil G, et al. Clinical performance of long axial field of view PET/CT: a head-to-head intra-individual comparison of the Biograph Vision Quadra with the Biograph Vision PET/CT. Eur J Nucl Med Mol Imaging 2021;1–10. https://doi.org/10.1007/s00259-021-05282-7.

11. Cherry SR, Badawi RD, Karp JS, et al. Total-body imaging: transforming the role of positron emission tomography. Sci Transl Med 2017;9(381). https://doi.org/10.1126/scitranslmed.aaf6169. eaaf6169.

12. Spencer BA, Berg E, Schmall JP, et al. Performance evaluation of the uEXPLORER Total-body PET/CT scanner based on NEMA NU 2-2018 with additional tests to characterize long axial field-of-view PET scanners. J Nucl Med 2021;62(6):861–70. https://doi.org/10.2967/jnumed.120.250597.

13. Badawi RD, Shi H, Hu P, et al. First human imaging studies with the EXPLORER total-body PET scanner*. J Nucl Med 2019;60(3):299–303.

14. Feng T, Zhao Y, Shi H, et al. Total-body quantitative parametric imaging of early kinetics of FDG. J Nucl Med 2021;62(5):738–44. https://doi.org/10.2967/jnumed.119.238113.

15. Vera DB, Schulte B, Henrich T, et al. First-in-human total-body PET imaging of HIV with 89Zr- VRC01 on the EXPLORER. J Nucl Med 2020;61(supplement 1):545.

16. Wang G, Parikh M, Nardo L, et al. Total-body dynamic PET of metastatic cancer: first patient results. J Nucl Med 2020;61(supplement 1):208.

17. Gunn RN, Gunn SR, Cunningham VJ. Positron emission tomography compartmental models. J Cereb Blood Flow Metab 2001;21(6):635–52.

18. Patlak CS, Blasberg RG, Fenstermacher JD. Graphical evaluation of blood-to-brain transfer Constants from multiple-time uptake data. J Cereb Blood Flow Metab 1983;3(1):1–7.

19. Watabe H, Ikoma Y, Kimura Y, et al. PET kinetic analysis—compartmental model. Ann Nucl Med 2006;20(9):583–8.

20. Hooker JM, Carson RE. Human positron emission tomography Neuroimaging. Annu Rev Biomed Eng 2019;21:551–81.

21. Dimitrakopoulou-Strauss A, Pan L, Sachpekidis C. Kinetic modeling and parametric imaging with dynamic PET for oncological applications: general considerations, current clinical applications, and future perspectives. Eur J Nucl Med Mol Imaging 2021;1–19. https://doi.org/10.1007/s00259-020-04843-6.

22. Eberl S, Anayat AR, Fulton RR. Evaluation of two population-based input functions for quantitative neurological FDG PET studies. Eur J Nucl Med 1997;24(3):299–304.

23. Gallezot J-D, Lu Y, Naganawa M, et al. Parametric imaging with PET and SPECT. IEEE Trans Radiat Plasma Med Sci 2020;4(1):1–23.

24. Zhang X, Cherry SR, Xie Z, et al. Subsecond total-body imaging using ultrasensitive positron emission tomography. Proc Natl Acad Sci U S A 2020;117(5):2265–7.

25. Mullani NA, Herbst RS, O'Neil RG, et al. Tumor blood flow measured by PET dynamic imaging of first-pass 18F-FDG uptake: a comparison with 15O-labeled water-measured blood flow. J Nucl Med 2008;49(4):517–23.

26. Abraham A, Nichol G, Williams KA, et al. ^{18}F-FDG PET imaging of myocardial viability in an experienced center with access to ^{18}F-FDG and integration with clinical Management teams: the Ottawa-FIVE Substudy of the PARR 2 trial. J Nucl Med 2010;51(4):567–74.

27. Chen DL, Cheriyan J, Chilvers ER, et al. Quantification of lung PET images: challenges and opportunities. J Nucl Med 2017;58(2):201–7.

28. Dimitrakopoulou-Strauss A, Strauss LG, Schwarzbach M, et al. Dynamic PET 18F-FDG studies in patients with Primary and Recurrent Soft-tissue Sarcomas: impact on diagnosis and correlation with Grading. J Nucl Med 2001;42(5):713–20.

29. Wang Y, Cherry S, Badawi R, et al. Effect of dual-input function and dispersion on lung FDG-PET kinetic quantification using the EXPLORER total-body PET/CT scanner. J Nucl Med 2020; 61(supplement 1):13.

30. Zuo Y, Cherry S, Badawi R, et al. Multiphase Patlak plot enabled by high temporal resolution total-body dynamic PET. J Nucl Med 2020;61(supplement 1): 207.

31. Cramer SP, Larsson HB. Accurate determination of blood–brain barrier permeability using dynamic contrast-enhanced T1-Weighted MRI: a simulation and in vivo study on healthy subjects and multiple Sclerosis patients. J Cereb Blood Flow Metab 2014;34(10):1655–65.

32. Wang G, Sarkar S, Kim E, et al. Time-varying kinetic modeling of high temporal- resolution dynamic 18F-FDG PET data for multiparametric imaging. J Nucl Med 2018;59(supplement 1):503.

33. Wang G, Spencer B, Sarkar S, et al. Quantification of glucose transport using high temporal resolution dynamic PET imaging. J Nucl Med 2019; 60(supplement 1):521.

34. Kadrmas DJ, Hoffman JM. Methodology for quantitative rapid multi-tracer PET tumor characterizations. Theranostics 2013;3(10):757–73.

35. Hanahan D, Weinberg RA. Hallmarks of cancer: the Next generation. Cell 2011;144(5):646–74.

36. Gunn RN, Sargent PA, Bench CJ, et al. Tracer kinetic modeling of the 5-HT1AReceptor ligand [carbonyl-11C]WAY-100635 for PET. NeuroImage 1998;8(4): 426–40.

37. Domingues I, Pereira G, Martins P, et al. Using deep learning techniques in medical imaging: a systematic review of applications on CT and PET. Artif Intell Rev 2020;53(6):4093–160.

38. Gong K, Berg E, Cherry SR, et al. Machine learning in PET: from photon detection to quantitative image reconstruction. Proc IEEE 2020;108(1):51–68.

39. Wang G, Corwin MT, Olson KA, et al. Dynamic PET of human liver inflammation: impact of kinetic modeling with optimization-derived dual-blood input function. Phys Med Biol 2018;63(15):155004.

40. Li E, Spencer BA, Schmall JP, Wang G, Cherry SR. Pulse-timing methods for time delay estimation in dynamic total-body PET kinetic modeling. In: Conference Proceeding of IEEE Nuclear Science Symposium and Medical Imaging Conference, 2020. (abstract only).

41. Keiding S. Bringing physiology into PET of the liver. J Nucl Med 2012;53(3):425–33.

42. Kuttner S, Wickstrøm KK, Lubberink M, et al. Cerebral blood flow measurements with ^{15}O-water PET using a non-invasive machine-learning-derived arterial input function. J Cereb Blood Flow Metab 2021. https://doi.org/10.1177/0271678X21991393. 0271678X2199139.

43. Wang L, Ma T, Yao S, et al. Direct estimation of input function based on Fine-tuned deep learning method in dynamic PET imaging. J Nucl Med 2020; 61(supplement 1):1394.

44. Burger C, Buck A. Tracer kinetic modelling of receptor data with mathematical metabolite correction. Eur J Nucl Med 1996;23(5):539–45.

45. Sanabria-Bohórquez SM, Labar D, Levêque P, et al. [11C]Flumazenil metabolite measurement in plasma is not necessary for accurate brain benzodiazepine receptor quantification. Eur J Nucl Med 2000;27(11): 1674–83.

46. Graham MM, Peterson LM, Hayward RM. Comparison of simplified quantitative analyses of FDG uptake. Nucl Med Biol 2000;27(7):647–55.

47. Feng DD, Chen K, Wen L. Noninvasive input function acquisition and simultaneous estimations with physiological parameters for PET quantification: a brief review. IEEE Trans Radiat Plasma Med Sci 2020; 4(6):676–83.

48. Golla SSV, Adriaanse SM, Yaqub M, et al. Model selection criteria for dynamic brain PET studies. EJNMMI Phys 2017;4(1):1–10.

49. Klyuzhin IS, Bevington CWJ, Cheng J-C, et al. Detection of transient neurotransmitter response using personalized neural networks. Phys Med Biol 2020;65(23):235004.

50. Fuller OK, Angelis GI, Meikle SR. Classification of neurotransmitter response in dynamic PET data using machine learning approaches. IEEE Trans Radiat Plasma Med Sci 2020;4(6):708–19.

51. Golish SR, Hove JD, Schelbert HR, et al. A fast nonlinear method for parametric imaging of myocardial perfusion by dynamic 13N-ammonia PET. J Nucl Med 2001;42(6):924–31.

52. Strauss LG, Pan L, Cheng C, et al. Shortened acquisition protocols for the quantitative assessment of the 2-tissue-compartment model using dynamic PET/CT 18F-FDG studies. J Nucl Med 2011;52(3):379–85.

53. Pan L, Cheng C, Haberkorn U, et al. Machine learning-based kinetic modeling: a robust and reproducible solution for quantitative analysis of dynamic PET data. Phys Med Biol 2017;62(9):3566.

54. Wang B, Ruan D, Liu H. Noninvasive estimation of macro-parameters by deep learning. IEEE Trans Radiat Plasma Med Sci 2020;4(6):684–95.

55. Wang G, Qi J. An optimization transfer algorithm for nonlinear parametric image reconstruction from dynamic PET data. IEEE Trans Med Imaging 2012; 31(10):1977–88.

56. Feng T, Zhao Y, Dong Y, et al. Acceleration of whole-body Patlak parametric image reconstruction using convolutional neural network. J Nucl Med 2019; 60(supplement 1):518.

57. Xie N, Gong K, Guo N, et al. Clinically translatable direct Patlak reconstruction from dynamic PET with motion correction using convolutional neural

network. In: Martel AL, Abolmaesumi P, Stoyanov D, et al, editors. Medical image computing and computer Assisted Intervention – MICCAI 2020. Vol 12267. Lecture Notes in computer Science. Cham, Switzerland: Springer International Publishing; 2020. p. 793–802. https://doi.org/10.1007/978-3-030-59728-3_77.

58. Zhou X, Belkin M. Semi-supervised learning. In: Theodoridis S, Chellappa R, Diniz P, Naylor P, Suykens J, editors. Academic press Library in signal processing, vol. 1. Cambridge, Massachusetts, USA: Elsevier; 2014. p. 1239–69. https://doi.org/10.1016/B978-0-12-396502-8.00022-X.

59. Jin X, Mulnix T, Gallezot J-D, et al. Evaluation of motion correction methods in human brain PET imaging-A simulation study based on human motion data: evaluation of human brain PET motion correction methods. Med Phys 2013;40(10):102503.

60. Bec J, Henry D, Kyme A, et al. Optical motion tracking for use with the EXPLORER total-body PET scanner. J Nucl Med. 2018, 59(supplement 1): 429.

61. Rahmim A, Olivier R, Habib Z. Strategies for motion tracking and correction in PET. PET Clin 2007;2(2): 251–66.

62. Lu Y, Naganawa M, Toyonaga T, et al. Data-driven motion detection and event-by-event correction for brain PET: comparison with vicra. J Nucl Med 2020;61(9):1397–403.

63. Ren S, Jin X, Chan C, et al. Data-driven event-by-event respiratory motion correction using TOF PET list-mode centroid of distribution. Phys Med Biol 2017;62(12):4741–55.

64. Lu Y, Gallezot J-D, Naganawa M, et al. Data-driven voluntary body motion detection and non-rigid event-by-event correction for static and dynamic PET. Phys Med Biol 2019;64(6):065002.

65. Li T, Zhang M, Qi W, et al. Motion correction of respiratory-gated PET images using deep learning based image registration framework. Phys Med Biol 2020;65(15):155003.

Role of Artificial Intelligence in Theranostics:
Toward Routine Personalized Radiopharmaceutical Therapies

Julia Brosch-Lenz, PhD[a], Fereshteh Yousefirizi, PhD[a],
Katherine Zukotynski, MD, PhD, FRCPC[b],
Jean-Mathieu Beauregard, MD, MSc, FRCPC[c,d], Vincent Gaudet, PhD, PEng[e],
Babak Saboury, MD, MPH, DABR, DABNM[f,g,h],
Arman Rahmim, PhD, DABSNM[a,i,j], Carlos Uribe, PhD, MCCPM[i,k,*]

KEYWORDS

- Theranostics • Radiopharmaceutical therapies • Dosimetry • Artificial intelligence
- Outcome prediction • Segmentation • Registration • Quantitative imaging

KEY POINTS

- AI has shown promising applications in quantitative imaging required for dosimetry.
- Segmentation of organs and tumors, the most time consuming task in the dosimetry workflow, can be automated using AI.
- Using the theranostic approach, AI models that predict absorbed dose and therapy outcomes might play a key role in personalizing RPTs.
- AI has significant potential to improve accuracy and reduce times for routine implementation of patient-specific dosimetry in RPTs.

INTRODUCTION

Radiopharmaceutical therapy (RPT) has shown promise in the treatment of various cancer types.[1] Metabolic processes or specific receptors serve as targets for the design of appropriate radiopharmaceuticals. The principle of "theranostics," in the context of nuclear medicine (**Fig. 1**), uses pairs of

a Department of Integrative Oncology, BC Cancer Research Institute, 675 West 10th Avenue, Vancouver, British Columbia V5Z 1L3, Canada; b Department of Medicine and Radiology, McMaster University, 1200 Main Street West, Hamilton, Ontario L9G 4X5, Canada; c Department of Radiology and Nuclear Medicine, Cancer Research Centre, Université Laval, 2325 Rue de l'Université, Québec City, Quebec G1V 0A6, Canada; d Department of Medical Imaging, Research Center (Oncology Axis), CHU de Québec - Université Laval, 2325 Rue de l'Université, Québec City, Quebec G1V 0A6, Canada; e Department of Electrical and Computer Engineering, University of Waterloo, 200 University Avenue West, Waterloo, Ontario N2L 3G1, Canada; f Department of Radiology and Imaging Sciences, Clinical Center, National Institutes of Health, 9000 Rockville Pike, Bethesda, MD 20892, USA; g Department of Computer Science and Electrical Engineering, University of Maryland Baltimore County, Baltimore, MD, USA; h Department of Radiology, Hospital of the University of Pennsylvania, 3400 Spruce Street, Philadelphia, PA 19104, USA; i Department of Radiology, University of British Columbia, 11th Floor, 2775 Laurel St, Vancouver, British Columbia V5Z 1M9, Canada; j Department of Physics, University of British Columbia, 325 - 6224 Agricultural Road, Vancouver, British Columbia V6T 1Z1, Canada; k Department of Functional Imaging, BC Cancer, 675 West 10th Avenue, Vancouver, British Columbia V5Z 1L3, Canada
* Corresponding author.
E-mail address: curibe@bccrc.ca

PET Clin 16 (2021) 627–641
https://doi.org/10.1016/j.cpet.2021.06.002

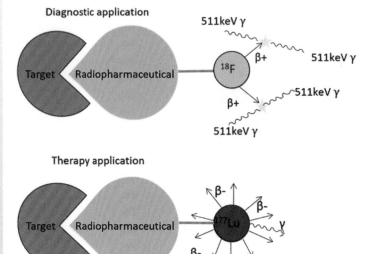

Diagnostic application

511keV γ

511keV γ

511keV γ

Therapy application

Fig. 1. An example of the principle of theranostics in nuclear medicine. Here, a radiopharmaceutical (*yellow*) developed to bind to the target (*blue*) can be labeled both with fluorine-18 (^{18}F) for diagnostic imaging purposes and lutetium-177 for therapeutic procedures.

radiopharmaceuticals to meet and explore both therapeutic and diagnostic purposes (ie, "theranostic"). The pharmaceuticals bind to the same target and can be radiolabeled with either a therapeutic (eg, beta or alpha emitting) or diagnostic imaging (eg, positron or gamma emitting) radionuclide.[2] This approach allows us to "see what we treat" and "treat what we see" at the molecular level.

Two examples of recent radiopharmaceutical developments include targeting (1) the somatostatin receptors for the diagnosis and treatment of neuroendocrine tumors (NET)[3] and (2) the prostate-specific membrane antigen (PSMA) to diagnose and treat metastatic castration-resistant prostate cancer (mCRPC)[4]; these are major frontiers in nuclear medicine, with significant existing and upcoming investments and efforts.[5] So far, the procedure guidelines from the International Atomic Energy Agency, the Society of Nuclear Medicine and Molecular Imaging, and the European Association of Nuclear Medicine have suggested the use of several cycles of a fixed therapeutic injection containing an activity of 7.4 GBq when lutetium-177 (^{177}Lu)-labeled compounds are used for NETs[6] or mCRPC treatments.[7] For NETs, [^{177}Lu]Lu-oxodotreotide has been approved by regulatory agencies to be used with a fixed activity of 7.4 GBq as the only option,[8] and a similar framework is expected for [^{177}Lu]Lu-PSMA-617 for mCRPC in the near future.

Treatment planning, however, should consider individual factors such as the patient's weight and height, the tumor burden, overall patient's health condition, as well as personal preferences

and values. The tolerance to radiation and function of organs at risk (OARs) as well as the patient-specific biological clearance and uptake of the radiopharmaceutical are further of substantial interest in personalized therapy. The key prerequisite for personalizing RPTs is routine and reliable dosimetry calculations. If dosimetry accompanies RPT, relationships between tumor and OAR radiation absorbed dose and therapy outcomes could be derived, providing evidence for adaptive treatment planning in clinical practice.[9]

The present state of RPTs (**Fig. 2**A) involves a diagnostic scan that is used by the physician to determine if a patient is suitable for therapy. If the patient expresses the target of interest, it is then referred to several cycles of therapy. Inter-therapy imaging is performed to qualitatively assess the performance of the treatment (eg, to visualize distribution of the therapeutic radiopharmaceutical). To date, the use of routine posttherapy dosimetry has been hindered by its complexity and immense workload for physicians, technologists, and medical physicists. Thus, to be adopted into routine clinical practice the technique needs to be not only accurate but also practical. Any development that simplifies, automates, or accelerates the steps within the dosimetry workflow would be likely to increase implementation of personalized medicine. Artificial intelligence (AI) may be a game changer in supporting and facilitating the dosimetry workflow.

Our vision for a comprehensive theranostics framework (**Fig. 2**B) involves the use of AI to simplify and motivate the personalization of RPTs. AI not only has direct applications in the

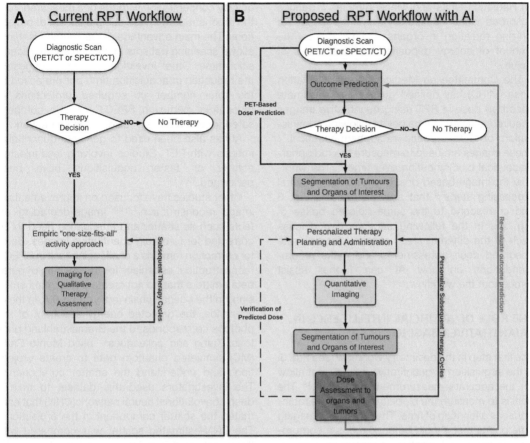

Fig. 2. (*A*) Current typical workflow of RPTs in which dosimetry is not routinely implemented. This workflow only requires a diagnostic examination to establish the suitability of a patient for therapy and possibly qualitative images to determine how good or bad the treatment is performing. (*B*) This diagram represents our vision for the whole theranostics approach. AI is a tool that can assist in every step in this workflow. Even more importantly, AI could predict outcomes and absorbed doses from pretherapy diagnostic scans to personalize the treatment starting from the first cycle.

different steps that form the dosimetry workflow (**Fig. 3**) but also could potentially be used to predict outcomes and absorbed doses.

In this work, we aim to highlight areas of importance on which AI can play a significant role in dosimetry using the theranostics approach. First, we focus on the current challenges of dosimetry after the administration of the therapeutic radiopharmaceutical and discuss the related AI applications.

Later, we describe our view on how AI can move us toward personalized RPTs making the theranostics workflow proposed in **Fig. 2**B a reality.

IMAGE-BASED DOSIMETRY IN RADIOPHARMACEUTICAL THERAPIES

The goal of internal dosimetry is to assess the radiation dose absorbed in healthy and malignant tissue. Report 85 of the International Commission

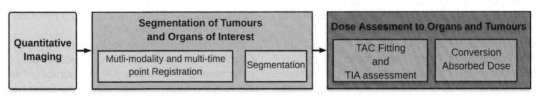

Fig. 3. Schematic representation of the dosimetry workflow for any image-based absorbed dose estimation for radiopharmaceutical therapy.

on Radiation Units and Measurements[10] defines absorbed dose caused by the interactions of ionizing radiation in organs and tumors as the amount of energy deposited per unit mass of tissue.

The Committee on Medical Internal Radiation Dose (MIRD) has defined guidelines to estimate absorbed dose in RPT using quantitative images acquired at different time points following administration of a therapeutic radiopharmaceutical.[11] These images are used to measure the radiopharmaceutical biodistribution over time.[12] The workflow for image-based dosimetry includes several processing steps[13] that are illustrated in **Fig. 3** and correspond to the same colored boxes of **Fig. 2B**. In the following sections, we discuss each of the different steps required for accurate absorbed dose assessments and make recommendations on how AI can further assist throughout the workflow.

THE ROLE OF ARTIFICIAL INTELLIGENCE IN QUANTITATIVE IMAGING

The first step in the dosimetry workflow (see **Fig. 3**) is the acquisition of quantitative images that allow for the accurate measurement of activity.[14] The goal is to measure the biodistribution of the radiotracer as a function of time. The number of imaging time points that should be acquired is a compromise between optimization of resources, simplification of protocols, and the accuracy for which the patient-specific effective half-life of the radiopharmaceutical can be estimated.[15] Quantitative imaging also implies the use of standardized acquisition protocols, image reconstruction parameters, and methods to determine the camera calibration factor.[11,16]

Both single-photon emission computed tomography (SPECT) and PET are quantitative imaging modalities that allow us to measure radioactivity distribution in the patient over time. Image acquisition and reconstruction parameters needed for accurate quantification is a topic of ongoing research.

Recent work has assessed the reduction in the number of acquired SPECT projections to reduce scan time without compromising quantitative accuracy or image quality. Rydén and colleagues[17] used a deep convolutional U-net-shaped neural network to generate intermediate ^{177}Lu SPECT projections (ie, projections that were not acquired). The investigators found that adding the projections generated by the U-net to the sparsely acquired projections provided similar visual image quality as the reference of a full set of projection data. Furthermore, they found comparable kidney

activity concentration with the one measured from the reconstructed image using a full set of projections. The main advantage of this method is that it allows scanning patients in a much shorter acquisition time. Other investigations have suggested the reduction in acquisition time per projection or the total number of acquired projections in myocardial perfusion SPECT may be compensated for using a deep residual neural network.[18]

AI has also been used to generate quantitative images with PET. Studies involving less injected activity or faster acquisitions have been performed.[19–21]

Other studies have focused on improvements in image reconstruction.[22–26] Image-degrading effects such as scatter and attenuation need to be corrected for to obtain quantitative images. Scatter correction remains a challenging task in SPECT reconstruction, especially for the imaging of pure-beta emitters that do not create any gamma emissions in their decay chain (eg, yttrium-90). In these scenarios, the detected energy spectrum of the photons corresponds to the Bremsstrahlung photons. Xiang and colleagues[27] used Monte Carlo (MC) simulated phantom data to create projections and understand the scatter components. The investigators used this dataset to train a deep convolutional neural network (CNN) that estimated the scatter component in the projections. The CNN-estimated scatter was compared with the one derived from MC simulations. The results were very similar between MC and CNN with the advantage that the latter required only a mere fraction of time compared with MC. The use of a fully connected CNN for SPECT reconstruction was investigated by Shao and colleagues[28] and outperformed conventional ordered subset expectation maximization SPECT reconstruction in terms of image resolution and quantitation.

In PET, new state-of-the-art reconstruction algorithms, such as the block sequential regularized expectation maximization algorithm, allow for a higher number of iterations without amplifying the image noise.[29] However, the increased number of iterations also increases the time needed to generate an image. AI has been used to speed up the reconstruction by generating images for intermediate iterations.[30] The improvements of reconstruction of newly introduced total body PET images using deep learning (DL) methods is subject to ongoing research.[31]

Image denoizing allows for the reconstruction of quantitative images with less injected activity, faster acquisition times, or a higher number of iterations in the reconstruction algorithm. There have been studies showing denoising methods using AI CNNs with scintillation camera data,[32] using generative adversarial networks (GAN)[33] for PET and using coupled U-nets for SPECT.[34]

The interest in targeted alpha therapies[35] is rapidly increasing, although the quantitative imaging remains a challenge.[36] AI methods could be applied to improve both image quantification accuracy and quality.

THE ROLE OF ARTIFICIAL INTELLIGENCE IN IMAGE REGISTRATION AND SEGMENTATION

The positioning of the patient during pretherapy and posttherapy scans is highly variable. To match the different organs and tumors' radiopharmaceutical uptake between imaging points, accurate image registration is required (see **Figs. 2** and **3**). Moreover, anatomic changes (eg, tumor shrinking or disease progress) between time points require nonrigid registration methods to fully account for those changes.

Multimodality and Multi–Time Point Registration

Medical image registration is necessary for subsequent segmentation, treatment planning, image-guided radiotherapy, and response assessment.[37] Different imaging modalities such as MR imaging, computed tomography (CT), PET, and SPECT exhibit differences in resolution and provide different complementary information (ie, anatomic vs functional). In addition to discrepancies of patient positioning, intra-abdominal organ movement can occur between the CT and the PET or SPECT acquisition within a single examination. Coregistration of serial and multimodality images, however, is a challenging task within the dosimetry workflow.

Conventional registration techniques such as rigid, nonrigid[38] and multiresolution approaches[39] can be used for this task. As image deformation may lead to changes in organ/tumor volumes, which get reflected in mass and activity measurements, it has a direct impact on the estimated absorbed dose. The registration method must be chosen and validated carefully. Significant differences have been shown in absorbed dose estimates, depending on whether manual, rigid, or deformable registration methods are applied.[38]

AI techniques have shown better accuracy and robustness compared with conventional registration methods and can be generalized better across different modalities.[40] Moreover, AI approaches can mitigate the effects of image artifacts on registration results.[41] Despite the fact that most AI-based registration techniques have not been developed specifically for RPT applications, they

have the potential to support the radiation therapy workflow.[42]

DL using CNNs has been used for medical image registration using supervised and unsupervised schemes. For instance, supervised training of a convolutional stacked autoencoder was proposed by Wu and colleagues[40] to learn discriminative features of images from different modalities. These features were then used in iterative deformable registration.

An unsupervised AI-based registration method was proposed by de Vos and colleagues[43] and Shan and colleagues[44] using a CNN without the need to include ground-truth labels. Liao and colleagues[45] proposed a method based on CNNs and reinforcement learning for CT to cone-beam CT registration. Studies on synthetic images (using GANs) with known labels to train a deep registration model without the need of annotated data also exist.[46] A 3D unsupervised network that uses a metabolic constraint function (MCF) and a multimodal similarity measure for PET/CT image registration was proposed by Yu and colleagues[47] (**Fig. 4**). The MCF is defined based on the standard uptake value (SUV) distribution of hypermetabolic regions to reduce the distortion on the displacement vector field (DVF). The DVF is estimated using a 3D CNN. 3D PET images are then wrapped to 3D CT images by a spatial transformer. The spatial and frequency domain similarity is then calculated based on the registered PET patches and the original CT patches. The loss function of the registration framework is the weighted sum of spatial and frequency similarity and a smoothness of DVF. A similar architecture could potentially be applied to the SPECT/CT data acquired during therapy (see **Fig. 2**) and to register diagnostic PET images to the therapeutic images.

Recent investigations by Guerra and colleagues[48] for radioembolization purposes used 2 different CNNs for automatic liver segmentation on MR and CT images and subsequently registered the segmentation results. We hypothesize that these AI approaches can be used in the future in an RPT context with multiple time point multimodality images by using CNNs for segmentation and subsequent VOI coregistration.

Segmentation of Organs and Tumors

The identification of OARs and tumors on images is important for absorbed dose estimation. The segmentation of tumors is required for tumor dosimetry, which is a critical component in determining the treatment response of RPT.[49] However, segmentation is the most time-consuming task in the dosimetry workflow (see **Figs. 2** and **3**)

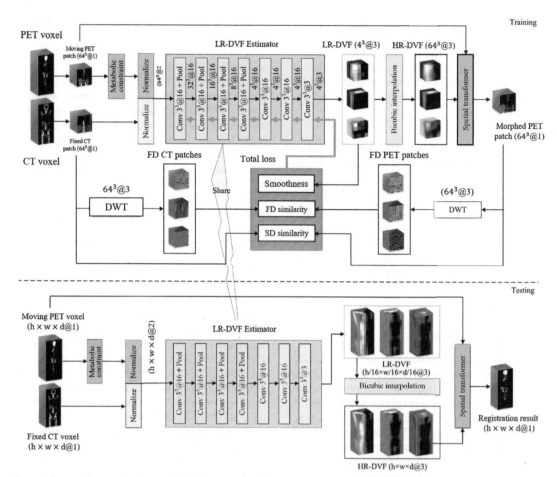

Fig. 4. The unsupervised 3D registration framework proposed by Yu and colleagues. (*From* Yu, H., et al., Unsupervised 3D PET-CT Image Registration Method Using a Metabolic Constraint Function and a Multi-Domain Similarity Measure. IEEE Access, 2020. 8: p. 63077-63089. The figure has already been published under the Creative Commons License which allows us to redistribute it in this document. A copy of the license can be found in https://creativecommons.org/licenses/by/4.0.)

because it often relies on manual delineation of volumes of interest (VOIs).[50–52] Segmentation allows the measurement of activity within each organ and tumor as well as the estimate of the corresponding mass of each VOI. Both quantities are required for accurate dosimetry calculations.

Compared with external beam radiotherapy, it is even more challenging for manual segmentation of tumor lesions for RPT, which specifically treats patients with metastatic cancer. Often patients may have a large number of lesions across the body, of heterogeneous sizes and tracer uptakes. Segmentation of all these lesions manually is not practical. Manual segmentation is also subject to intraobserver[53] and interobserver variability.[54] Validated AI-based models for fully automated, robust, accurate segmentation of organs/lesions in PET, PET/CT, and SPECT/CT images can help delineate OARs and lesions to achieve a personalized dosimetry framework. Normal organ segmentation approaches using DL models could use CT data,[55,56] or combined image data such as PET/CT.[57,58] Wang and colleagues[59] segmented normal organs based on CT images using a multi-atlas method and refined the segmentation on the PET images. A triple-combining 2.5D U-net, which simultaneously extracts features from axial, coronal, and sagittal planes, has been developed to mimic the workflow of physicians for the automated characterization of lesions on PSMA PET.[60]

Diagnostic PET images can be expected to have similar intensity profiles as SPECT images acquired in therapy because they are targeting the same receptors; this allows using transfer-learning approaches for segmentation. Diagnostic PET images should be smoothed in this regard to account for the differences in resolution with respect to SPECT. The quality of CT images is the same or very similar between PET/CT and SPECT/CT modalities. AI models can be pretrained on PET/CT images and then "tuned" using SPECT/CT data. The cross-modality knowledge transfer for lesion segmentation in SPECT images using PET segmentations can be done using unsupervised adversarial training to learn feature mapping between domains (PET and SPECT) as previously shown for domain adaptation from MR imaging to CT.[61] The probability map (PM) based on diagnostic PET images can be estimated and added to the segmentation model for SPECT/CT images. This learnt PM captures the probability that a voxel in a SPECT image belongs to a tumor or OAR. The PM may not be accurate enough to fully segment SPECT/CT images (as tumors can change over time) but can be used as initial guidance (eg, increase probability of detection for smaller tumors).

In the direct context of segmentation for dosimetry, Jackson and colleagues[62] showed promising results when using a 3D CNN for kidney segmentation on the low-dose CT from posttherapy [177Lu]Lu-PSMA SPECT/CT against manual organ delineation for renal absorbed dose estimation. In addition, a 3D U-net model was proposed for kidney segmentation for uptake quantification.[63] Tang and colleagues[64] suggested that a CNN model for liver segmentation be used for personalized liver radioembolization.

Besides intratherapy cycle image registration and segmentation, the possibility to transfer VOIs to subsequent cycles should be investigated. AI could further assist in registering and segmenting intra-abdominal organ movement and tumor shrinkage or disease progress between therapy cycles.

THE ROLE OF ARTIFICIAL INTELLIGENCE IN TIME ACTIVITY CURVE ASSESSMENT AND TIME INTEGRATION OF ACTIVITY

Following registration and segmentation, the next step of the dosimetry workflow pertains to the fit of a model function to the time activity curve (TAC) (see **Fig. 3**) on an organ or voxel level. This model function must be chosen carefully to describe the pharmacokinetics of the radiopharmaceutical under investigation. Typically, monoexponential or biexponential functions are used (**Fig. 5**), but triexponential functions have also been found in the literature.[65] Also, there are situations in which the initial uptake is approximated using a trapezoid. The subsequent calculation of the time-integrated activity (TIA) can be performed on an organ or voxel level. The latter yields a 3D

time-integrated activity map (TIAM),[66] from which a 3D absorbed dose estimation can be completed.

The fit function describes the pharmacokinetics of the radiopharmaceutical. Sarrut and colleagues[66] described a multimodal fitting approach on the voxel level for multiple fitting models using nonlinear least-square optimization. The best fitting model per voxel was then chosen based on the Akaike information criterion similar to the proposed one in the NUKFIT software by Kletting and colleagues.[67] The applicability of a particle filter to denoise TACs on the voxel level was proposed by Götz and colleagues[68] with promising results. Kost and colleagues[69] on the contrary used a different approach of first generating absorbed dose rate maps on each of the serial quantitative activity images at the voxel level followed by pharmacokinetic modeling.

AI remains to be actively used for TAC or TIA estimation with great potential in this step of the dosimetry workflow both in organ- and voxel-level approaches. Possible applications could include investigation of CNNs that use information of serial quantitative images to predict TIAs using only a single posttherapy scan. Moreover, data from the diagnostic imaging could be used in conjunction with the single therapeutic image acquisition to improve the TAC and thus have higher confidence in the absorbed dose results further down the workflow. Last, AI can use the information from the diagnostic scans and therapeutic cycles together to improve the TIA of subsequent therapy cycles. Reducing the number of posttherapy scans is advantageous for the patients' comfort and decreases the workload for clinical personnel. Advances in image coregistration and reconstruction may further enhance progress in minimizing error from voxelwise fitting due to image artifacts in individual voxels.

THE ROLE OF ARTIFICIAL INTELLIGENCE IN CONVERSION TO ABSORBED DOSE

The last step of the workflow entails the conversion of TIA into absorbed dose (see **Fig. 3**). Dosimetry can be performed on an organ[70] or voxel level,[71,72] each associated with different degrees of accuracy and complexity.

Organ-level absorbed dose estimation according to MIRD[70] uses organ- and radionuclide-specific S-values derived from simulations with reference human phantoms. These S-values yield the absorbed dose in a target organ per decay in a source organ. The radiation-absorbed dose to an organ is hence derived from the sum of all sources to target combinations of TIAs multiplied by the respective S-values.

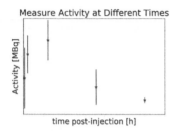
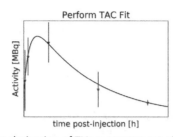
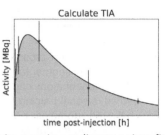

Fig. 5. Simplified representation of the derivation of TIA: measurement of activity over time at discrete points; fit of monoexponential decay function to data points; calculation of the area under the curve, that is, TIA.

Similarly, voxel S-value kernels are simulated for a specific tissue composition and radionuclide. Kernels are then convolved with the TIAM to create 3D absorbed dose maps.[71] MC simulations use the patient-individual 3D CT and TIAM to precisely model the absorbed dose for heterogeneous tissues and activity distributions.[72] Although MC simulation-based dosimetry taking into account heterogeneous activity and tissue distributions is still the gold standard against to which other methods are validated,[73,74] this is the most complex, computationally demanding, and time-consuming dosimetry method. AI offers the potential to maintain accuracy of MC dosimetry while reducing the time required. **Table 1** summarizes the different assumptions made when different dosimetry approaches are used.

Image-based organ- or voxel-level dosimetry approaches yield macroscopic absorbed doses. However, there is increasing interest in describing the radiation damage on smaller region of an organ or tumor or even at the cellular level.[75] Knowing this can provide a better understanding of the underlying radiobiological effects during RPT.[76–78] At present, RPTs are limited to absorbed doses based on the experience of external beam radiation therapies (EBRT). However, differences in absorbed dose rates and number of cycles of RPT compared with EBRT has led us to think that different absorbed dose limits should be set for internal radiation therapies. As an example, the absorbed dose to kidneys is commonly limited

to 23 Gy. However, absorbed doses of up to 40 Gy have been shown to be tolerated by patients without risk factors.[79] AI can potentially be used to combine multiscale dosimetry knowledge for accurate effective dose modeling. AI may unveil the complex relationship between pretherapy patient data, such as imaging, demographic data, laboratory test results, and the radiation dose distribution to be obtained during therapy, which is a problem too complicated to be described by conventional mathematical modeling approaches. GANs attempt to model the posttherapy voxel-wise dosimetry directly from pretherapy imaging.

The prediction of deposited energy distribution and voxel-based dosimetry using a deep neural network was assessed by Akhavanallaf and colleagues[51] as illustrated in **Fig. 6**. Their approach used whole-body 3D density maps (derived from patient CT images) and 3D absorbed dose maps (generated with MC simulations) as input to train a deep neural network to generate tissue-specific S-value kernels. Their method has the potential to overcome the general limitation of voxel S-value kernels that assume homogeneous tissue and typically water density. Götz and colleagues[80] used a CNN to predict density-specific voxel S-value kernels.

As alternative to MC dosimetry, Lee and colleagues[81] studied the use of a CNN for dosimetry estimation at a voxel level. Their network was trained to yield absorbed dose rate maps for activity and tissue distributions of gallium-68 (^{68}Ga)

Table 1			
Different assumptions per dosimetry method and yielded absorbed dose result (ie, organ or voxel level)			
	Organ S-Value	**Voxel S-Value**	**MC Dosimetry Simulation**
Activity distribution	Homogeneous	Heterogeneous	Heterogeneous
Tissue composition	Homogeneous medium	Homogeneous medium	Heterogeneous patient anatomy using CT
Dose output	Mean absorbed dose	3D absorbed dose map	3D absorbed dose map

The complexity and accuracy of dosimetry methods increases from left to right.

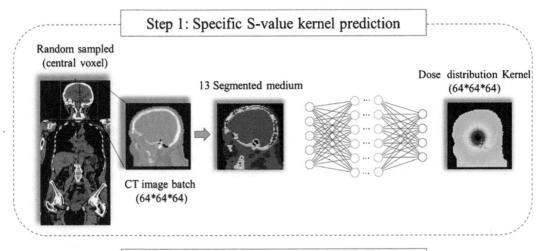

Step 1: Specific S-value kernel prediction

Random sampled (central voxel)

13 Segmented medium

Dose distribution Kernel (64*64*64)

CT image batch (64*64*64)

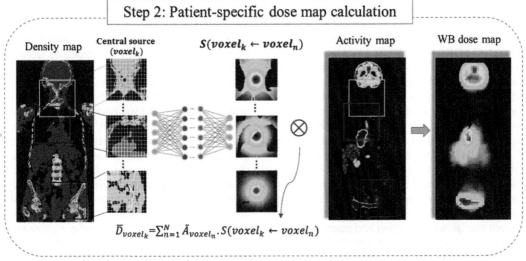

Step 2: Patient-specific dose map calculation

Density map

Central source $(voxel_k)$

$S(voxel_k \leftarrow voxel_n)$

Activity map

WB dose map

$$\overline{D}_{voxel_k} = \sum_{n=1}^{N} \tilde{A}_{voxel_n} \cdot S(voxel_k \leftarrow voxel_n)$$

Fig. 6. Diagram of the procedure used by Akhavanallaf and colleagues in which a dose kernel is generated using a deep neural network. The kernel can then be convolved with the TIAM to generate an absorbed dose distribution. (*From* Akhavanallaf, A., et al., Whole-body voxel-based internal dosimetry using deep learning. European Journal of Nuclear Medicine and Molecular Imaging, 2021. **48**(3): p. 670-682. The figure has been already published under the Creative Commons Attribution 4.0 that allows us to redistribute it in this document. A copy of the license can be found in https://creativecommons.org/licenses/by/4.0.)

[^{68}Ga]Ga-NOTARGD PET/CT based on ground-truth MC simulation-derived absorbed dose rate maps. The dose difference of CNN-derived absorbed dose rate maps against MC was less than 2% with a time effort of less than 4 minutes compared with more than 235 hours computation time of the MC simulation. Similarly, Götz and colleagues[82] trained a CNN with MC reference absorbed dose maps to generate voxel absorbed dose maps on the input of density maps from CT and TIAMs from serial ^{177}Lu SPECT/CT. The predicted absorbed dose maps from the model outperformed the use of a soft tissue voxel S-value kernel when compared with MC-generated absorbed dose maps.

ARTIFICIAL INTELLIGENCE AND THE FUTURE OF PERSONALIZED RADIOPHARMACEUTICAL THERAPY: RADIOMICS, DOSIOMICS, AND OUTCOME PREDICTION

Improved therapeutic absorbed dose estimation directly translates into the possibility of correlating absorbed dose with tumor response or normal organ toxicities. Knowledge of absorbed dose-response relationships might enable us to personalize activity planning for subsequent therapy cycles. Combined analysis of diagnostic imaging and therapeutic radiation absorbed doses might then allow for therapy outcome prediction.

Because of the theranostics approach, the outcome prediction could potentially be implemented with the diagnostic scans even before the RPT. This prediction can then be verified and updated in combination with additional information collected in subsequent therapy cycles (see **Fig. 2B**). Studies like the one performed by Xue and colleagues[83] have already used voxelwise absorbed dose prediction for [^{177}Lu]Lu-PSMA therapy based on pretherapeutic PSMA PET/CT. The investigators trained GANs using the diagnostic [^{68}Ga]Ga-PSMA PET/CTs and 3D absorbed dose maps. This described approach in combination with known dose-response relationships could assist the physicians in making the best therapy decision (see **Fig. 2B**). AI has shown the capability to discover effective predictive biomarkers for treatment outcome and long-term survival. There is an untapped potential to apply radiomics analysis to molecular imaging (both from pretherapy and posttherapy images) that can contain biological information. Moreover, there might be features detectable from within the 3D absorbed dose maps that can also show value toward better understanding of therapy response and outcome, enabling further personalization of therapies. We refer to the analysis performed on the 3D absorbed dose maps using the term dosiomics. The combination of radiomic features from CT, PET, MR imaging, and SPECT with dosiomic features from the absorbed dose maps can be used to train AI models that can better guide physicians with treatment planning and absorbed dose predictions. Moreover, DL approaches using different modalities of imaging and absorbed dose maps can inherently find features that are good predictors of outcome.

To develop robust outcome prediction models based on radiomics and dosiomics, the datasets must be representative of the disease and contain variant types and severities of it. Standardized imaging protocols and preprocessing steps are important to ensure consistent image quality.[84] An array of features can be used as input to the models for outcome prediction. For example, (1) absorbed dose-volume histogram measures could be computed from segmented 3D absorbed dose maps and are increasingly available in radiomics software packages. Such measures could also be correlated with tumor control probability and potential normal tissue toxicity. (2) Quantitative features from diagnostic scans such as SUV_{mean}, SUV_{max}, SUV_{peak}, molecular tumor volume, total lesion activity (TLA), and total lesion fraction (ie, TLA divided by body weight) could further serve as input for outcome prediction models. Analysis can be performed using PET-only, SPECT-only, and PET/SPECT. The subtraction of these parameters between cycles could be applied for outcome prediction.[85,86] (3) The analysis can include an array of radiomics features, beyond the above-mentioned simpler metrics. It has been shown that radiomic features at PET resolution can preserve their value at lower SPECT resolution.[87]

Investigations can include the detection of radiomic features in relation to biomarkers for disease staging[88] and could be extended to use of neural networks (NNs) or CNNs to predict the outcome of therapy.[89–91] In addition, NNs can model nonlinear survival data by classifications.[92] A deep network can directly extract and identify the most predictive radiomic features and could further learn unique features that may not be captured by handcrafted radiomics. The new paradigms of fusion radiomics have been investigated on PET/CT in head and neck cancer[93,94] and could be extended to SPECT/CT scans. Furthermore, subsequent therapy cycles could involve adapted therapy planning based on available dosimetry and outcome modeling.

As technology keeps improving, it also expands the possibilities of data collection. For example, recently developed total-body PET scanners[95,96] would enable the collection of dynamic whole-body data[97,98] of the diagnostic radiopharmaceutical; this allows for the generation of parametric images that also provide information about the biokinetics of the radiopharmaceutical.[99] Although there are limitations related to the early acquisition time and shorter half-life of diagnostic radionuclides compared with therapeutic radionuclides, AI can play an important role in understanding the dynamic scans and can possibly predict the uptake of the radiopharmaceutical in the therapy cycle.

In addition, the denoising examples mentioned before, in combination with more sensitive scanners, can allow us to perform the diagnostic scan at much later times that might correspond to the washout phase of the radiotracer. For example, it has been reported that the new EXPLORER total-body PET scanner has the ability to image a patient injected with fludeoxyglucose F 18 up to 5 half-lives after injection,[96] something unthinkable with current limited axial field of view scanners. Also, longer half-life PET radionuclides such as copper-64 (^{64}Cu) (12.7 h half-life) or zirconium-89 (^{89}Zr) (78.4 h half-life) that are used to label theranostic pairs could provide the data required to predict absorbed doses and outcomes for which AI is a fantastic tool to explore with currently existing scanners.

Benefiting of the emerging research and applications of AI in the fields of quantitative imaging, segmentation, registration absorbed dose prediction, and outcome modeling we believe personalized therapies can easily be implemented in the clinical setting.

SUMMARY

For adaptive RPT planning and personalized activity prescription, predictive dosimetry before treatment as well as absorbed dose verification is required to optimize therapy. For that, it is mandatory to have standardized protocols and reliable absorbed dose values first. Hence, efforts should concentrate on accuracy improvements of any of the steps within the dosimetry workflow. Cancer treatments are often difficult and complex, but the nuclear medicine community can incorporate the technological advancements of AI to make dosimetry a feasible task in the clinical setting; this includes applications for image quantification, registration, segmentation, biodistribution modeling, and absorbed dose value calculation. Predictive modeling of therapy outcome and absorbed doses following a therapeutic injection can assist in treatment planning and benefit patients from personalized RPTs.

The future of personalized RPT will likely benefit from active use of AI methods in the field of theranostics. This work highlighted different possible applications of AI, with the hope of motivating the community to expand and align efforts toward routine and reliable personalization of RPTs.

CLINICS CARE POINTS

- RPTs have shown promising results in the treatment of several diseases.

- Current RPTs use a fixed injected activity for all patients without accounting for individual factors such as the patient's weight, height, tumor burden, health condition, and physiological differences.

- For adaptive RPT planning and personalized activity prescription, predictive dosimetry before treatment as well as absorbed dose verification is required to optimize therapy.

- However, more evidence showing dose-response relationships in RPTs are still needed.

- AI has the potential of enabling fast and reliable personalized dosimetry in routine clinical practice prescribed activities for RPTs.

ACKNOWLEDGMENTS

This work was in part supported by the Natural Sciences and Engineering Research Council of Canada (NSERC) Discovery Grants RGPIN-2019-06467 and RGPIN-2021-02965.

DISCLOSURE

The authors have nothing to disclose.

REFERENCES

1. Sgouros G, Bodei L, McDevitt M, et al. Radiopharmaceutical therapy in cancer: clinical advances and challenges. Nat Rev Drug Discov 2020;19(9): 589–608.
2. Yordanova A, Eppard E, Kürpig S, et al. Theranostics in nuclear medicine practice. OncoTargets Ther 2017;10:4821.
3. Kaemmerer D, Peter L, Lupp A, et al. Molecular imaging with 68 Ga-SSTR PET/CT and correlation to immunohistochemistry of somatostatin receptors in neuroendocrine tumours. Eur J Nucl Med Mol Imaging 2011; 38(9):1659.
4. Benešová M, Schäfer M, Bauder-Wüst U, et al. Preclinical evaluation of a tailor-made DOTA-conjugated PSMA inhibitor with optimized linker moiety for imaging and endoradiotherapy of prostate cancer. J Nucl Med 2015;56(6):914–20.
5. Herrmann K, Schwaiger M, Lewis J, et al. Radiotheranostics: a roadmap for future development. Lancet Oncol 2020;21(3):e146–56.
6. Zaknun JJ, Bodei L, Mueller-Brand J, et al. The joint IAEA, EANM, and SNMMI practical guidance on peptide receptor radionuclide therapy (PRRNT) in neuroendocrine tumours. Eur J Nucl Med Mol Imaging 2013;40(5):800–16.
7. Kratochwil C, Fendler W, Eiber M, et al. EANM procedure guidelines for radionuclide therapy with 177 Lu-labelled PSMA-ligands (177 Lu-PSMA-RLT). Eur J Nucl Med Mol Imaging 2019;46(12):2536–44.
8. Strosberg J, El-Haddad G, Wolin E, et al. Phase 3 trial of 177Lu-Dotatate for midgut neuroendocrine tumors. N Engl J Med 2017;376(2):125–35.
9. Strigari L, Konijnenberg M, Chiesa C, et al. The evidence base for the use of internal dosimetry in the clinical practice of molecular radiotherapy. Eur J Nucl Med Mol Imaging 2014;41(10):1976–88.
10. Seltzer S, Bartlett D, Burns D, et al. ICRU report 85 fundamental quantities and units for ionizing radiation. J ICRU 2011;11(1):1–31.
11. Dewaraja YK, Frey EC, Sgouros G, et al. MIRD pamphlet no. 23: quantitative SPECT for patient-specific 3-dimensional dosimetry in internal radionuclide therapy. J Nucl Med 2012;53(8):1310–25.
12. Sgouros G, Frey E, Wahl R, et al. Three-dimensional imaging-based radiobiological dosimetry. In:

Seminars in nuclear medicine. Elsevier; Semin Nucl Med 2008; 38(5):321-334

13. Mora-Ramirez E, Santoro L, Cassol E, et al. Comparison of commercial dosimetric software platforms in patients treated with 177Lu-DOTATATE for peptide receptor radionuclide therapy. Med Phys 2020; 47(9):4602–15.

14. Li T, Ao E, Lambert B, et al. Quantitative imaging for targeted radionuclide therapy dosimetry-technical review. Theranostics 2017;7(18):4551.

15. Siegel JA, Thomas SR, Stubbs JB, et al. MIRD pamphlet no. 16: techniques for quantitative radio-pharmaceutical biodistribution data acquisition and analysis for use in human radiation dose estimates. J Nucl Med 1999;40(2):37S–61S.

16. Uribe CF, Esquinas PL, Tanguay J, et al. Accuracy of 177 Lu activity quantification in SPECT imaging: a phantom study. EJNMMI Phys 2017;4(1):1–20.

17. Rydén T, Van Essen M, Marin I, et al. Deep-learning generation of synthetic intermediate projections improves 177Lu SPECT images reconstructed with sparsely acquired projections. J Nucl Med 2021; 62(4):528–35.

18. Shiri I, Sabet K, Arabi H, et al. Standard SPECT myocardial perfusion estimation from half-time acquisitions using deep convolutional residual neural networks. J Nucl Cardiol 2020;1–19.

19. Katsari K, Penna D, Arena V, et al. Artificial intelligence for reduced dose 18F-FDG PET examinations: a real-world deployment through a standardized framework and business case assessment. EJNMMI Phys 2021;8(1):1–15.

20. Xiang L, Qiao Y, Nie D, et al. Deep auto-context convolutional neural networks for standard-dose PET image estimation from low-dose PET/MRI. Neurocomputing 2017;267:406–16.

21. Le V, Frye S, Botkin C, et al. Effect of PET scan with count reduction using AI-based processing techniques on image quality. J Nucl Med 2020; 61(supplement 1):3095.

22. Wang T, Lei Y, Fu Y, et al. Machine learning in quantitative PET: a review of attenuation correction and low-count image reconstruction methods. Phys Med 2020;76:294–306.

23. Shi L, Onofrey JA, Liu H, et al. Deep learning-based attenuation map generation for myocardial perfusion SPECT. Eur J Nucl Med Mol Imaging 2020;1–13.

24. Hwang D, Kang SK, Kim KY, et al. Generation of PET attenuation map for whole-body time-of-flight 18F-FDG PET/MRI using a deep neural network trained with simultaneously reconstructed activity and attenuation maps. J Nucl Med 2019;60(8):1183–9.

25. Shiri I, Arabi H, Geramifar P, et al. Deep-JASC: joint attenuation and scatter correction in whole-body 18 F-FDG PET using a deep residual network. Eur J Nucl Med Mol Imaging 2020;47:2533–48.

26. Dietze MM, Branderhorst W, Kunnen B, et al. Accelerated SPECT image reconstruction with FBP and an image enhancement convolutional neural network. EJNMMI Phys 2019;6(1):1–12.

27. Xiang H, Lim H, Fessler JA, et al. A deep neural network for fast and accurate scatter estimation in quantitative SPECT/CT under challenging scatter conditions. Eur J Nucl Med Mol Imaging 2020;1–12.

28. Shao W, Pomper MG, Du Y. A learned reconstruction network for SPECT imaging. IEEE Trans Radiat Plasma Med Sci 2020;5(1):26–34.

29. Ahn S, Ross SG, Asma E, et al. Quantitative comparison of OSEM and penalized likelihood image reconstruction using relative difference penalties for clinical PET. Phys Med Biol 2015;60(15):5733.

30. Cheng L, Ahn S, Ross SG. Accelerated iterative image reconstruction using a deep learning based leapfrogging strategy. In International conference on fully three-dimensional image reconstruction in radiology and nuclear medicine. 2017. pp. 715–720.

31. Ma R, Sari H, Xue S, et al. Total-body PET images reconstruction optimization using deep learning. Nuklearmedizin 2021;60(02):V45.

32. Minarik D, Enqvist O, Trägårdh E. Denoising of scintillation camera images using a deep convolutional neural network: a Monte Carlo simulation approach. J Nucl Med 2020;61(2):298–303.

33. Wang Y, Yu B, Wang L, et al. 3D conditional generative adversarial networks for high-quality PET image estimation at low dose. Neuroimage 2018;174:550–62.

34. Liu J, Yang Y, Wernick MN, et al. Deep learning with noise-to-noise training for denoising in SPECT myocardial perfusion imaging. Med Phys 2021;48(1):156–68.

35. Yadav MP, Ballal S, Sahoo RK, et al. Efficacy and safety of 225Ac-PSMA-617 targeted alpha therapy in metastatic castration-resistant Prostate Cancer patients. Theranostics 2020;10(20):9364.

36. Gosewisch A, Schleske M, Gildehaus FJ, et al. Image-based dosimetry for 225 Ac-PSMA-I&T therapy using quantitative SPECT. Eur J Nucl Med Mol Imaging 2021;48(4):1260–1.

37. Brock KK, Mutic S, McNutt TR, et al. Use of image registration and fusion algorithms and techniques in radiotherapy: report of the AAPM radiation therapy committee task group No. 132. Med Phys 2017;44(7):e43–76.

38. Grassi E, Fioroni F, Berenato S, et al. Effect of image registration on 3D absorbed dose calculations in 177Lu-DOTATOC peptide receptor radionuclide therapy. Phys Med 2018;45:177–85.

39. Dandois F, De Buck S, Beckers L, et al. SCreg: a registration-based platform to compare unicondylar knee arthroplasty SPECT/CT scans. BMC Musculoskelet Disord 2020;21(1):1–8.

40. Wu G, Kim M, Wang Q, et al. Scalable high-performance image registration framework by unsupervised deep feature representations learning. IEEE Trans Biomed Eng 2015;63(7):1505–16.

41. Huynh E, Hosny A, Guthier C, et al. Artificial intelligence in radiation oncology. Nat Rev Clin Oncol 2020;17(12):771–81.

42. Kearney V, Haaf S, Sudhyadhom A, et al. An unsupervised convolutional neural network-based algorithm for deformable image registration. Phys Med Biol 2018;63(18):185017.

43. de Vos BD, Berendsen FF, Viergever MA, et al. End-to-end unsupervised deformable image registration with a convolutional neural network. In: Deep learning in medical image analysis and multimodal learning for clinical decision support. Springer; 2017. p. 204–12.

44. Shan S, Yan W, Guo X, et al. Unsupervised end-to-end learning for deformable medical image registration 2017. arXiv preprint arXiv:1711.08608.

45. Liao R, Miao S, de Tournemire P, et al. An artificial agent for robust image registration. in Proceedings of the AAAI conference on artificial intelligence. 2017;31:(1).

46. Mahapatra D, Antony B, Sedai S, et al. Deformable medical image registration using generative adversarial networks. in 2018 IEEE 15th international symposium on biomedical imaging (ISBI 2018). 2018.IEEE.p. 1449-1453.

47. Yu H, Jiang H, Zhou X, et al. Unsupervised 3D PET-CT image registration method using a metabolic constraint function and a multi-domain similarity measure. IEEE Access 2020;8:63077–89.

48. Guerra JM, Mustafa M, Krönke M, et al. Novel low-dose CT based automatic segmentation and registration framework for liver radioembolization planning. Nuklearmedizin 2021;60(02):P38.

49. Violet J, Jackson P, Ferdinandus J, et al. Dosimetry of (177)Lu-PSMA-617 in metastatic castration-resistant prostate cancer: correlations between pre-therapeutic imaging and whole-body tumor dosimetry with treatment outcomes. J Nucl Med 2019; 60(4):517–23.

50. Lee MS, Kim JH, Paeng JC, et al. Whole-body voxel-based personalized dosimetry: the multiple voxel S-value approach for heterogeneous media with nonuniform activity distributions. J Nucl Med 2018; 59(7):1133–9.

51. Akhavanallaf A, Shiri I, Arabi H, et al. Whole-body voxel-based internal dosimetry using deep learning. Eur J Nucl Med Mol Imaging 2021;48(3):670–82.

52. Vinod SK, Jameson MG, Min M, et al. Uncertainties in volume delineation in radiation oncology: a systematic review and recommendations for future studies. Radiother Oncol 2016;121(2):169–79.

53. Starmans MP, van der Voort SR, Tovar JM, et al. Radiomics: data mining using quantitative medical image features. In: Handbook of medical image computing and computer assisted intervention. Elsevier; 2020. p. 429–56.

54. Gudi S, Ghosh-Laskar S, Agarwal JP, et al. Interobserver variability in the delineation of gross tumour volume and specified organs-at-risk during IMRT for head and neck cancers and the impact of FDG-PET/CT on such variability at the primary site. J Med Imaging Radiat Sci 2017;48(2):184–92.

55. Bieth M, Peter L, Nekolla SG, et al. Segmentation of skeleton and organs in whole-body CT images via iterative trilateration. IEEE Trans Med Imaging 2017;36(11):2276–86.

56. Yu Y, Decazes P, Gardin I, et al. 3D lymphoma segmentation in PET/CT images based on fully connected CRFs. In: Molecular imaging, reconstruction and analysis of moving body organs, and stroke imaging and treatment. Springer; 2017. p. 3–12.

57. Xu L, Tetteh G, Lipkova J, et al. Automated whole-body bone lesion detection for multiple Myeloma on 68Ga-pentixafor PET/CT imaging using deep learning methods. Contrast Media Mol Imaging 2018;2018:11.

58. Hu X, Guo R, Chen J, et al. Coarse-to-Fine adversarial networks and zone-based uncertainty analysis for NK/T-cell lymphoma segmentation in CT/PET images. IEEE J Biomed Health Inform 2020;24(9):p. 2599–608.

59. Wang H, Zhang N, Huo L, et al. Dual-modality multi-atlas segmentation of torso organs from [18 F] FDG-PET/CT images. Int J Comput Assist Radiol Surg 2019;14(3):473–82.

60. Zhao Y, Gafita A, Vollnberg B, et al. Deep neural network for automatic characterization of lesions on (68)Ga-PSMA-11 PET/CT. Eur J Nucl Med Mol Imaging 2020;47(3):603–13.

61. Duo Q, Ouyang C, Chen C, et al. Unsupervised cross-modality domain adaptation of convnets for biomedical image segmentations with adversarial loss 2018. arXiv preprint arXiv:1804.10916.

62. Jackson P, Hardcastle N, Daw N, et al. Deep learning renal segmentation for fully automated radiation dose estimation in unsealed source therapy. Front Oncol 2018;8:215.

63. Rydén T, van Essen M, Svensson J, et al. Deep learning-based SPECT/CT quantification of 177Lu uptake in the kidneys. J Nucl Med 2020; 61(supplement 1):1401.

64. Tang X, Rangraz EJ, Coudyzer W, et al. Whole liver segmentation based on deep learning and manual adjustment for clinical use in SIRT. Eur J Nucl Med Mol Imaging 2020;47(12):2742–52.

65. Jackson PA, Beauregard J-M, Hofman MS, et al. An automated voxelized dosimetry tool for radionuclide therapy based on serial quantitative SPECT/CT imaging. Med Phys 2013;40(11):112503.

66. Sarrut D, Halty A, Badel JN, et al. Voxel-based multi-model fitting method for modeling time activity curves in SPECT images. Med Phys 2017;44(12): 6280–8.

67. Kletting P, Schimmel S, Kestler HA, et al. Molecular radiotherapy: the NUKFIT software for calculating the time-integrated activity coefficient. Med Phys 2013;40(10):102504.

68. Götz TI, Lang EW, Schmidkonz C, et al. Particle filter de-noising of voxel-specific time-activity-curves in personalized 177Lu therapy. Z Med Phys 2020; 30(2):116–34.

69. Kost SD, Dewaraja YK, Abramson RG, et al. VIDA: a voxel-based dosimetry method for targeted radionu-clide therapy using Geant4. Cancer Biother Radio-pharm 2015;30(1):16–26.

70. Snyder WS, Ford MR, Warner GG, et al. MIRD pamphlet no. 11. New York: The Society of Nuclear Medicine; 1975. p. 92–3.

71. Bolch WE, Bouchet LG, Robertson JS, et al. MIRD pamphlet no. 17: the dosimetry of nonuniform activ-ity distributions—radionuclide S values at the voxel level. J Nucl Med 1999;40(1):11S–36S.

72. Sarrut D, Bardiès M, Boussion N, et al. A review of the use and potential of the GATE Monte Carlo simu-lation code for radiation therapy and dosimetry ap-plications. Med Phys 2014;41(6Part1):064301.

73. Brosch-Lenz J, Uribe C, Gosewisch A, et al. Influ-ence of dosimetry method on bone lesion absorbed dose estimates in PSMA therapy: application to mCRPC patients receiving Lu-177-PSMA-I&T. EJNMMI Phys 2021;8(1):1–17.

74. Dieudonné A, Hobbs RF, Lebtahi R, et al. Study of the impact of tissue density heterogeneities on 3-dimensional abdominal dosimetry: comparison be-tween dose kernel convolution and direct Monte Carlo methods. J Nucl Med 2013;54(2):236–43.

75. Hobbs RF, Song H, Huso DL, et al. A nephron-based model of the kidneys for macro-to-micro α-particle dosimetry. Phys Med Biol 2012;57(13):4403.

76. Vaziri B, Wu H, Dhawan AP, et al. MIRD pamphlet no. 25: MIRDcell V2. 0 software tool for dosimetric anal-ysis of biologic response of multicellular popula-tions. J Nucl Med 2014;55(9):1557–64.

77. Lampe N, Karamitros M, Breton V, et al. Mechanistic DNA damage simulations in Geant4-DNA part 1: a parameter study in a simplified geometry. Phys Med 2018;48:135–45.

78. Alocer-Ávila ME, Ferreira A, Quinto MA, et al. Radia-tion doses from 161 Tb and 177 Lu in single tumour cells and micrometastases. EJNMMI Phys 2020;7: 1–9.

79. Bodei L, Cremonesi M, Ferrari M, et al. Long-term evaluation of renal toxicity after peptide receptor radionuclide therapy with 90 Y-DOTATOC and 177 Lu-DOTATATE: the role of associated risk factors. Eur J Nucl Med Mol Imaging 2008; 35(10):1847–56.

80. Götz TI, Lang EW, Schmidkonz C, et al. Dose voxel kernel prediction with neural networks for radiation dose estimation. Z Med Phys 2021;31(1):23–36.

81. Lee MS, Hwang D, Kim JH, et al. Deep-dose: a voxel dose estimation method using deep convolutional neural network for personalized internal dosimetry. Sci Rep 2019;9(1):1–9.

82. Götz TI, Schmidkonz C, Chen S, et al. A deep learning approach to radiation dose estimation. Phys Med Biol 2020;65(3):035007.

83. Xue S, Gafita A, Afshar-Oromieh A, et al. Voxel-wise prediction of post-therapy dosimetry for 177Lu-PSMA I&T therapy using deep learning. J Nucl Med 2020;61(supplement 1):1424.

84. Fournier L, Costaridou L, Bidaut L, et al. Incorpo-rating radiomics into clinical trials: expert consensus endorsed by the European Society of Radiology on considerations for data-driven compared to biologi-cally driven quantitative biomarkers. Eur Radiol 2021;1–12.

85. Beauregard J-M, Cadieux P, Buteau F-A, et al. Development of Theranostic response criteria in solid tumors (THERCIST) and tumor burden quantifi-cation methods for 68Ga-PET/CT and 177Lu-QSPECT/CT. J Nucl Med 2019;60(supplement 1): 626.

86. Beauregard J-M, Forget V, Desy A, et al. Quantita-tive 177Lu-SPECT (QSPECT) during second cycle predicts 68Ga-octreotate-PET/CT molecular response to 177Lu-octreotate PRRT. J Nucl Med 2020;61(supplement 1):411.

87. Blinder SA, Klyuzhin I, Gonzalez M, et al. Texture and shape analysis on high and low spatial resolu-tion emission images. In: 2014 IEEE Nuclear Sci-ence Symposium and Medical Imaging Conference (NSS/MIC). 2014. p. 1–6.

88. Klyuzhin IS, Fu JF, Shenkov N, et al. Use of genera-tive disease models for analysis and selection of ra-diomic features in PET. IEEE Trans Radiat Plasma Med Sci 2018;3(2):178–91.

89. Ypsilantis P-P, Siddique M, Sohn H-M, et al. Predict-ing response to neoadjuvant chemotherapy with PET imaging using convolutional neural networks. PLoS one 2015;10(9):e0137036.

90. Amyar A, Ruan S, Gardin I, et al. 3-d rpet-net: devel-opment of a 3-d pet imaging convolutional neural network for radiomics analysis and outcome predic-tion. IEEE Trans Radiat Plasma Med Sci 2019;3(2): 225–31.

91. Baek S, He Y, Allen BG, et al. Deep segmentation networks predict survival of non-small cell lung can-cer. Sci Rep 2019;9(1):1–10.

92. Katzman JL, Shaham U, Cloninger A, et al. Deep-Surv: personalized treatment recommender system

using a Cox proportional hazards deep neural network. BMC Med Res Methodol 2018;18(1):1–12.

93. Lv W, Ashrafinia S, Ma J, et al. Multi-level multimodality fusion radiomics: application to PET and CT imaging for prognostication of head and neck cancer. IEEE J Biomed Health Inform 2019;24(8): 2268–77.

94. Lv W, Yuan Q, Wang Q, et al. Radiomics analysis of PET and CT components of PET/CT imaging integrated with clinical parameters: application to prognosis for nasopharyngeal carcinoma. Mol Imaging Biol 2019;21(5):954–64.

95. Cherry SR, Jones T, Karp JS, et al. Total-body PET: maximizing sensitivity to create new opportunities

for clinical research and patient care. J Nucl Med 2018;59(1):3–12.

96. Badawi RD, Shi H, Hu P, et al. First human imaging studies with the EXPLORER total-body PET scanner. J Nucl Med 2019;60(3):299–303.

97. Vandenberghe S, Moskal P, Karp JS. State of the art in total body PET. EJNMMI Phys 2020;7:1–33.

98. Zhang X, Berg E, Bec J, et al. First pre-clinical study of total-body dynamic PET imaging using the mini-EXPLORER scanner. J Nucl Med 2017; 58(supplement 1):394.

99. Wang G, Rahmim A, Gunn RN. PET parametric imaging: past, present, and future. IEEE Trans Radiat Plasma Med Sci 2020;4(6):663–75.

Equitable Implementation of Artificial Intelligence in Medical Imaging: What Can be Learned from Implementation Science?

Reza Yousefi Nooraie, PhD, MD[a],*, Patrick G. Lyons, MD, MSc[b,c],
Ana A. Baumann, PhD[d], Babak Saboury, MD, MPH, DABR, DABNM[e,f,g]

KEYWORDS

• Artificial intelligence • Medical imaging • Implementation science • Health equity

KEY POINTS

- An equity-focused dissemination and implementation lens can inform the scaling up and institutionalization of AI in medical imaging.
- Barriers to AI implementation present at individual (eg, transparency, evaluation, clinician accountability), organizational (eg, modification of workflows, availability of resources, workforce training), and broader contextual levels (eg, regulations and standards, financial support, and the culture of trust).
- Implementation of AI could be enhanced through sensitizing the processes, engagement of stakeholders, and recognizing the emergent and evolving nature of AI implementation.
- Incorporating implementation into earlier-stage translational research to develop AI technologies that are sensitive, responsive, and adaptable is recommended.

INTRODUCTION

Broadly, artificial intelligence (AI) can be defined as a branch of computer science that attempts to understand and build automated entities that imitate human action, behavior, or performance, which might be indistinguishable from a human (Turing test).[1] Within the context of medicine, AI represents computational approaches toward automating various tasks through supervised or unsupervised learning from data, with the ultimate goal of improving performance.[2] Because evidence-based medical care often is based on many changing and complex decision tools, AI has been rapidly adopted in many specialties to support encoding higher-order interactions among different pieces of knowledge available to providers.[3] Within radiology and medical imaging, applications of AI run the gamut from radiopharmaceutical development and radiochemical

[a] Department of Public Health Sciences, University of Rochester School of Medicine and Dentistry, 265 Crittenden Blvd, Rochester, NY 14642, USA; [b] Department of Medicine, Division of Pulmonary and Critical Care Medicine, Washington University School of Medicine in St Louis, 660 South Euclid Avenue, MSC 8052-43-14, St. Louis, MO 63110-1010, USA; [c] Healthcare Innovation Lab, BJC HealthCare, St Louis, MO, USA; [d] Brown School of Social Work, Washington University in St. Louis, 600 S. Taylor Ave, MSC:8100-0094-02, St. Louis, MO 63110, USA; [e] Department of Radiology and Imaging Sciences, Clinical Center, National Institutes of Health, 9000 Rockville Pike, Building 10, Room 1C455, Baltimore, MD 20892, USA; [f] Department of Computer Science and Electrical Engineering, University of Maryland, Baltimore County, Baltimore, MD, USA; [g] Department of Radiology, Hospital of the University of Pennsylvania, Philadelphia, PA, USA
* Corresponding author.
E-mail address: reza_yousefi-nooraie@urmc.rochester.edu

PET Clin 16 (2021) 643–653
https://doi.org/10.1016/j.cpet.2021.07.002

synthesis to patient scheduling, image reconstruction and enhancement, and data processing (eg, radiomics and lesion detection) to communication with the requesting physician (eg, enhanced reporting and follow-up recommendations). Of particular relevance to this discussion is the field of molecular imaging and PET imaging, which demonstrates rapidly growing academic and commercial interest in AI.

Historically, the implementation of AI in routine medical practice has been slow, limited periodically by important roadblocks. During the past 65 years, since the Dartmouth Summer Research Project on Artificial Intelligence, AI experienced 2 periods of reducing funding and interests (henceforth called *AI winters*).[4] These disappointments occurred due to slow progress in computing capabilities, the complex nature of AI research that requires close collaboration between investigators at various stages of translational research, and challenges with public trust.[5] Currently, the field of AI is progressing rapidly with various frontiers opening for routine use of AI in preclinical, clinical, and administrative health care; and promising evidence is being collected on its advantages to current practice. Unprepared and inequitable implementation and scale-up of AI in health care, however, may pose new challenges, potentially leading to another chain reaction of criticism, pessimism, distrust, funding cuts, and ultimately the third winter.[6] To prevent such a possible destiny, a focus on implementation science and health equity could be utilized to describe the complex process of AI implementation in health care settings, predict and diagnose the pitfalls, and propose the appropriate interventions.

The field of implementation science typically aims to narrow the evidence-to-practice gap that slows the reach of evidence-based interventions in usual care.[7] Implementation is the processes through which evidence-based practices are adopted and integrated in clinical and community settings.[8] This article focuses on AI as a case example of interventions implemented in health care systems; how an implementation framework and an equity lens can inform the implementation and scale up of AI in health care is described.

THE PROMISE OF ARTIFICIAL INTELLIGENCE IN MEDICAL IMAGING

AI provides several potentials to improve the practice of diagnostic imaging. Highly accurate AI algorithms can detect lesions that might be missed and facilitate standardization (improvement on variability between human operators as well as instruments). Increased accuracy can decrease mental burden on operators and physicians and the need for mundane and repetitive tasks through automation of protocols and localizations of abnormalities. AI also has the potential to increase efficiency through its ability to detect same signals with less data (hence decreasing the time or imaging and the radiation emitted to a patient's body).

At the time of the writing of this article, there are 122 Food and Drug Administration (FDA)-cleared AI applications in the realm of radiology ("medical imaging software as a medical device" products). This growth is occurring at a rapid pace from 2008 through 2020 with approximately 75% of these receiving clearance in the past 2 years. These tools demonstrate robust performance satisfying the claims submitted to regulatory agencies. Among them, 1 application is reimbursed by the Centers for Medicare & Medicaid Services through New Technology Add-On Payments. Viz.ai automatically detects large vessel occlusion on CT scan with a sensitivity of 96% and specificity of 94%. Through this innovative measure, the stroke care delivers much faster, as seconds are important to save the brain.[9,10]

Saving time through more efficient AI solutions facilitates making faster critical decisions for time-sensitive tasks, such as in pulmonary embolism, and saving costs by reducing scanner table times (such as faster PET imaging for the same quality by image reconstruction improvement) and freeing up operator and clinician times (to visit more patients).

ARTIFICIAL INTELLIGENCE AS A COMPLEX INTERVENTION

Because medical AI involves complex decision tools, a dynamic basic, translational, and clinical evidence base, and several direct interactions with different stakeholders, it can be defined as a complex intervention.

Composed of several active ingredients, complex interventions are interwoven delicately and work together in relation to multiple individual, contextual, and systemic factors.[11] Complexity may be presented in the multiplicity of intervention components (eg, an innovation involving various inter-related activities and technologies), complicated or nonlinear causal pathways, complexity of targeted populations and players (ie, the intervention may require interaction between various players and stakeholders), complexity of implementation in routine care (ie, requiring multifaceted adoption, uptake, or integration strategies), or the complexity of contexts in which the intervention is used.

Successful implementation of complex interventions requires both recognizing this intricacy and developing solutions and adapting them to multi-level barriers. The authors argue that AI imaging is by nature a complex intervention, as manifested by its advanced and hard-to-interpret technologies, the complexity of its integration in workflows and decision-making processes, the required skill set and equipment for its proper operation and interpretation, and the complexity of context in relation to broader public understanding toward AI and potential ethical, legal, and financial implications. AI imaging as a complex intervention involves the technology (eg, PET imaging), AI algorithms, integration into clinical care (ie, patient eligibility and diagnostic and therapeutic decision making), and billing and financial aspects. This multicomponent interacting system makes the success of implementation conditional to the selection of proper patients, existence of proper technology, competency of certain AI solutions, proper integration of findings to certain clinical decisions, and development of proper reimbursement mechanisms.

The complexity of AI imaging is even doubled due to the dynamic nature of AI, as it learns to respond to the data they process, meaning that the choice of population and clinical condition determines the suitability of solutions over time. Because AI algorithms must be *trained* before use, they inherently are limited by the quality and breadth of these training data sets. This inherent characteristic of AI has several potentially unintended consequences. Data represent human decisions that already have been made, which also includes suboptimal decisions, which affects the quality of outputs (counterfactual information not readily available),[12] and the data frequently are influenced by societal/historical inequities.[13–15] In addition, all models are overfit (ie, the algorithm inappropriately recognizes *noise* as *signal*) to some degree; the extent to which this occurs depends on the size of the training data, the complexity (how many degrees of freedom) in the model, and the data's representativeness of real-life.[16]

THE SCIENCE OF IMPLEMENTATION

Implementing AI imaging in clinical settings, akin to many other evidence-based interventions, may face challenges that need to be recognized, addressed, and evaluated proactively.[17–19] Data have indicated that it takes approximately 17 years for only a small percentage of evidence-based interventions, practices, or guidelines to be incorporated in practice, whereas many evidence-based interventions never are implemented.[20,21] Regardless of their novelty or strong evidence base, health interventions face barriers in real practice,

many of which are rooted in interaction of individuals (ie, health care providers or patients) with the intervention (eg, Do healthcare professionals know about it? Do they like it? Do they feel capable adopting it? Do they have motivation?), and the ways the intervention is embedded in various social, organizational, and ecological contexts (eg, does it fit? Is the organization ready to change? Is it supported by leadership? Does it conform to the norms? Do enough resources exist and could be repurposed?). Failing to recognize and address these complexities may explain the inconsistencies of implementation success across studies. For example, a systematic review by Jones and colleagues (2014)[22] showed that inattention to context and implementation may explain inconsistencies in the effectiveness health information technology interventions. According to a systematic review by Kruse and colleagues (2016),[23] staff competencies and resistance to change are more prominent barriers to implement telemedicine than the cost and technological requirement. At the time of writing this article, the Untied States is struggling with the lack of adoption of state of the art COVID-19 vaccines, which already have been tested in several international trials,[24,25] mostly due to misinformation or lack of trust.[26]

The field of implementation science typically aims to narrow the evidence-to-practice gap that slows the reach and adoption of evidence-based interventions[27]. Implementation is the process of systematic uptake of health interventions into routine practice.[8,28] The process of implementation is far from linear and straightforward. The barriers of implementing a new intervention in a health care system may happen at various levels,[29] including individuals (eg, how doctors feel interested and competent in using the intervention or whether they find the intervention adaptable to their needs and values), interindividual (eg, how negative group norms and styles of practice impede implementation), organizational (eg, if implementing an intervention will increase workload or whether the required infrastructures exist), or broader contexts (eg, Is the intervention compatible with the financial, cultural, and societal norms and constraints?).

Implementation scientists use models and frameworks to make sense of the complexity of the implementation process.[30] The choice of the model/framework depends on the nature of the intervention, implementers, and contexts of implementation. To frame this discussion of the challenges of implementing AI in imaging, **normalization process theory (NPT)** is used, which has been developed and applied to guide the implementation of complex interventions.[31,32] It includes components pertaining to both the process of implementation (similar to knowledge-to-action framework[33]) as well as determinants of implementation success (similar to the Consolidated Framework for Implementation Research[29]).

CHALLENGES IN IMPLEMENTING ARTIFICIAL INTELLIGENCE

Normalization of health interventions is the collective action of incorporating them into everyday practice so they become institutionalized (or normalized, hence disappear from view[32]). Embedding AI in health care routine health care is the result of various interacting mechanisms. According to NPT, the process of implementation involves various interconnected (and nonlinear) steps (**Fig. 1**): users relate to and make sense of the new intervention (coherence building), develop collective commitment to use it (cognitive participation), collectively engage in the act of implementing (collective action), and continuously evaluate and reconfigure it (reflexive monitoring). This process happens within complex contexts (norms, social roles, and material and informational resources); They shape users' coherence building and cognitive participation and provide resources to help users interact with intervention components (workability) and integrate them in their social system, during their collective action. In the following sections, as we discuss main constructs of NPT in relation to the implementation of AI (**Fig. 1**), we will describe how a health equity lens can sensitize implementation planning and evaluation of AI implementation.

Coherence building is the process of sense-making work that people do individually and collectively. It involves differentiating the new intervention from other practices and development of a collective understanding of the purpose of the intervention, its values and expected benefits, and how it will affect the nature of their work.

The clarity of the intervention and its components to the users is an important factor influencing the coherence-building process. Clarity is challenging in the context of AI because of the unique ways that machines work (ie, algorithmic opacity). Such lack of clarity in many AI solutions results in a black box phenomenon in which the process is not transparent and the user has limited abilities to make sense and personally validate it.[34]

Limited transparency of AI to the users may present itself at various levels, including transparent and reproducible reporting of scientific evidence (what should be reported in scientific studies), transparency in approval processes by regulating bodies (such as the FDA), and transparency of the processes for end users.[35] The novelty of AI imaging and its argued superiority to current solutions, which resulted in incidental and unexpected diagnoses,[36] have limited the possibility of diagnostic accuracy studies, which could be interpreted as lack of evidence for effectiveness. Recently, guidelines aim to harmonize reporting of AI evidence of effectiveness[37,38] and improve methodological quality of studie,[39] access to codes and raw data,[40] and development of regulatory standards for AI in medicine.[41] Existing opacities in scientific reports, regulatory standards, and the actual AI mechanisms, however, have impeded coherence building in end users.

Cognitive participation is the relational work that people do to build and sustain a community around a complex intervention, because the normalization process always is a collective action (ie, not done in silos). Cognitive participation of users in normalization involves the engagement of champions and opinion leaders, legitimizing the intervention, and development of collective commitment toward implementation. Threats to successful participation of clinicians, patients, and health systems in AI implementation include loss of human interaction; ethical, accountability, and patient safety concerns; and data privacy, especially with regard to insurance payers, employers, and potential misuses.[42,43]

AI solutions interact with clinician's agency and may invoke concerns related to accountability, liability, and legal consequences (eg, Should AI creators or maintainers bear liability for adverse outcomes related to false-positive or negative AI result?) and has been the subject of heated ongoing discussions on the notion of the responsibility and AI ethics.[6] These potential legal and ethical challenges highlights the need for development of field-specific ethical standards of practice,[44] training clinicians to understand and communicate uncertainties and implications for patients, and competent regulatory and quality-control mechanisms.[45]

In addition to the cognitive participation of individual care providers, health systems and insurance companies are other important stakeholders of AI implementation. Their motivation and commitment in supporting the implementation and institutionalization of AI are the result of a complicated network of factors, including norms of practice, evidence of accuracy, cost saving, and ultimate patient outcomes.[46]

Reflexive monitoring is the appraisal work that people do to assess and understand the ways that a new set of practices affect them and others around them. Appraising involves conducting formal effectiveness studies or less formal and

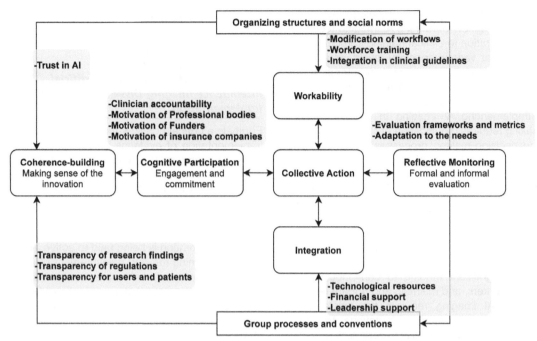

Fig. 1. NPT and implementation of AI. (*Adapted from* May CR, Cummings A, Girling M, et al. Using Normalization Process Theory in feasibility studies and process evaluations of complex healthcare interventions: a systematic review. *Implementation Science.* 2018;13(1):80. This article is distributed under the terms of the Creative Commons Attribution 4.0 International License (http://creativecommons.org/licenses/by/4.0/).)

more localized continuous evaluations. After effectiveness is established, appraisal may lead to gradual adaptation and reconfiguration of the intervention for different contexts.

Evaluating the effectiveness and impact of implementing AI imaging in health care settings comes with its own challenges, given the lack of proper controls (ie, gold standards, because it is argued that AI solutions may behave better than the existing diagnostic tools), the need for advanced diagnostic metrics, the challenges of generalizability (because a model may behave perfectly on 1 set of data, which is not generalizable), and that the evaluation of the performance of AI imaging solutions is challenging,[47] given the complexity of research methods, lack of standardized metrics, and external validity issues. In addition to the performance and accuracy challenges, the evidence supporting whether AI solutions bring added value to patients and health systems, hence are worth the investment, has not been established.[48]

The contexts of implementation are complex transaction spaces that enable or impede the implementation of AI. They include social norms, social roles and identities, and material and informational resources. The contexts influence the capabilities that enables the users interact with the intervention. In the NPT, these capabilities are categorized into workability and integration.

Workability and integration involve the development, modification, and propagation of skill sets and workflows that enables individuals and communities to continuously engage with the intervention (collective action). These include how communities of users trust and support the intervention, obtain skill sets to operationalize it, and mobilize resources to integrate the intervention into daily work.

An important challenge in implementing AI is the widespread belief about its biased nature and its role in replicating status quo and deepening health inequities.[49] Biases may happen through various phases of model design (labels that mean differently for various groups), model training (relying on easily available data sets that do not represent all groups or fewer data may be available for underrepresented populations due to limited access), and interaction with clinicians (over-reliance on results that are not generalizable to specific populations, ignoring possible discrepancies, or allocation bias[50]). These potential biases, concerns related to data privacy and AI, and the concern that unique characteristics, circumstances, and symptoms will be neglected by AI solutions compared with human providers, can contribute to a negative public attitude toward AI.[51]

Proper operation and interpretation of AI in imaging require multifaceted training and preparation of a diverse workforce. The training may involve technical aspects of running AI imaging technologies, integration to clinical training curriculums for clinicians at various specialty levels, and patient education and empowerment programs to be involved more actively in clinical decisions facilitated through AI results.[48]

Implementing AI imaging in clinical decision making requires modification of current workflows and decision-making processes at provider and health system levels. AI imaging could be used to screen and triage or to replace radiologists or be applied to certain patients with specific criteria. Development and modification of diagnostic and treatment workflows require coordination and collaboration of different clinical roles and proper integration in medical data systems.[52]

Maintenance and advancement of AI solutions require significant funding to continuously train health workers, and maintain and update technologies.[48] AI imaging requires the existence of advanced imaging and computational technologies, limiting its accessibility to certain clinical contexts, which may exacerbate disparities.

The contexts are not static. Throughout the process of implementation, users negotiate and restructure the contexts through reinforcing and balancing mechanisms to maximize workability and integration of the interventions. The supply-demand balance for AI-imaging will evolve in nonlinear fashion, as a result of complex feedback loops and causal pathways. For example, if evidence shows that AI-imaging will save lives and money, the increasing demand will increase its accessibility through facilitated reimbursement and capacity-building. More accessible AI technology will influence target populations, eligible clinical settings, and diseases, which themselves influence the AI learning process through shifting data and so forth. Social norms and conventions related to AI also are evolving constantly, both in health care and in broader societies. The notion of trust in AI and collective capacities in incorporating it in daily practice are changing quickly.

As discussed previously, equitable implementation of AI may face roadblocks at various stages of the implementation process and various levels of health care, social, and financial contexts that surround medical imaging practice. An equity-focused approach to implementation of AI will provide solutions to address these challenges. As discussed, solutions are categorized into the following recommendations: reframing implementation with an equity lens, active and inclusive engagement of stakeholders, recognizing the iterative nature of implementation and evaluation, and integrating implementation into early-stage AI research and development.

RECOMMENDATIONS
Equity Is a Critical Aspect of Artificial Intelligence Imaging Dissemination and Implementation

Equity is a critical consideration in the process of implementation of evidence-based interventions; because many of the mentioned barriers, discussed previously, may exist in the very settings most in need of a particular intervention. Moreover, neglecting equity through the process of implementation may deepen existing disparities in quality access and care. Consequently, increasing attention is being paid to active awareness of, planning for, and measurement of equity in implementation of health care innovations.[53]

Health equity means that everyone has a fair and just opportunity to be as healthy as possible, experiencing no unfair and avoidable or remediable differences in health,[54] regardless of social, economic, demographic, or geographic differences.[55] Health inequity often is defined as unjust access to and delivery of care. A health equity lens can sensitize implementation processes and activities to consciously recognize disparities as potential barriers to implement and to choose implementation strategies and evaluation metrics aiming to achieve an equitable implementation.[56] Given the very nature of AI, its complexity and constantly changing nature, defining equity in AI is challenging because it will be context bounded by the new technology, the new data, and the setting in which it is being deployed.[57]

Several aspects of AI implementation have direct consequences and implications for health equity. First, the biased nature of training data may make AI solutions less relevant, or even harmful, to underrepresented populations. Second, a lack of trust in AI and subsequent hesitation to act on insights generated from AI interventions may be more prominent in populations with higher baseline mistrust in health care systems. Clinicians in community-based, rural, and under-resourced systems may not have resources for training on how to effectively interpret AI data, perhaps resulting in misinterpretation of the results, and deficient communication with patients about the results and their implications. Third, clinicians' concerns regarding accountability of the data imputed in AI may bias the population of AI users against patients with complex medical issues and multimorbidities. Fourth, lack of resources may also present themselves in availability of less advanced infrastructure and technologies in the hospitals. All these factors may invoke a negative feedback loop through which AI solutions are faced with bias and not well implemented—potentially increasing inequities in the health care system.

Baumann and Cabassa (2020)[53] developed recommendations for reframing the science of implementation to consider and address health equity at the forefront. These recommendations are adapted to the context of AI within medical imaging:

1. **Focus on reach from the very beginning:** the notions of reach and relevance are critical in AI science, because the end results of the AI algorithmics are directly responsive to the input data for training and testing the solutions. The authors recommend that underrepresented populations and conditions be prospectively considered in effectiveness studies, cross-institution standard data sets be created with diversity in mind, and generalizability of study findings be elaborated clearly in AI research. This is a crucial step because the data feeding AI algorithms is not just about numbers— data are not neutral but rather embedded in social, cultural, and institutional biases.[58,59] In addition to diversifying and carefully increasing the reach of historically underserved populations in effectiveness studies, the authors advocate for increasing the reach and diversifying the research and implementation teams in charge of inputting the data and training AI algorithmics.[60]

2. **Design and select interventions for vulnerable populations and low-resource communities with implementation in mind.** Planning for equitable implementation of AI may include development of inclusive insurance coverage solutions, development of data sharing platforms to facilitate access for under-resourced settings by connection to hubs, develop plans for efficient and equitable use of freed-up time and resources due to implementing AI, and active planning for adaptation of AI solutions for various contexts and needs. An example of designing an AI intervention with equity in mind is the AI-assisted translation technology to provide examination and imaging instructions to patients with limited English proficiency in their native language.[61]

3. **Implement what works and develop implementation strategies that can help reduce inequities in care.** Operators and clinicians should be trained to be competent in understanding the uncertainties of the algorithms,[62] to address patients' hesitations and concerns and to conduct proper data collection and report undesirable results in underrepresented patients. Workflows and clinical pathways should be adaptively revised to integrate AI in clinical care while preserving the agency and accountability of clinicians,[63] especially in busy contexts.

4. **Develop the science of adaptations.** Various components of AI solutions could be adapted to local settings and different target populations. Little is known about the core components of AI imaging and what could be adapted. The process of adaptation should be participatory and should be prospectively documented.[64]

5. **Use an equity lens for implementation outcomes.** Implementation science provides evaluation frameworks (such as RE-AIM[65]) that have been adapted to address equity and sustainability issues.[66] These indicators include the reach (eg, who is in need of the intervention but does not have access), effectiveness (eg, is the clinical effectiveness of AI different across groups?), adoption (eg, which factors facilitate the engagement of new settings and professional groups in learning about and building capacity for AI), implementation (eg, which factors facilitate successful addition and integration of AI imaging to routine practice), and maintenance/sustainment (eg, which factors facilitate sustained formation and modifications of processes, skill sets, communities of practice, and incentives for long-term integration of AI in routine practice).

6. **Develop a supportive context of equitable implementation.** Health inequities happen in complex and intersecting contexts. Likewise, equitable implementation requires supportive contexts, that usually are beyond control of individual implementers (eg, health care providers or health care systems). An example of such contextual support is providing legal consultation and representation to patients using AI interventions. This subsidized access to legal protection can improve the sense of agency and safety in vulnerable patients when the intervention is still experimental.

Engage Stakeholders in Implementation and Evaluation

Stakeholder engagement is critical in conception and planning, implementation, and evaluation of complex interventions.[67] It is important particularly in the context of AI,[50] in which there are several misconceptions and also valid concerns in relation to trustworthiness, privacy, and potentials for discrimination and disparities in design and utilization of AI solutions. Clinicians themselves have several potential concerns, in addition to challenges discussed previously, including lack of competence in using the technology, and negative perceptions regarding the potentials of AI to replace humans. Policy makers and health system administrators also may have concerns regarding potential legal consequences, overall added value of the technology, and the need for initial investments.

Stakeholders who are actively involved and engaged in the processes of implementation may feel more invested in helping implement and sustain the intervention, are more committed to using it, may identify localized or context-specific barriers that might have been neglected, may provide feedback on whether the intervention is working and the need for refinements and adaptations, and can enhance relevance and fit.[68]

The dynamic nature of AI evolution necessitates rapid cycle, flexible design methods. The risks of biases and inequities in access and relevance necessitate meaningful stakeholder engagement in a continuous way;[69] and the complexity of AI systems, accompanied by knowledge silos (subject matter experts), may be best addressed by codesign/participatory methods.

Recognizing the multicomponent nature of the AI imaging interventions means that various implementation strategies may be needed to address barriers to each component and their interactions. Participatory methods, such as implementation mapping[70] and group model building,[71] can help development of sensitive and adaptive implementation strategies.

Implementation Is Iterative

Addressing multilevel and emergent barriers to implement and scale up of AI requires responsive, participatory, and tailored strategies that should be considered by implementers and be studied by scientists. Due to its quick pace of evolution, and changing nature of the intervention, implementation of AI imaging requires rapid cycles of planning-implementation-evaluation. Participatory design methods, such as those within human-centered design, are a possible approach to ensuring stakeholder-engaged, rapid-cycle design and testing of solutions.[72] As discussed previously, however, these qualities are necessary but insufficient for ensuring equity within a new AI implementation.

Evaluation is not a 1-time process in implementation; it is an iterative, ongoing activity that is responsive to the evolution of scientific evidence and also to societal, cultural, and financial changes.[73,74] Dissemination and implementation evaluation frameworks, such as RE-AIM, can be iteratively applied to track where inequities and implementation roadblocks happen and to inform subsequent adaptations.[66,74] Adaptation also is an iterative process and could be incorporated into routine practice in an ongoing and participatory manner, informed by novel frameworks for iterative adaptation.[73]

Integrate Equity and Implementation Science in Early-stage Artificial Intelligence Research

AI is a rapidly emerging field of research. The evidence base for its effectiveness and best practices to ensure optimal performance are being developed continuously. AI imaging by nature is a translational research field that bridges various scientific disciplines of data science, computer science, mathematics, health sciences, and clinical medicine. With recent expansions and new applications, it has potential to also bridge into public health and social sciences. The success of translational science is determined by the level of engagement and dynamic dialogues between people from various disciplines. Implementation science increasingly is recognized as a pillar of translational research.[75] Traditionally, implementation has been placed at the later stages of translational spectrum, when the basic sciences and clinical effectiveness are established. Equity also usually is an afterthought and a subject for scientists to show and measure.

There are increasing calls for integration of implementation into earlier stages of translational research.[75] Dissemination and implementation science can provide insights into ultimate application and scale up, with implications for development of solutions at earlier stages of AI research pipeline. Novel AI technologies could be developed to improve the implementation processes (as explained through NPT implementation model),[32] to add to transparency and facilitate quality control. Equity also should be considered at earlier stages of AI science. This could be through sensitizing and educating AI researchers about the discriminatory implications of AI and how to address them through innovative technologies.[76]

The cyclical process of translational partnership implies that as AI is implemented in the field and new barriers and challenges are to become known, they will pose new tasks for early-stage researchers to think about innovations responsive to those later stage challenges.

SUMMARY

This article applies an equity-focused dissemination and implementation lens to explore various barriers that impede scaling up and institutionalization of AI in medical imaging. These barriers are mapped onto stages of implementation (eg, transparency and complexity of AI, challenges with evaluation and research validity, clinician accountability, modification of workflows, and formation of communities of support and learning) and multilayered contexts in which the implementation is embedded (eg, availability of resources and infrastructure, workforce training and curriculum modification, regulations and standards, financial support, and the culture of trust in AI). These barriers have several implications for health equity, which may invoke the vicious cycle of augmenting biases of AI findings (due to limited access of and relevance to vulnerable populations), influencing the suitability of AI solutions, hence enhancing the barriers, through feedback loops. General recommendations are provided for a more equity-conscious implementation, through sensitizing the processes with equity lens, engagement of stakeholders in planning and evaluation, recognizing the emergent and evolving nature of AI implementation through iterative assessment and adaptation, and incorporating implementation into earlier-stage translational research to develop AI technologies that are sensitive, responsive, and adaptable.

AUTHORS' CONTRIBUTIONS

All authors contributed in conceptualization and development of the article and reviewing various versions. All authors reviewed and approved the final version.

ACKNOWLEDGMENTS AND FUNDING

R.Yousefi Nooraie's efforts are supported by UL1 TR002001, U24 TR002260 from the National Center for Advancing Translational Sciences (NCATS) of the National Institutes of Health. P.G Lyons is supported by Grant 2015215 from the Doris Duke Charitable Foundation and KL2 TR002346 from NCATS. A.A. Baumann is supported by UL1TR002345, 5U24HL136790, P50 CA-244431, 3D43TW011541-01S1, 1U24HL154426-01, 5U01HL133994-05, 3R01HD091218, and 1 P50 MH122351-01A1. The content is solely the responsibility of the authors and does not necessarily represent the official views of the National Institutes of Health and other supporting organizations.

DISCLOSURE

The authors have nothing to disclose.

REFERENCES

1. Yu K-H, Beam AL, Kohane IS. Artificial intelligence in healthcare. Nat Biomed Eng 2018;2(10):719–31.
2. Sadegh-Zadeh K. Machine over mind. Artif Intell Med 1989;1(1):3–10.
3. Buch VH, Ahmed I, Maruthappu M. Artificial intelligence in medicine: current trends and future possibilities. Br J Gen Pract 2018;68(668):143–4.
4. Roski J, Maier EJ, Vigilante K, et al. Enhancing trust in AI through industry self-governance. J Am Med Inform Assoc 2021.
5. Kaul V, Enslin S, Gross SA. History of artificial intelligence in medicine. Gastrointest Endosc 2020;92(4): 807–12.
6. Morley J, Machado CCV, Burr C, et al. The ethics of AI in health care: a mapping review. Soc Sci Med 2020;260:113172.
7. Shelton RC, Lee M, Brotzman LE, et al. What is dissemination and implementation science?: an introduction and opportunities to advance behavioral medicine and public health globally. Int J Behav Med 2020;27(1):3–20.
8. Glasgow RE, Vinson C, Chambers D, et al. National Institutes of health approaches to dissemination and implementation science: current and future directions. Am J Public Health 2012;102(7):1274–81.
9. Paz D, Yagoda D, Wein T. Single Site performance of AI software for stroke detection and Triage. medRxiv 2021. 2021.2004.2002.21253083.
10. Froehler MT, Saver JL, Zaidat OO, et al. Interhospital transfer before thrombectomy is associated with delayed treatment and worse outcome in the STRATIS registry (systematic evaluation of patients treated with neurothrombectomy devices for acute ischemic stroke). Circulation 2017;136(24):2311–21.
11. Guise J-M, Chang C, Butler M, et al. AHRQ series on complex intervention systematic reviews—paper 1: an introduction to a series of articles that provide guidance and tools for reviews of complex interventions. J Clin Epidemiol 2017;90:6–10.
12. Richens JG, Lee CM, Johri S. Improving the accuracy of medical diagnosis with causal machine learning. Nat Commun 2020;11(1):3923.
13. Obermeyer Z, Powers B, Vogeli C, et al. Dissecting racial bias in an algorithm used to manage the health of populations. Science 2019;366(6464):447–53.
14. Ashana DC, Anesi GL, Liu VX, et al. Equitably allocating resources during crises: racial differences in mortality prediction models. Am J Respir Crit Care Med 2021. https://doi.org/10.1164/rccm.202012-4383OC.
15. Adamson AS, Smith A. Machine learning and health care disparities in dermatology. JAMA Dermatol 2018;154(11):1247–8.
16. Steyerberg E. Clinical prediction models: a practical approach to development, validation, and updating. Springer-Verlag New York; 2008.

17. Bach-Mortensen AM, Lange BCL, Montgomery P. Barriers and facilitators to implementing evidence-based interventions among third sector organisations: a systematic review. Implementation Sci 2018;13(1):103.

18. Li S-A, Jeffs L, Barwick M, et al. Organizational contextual features that influence the implementation of evidence-based practices across healthcare settings: a systematic integrative review. Syst Rev 2018;7(1):72.

19. Waltz TJ, Powell BJ, Fernández ME, et al. Choosing implementation strategies to address contextual barriers: diversity in recommendations and future directions. Implementation Sci 2019;14(1):42.

20. Morris ZS, Wooding S, Grant J. The answer is 17 years, what is the question: understanding time lags in translational research. J R Soc Med 2011; 104(12):510–20.

21. Khan S, Chambers D, Neta G. Revisiting time to translation: implementation of evidence-based practices (EBPs) in cancer control. Cancer Causes Control 2021;32(3):221–30.

22. Jones SS, Rudin RS, Perry T, et al. Health information technology: an updated systematic review with a focus on meaningful use. Ann Intern Med 2014; 160(1):48–54.

23. Scott Kruse C, Karem P, Shifflett K, et al. Evaluating barriers to adopting telemedicine worldwide: a systematic review. J Telemed Telecare 2016;24(1): 4–12.

24. Baden LR, El Sahly HM, Essink B, et al. Efficacy and safety of the mRNA-1273 SARS-CoV-2 vaccine. N Engl J Med 2021;384(5):403–16.

25. Mulligan MJ, Lyke KE, Kitchin N, et al. Phase I/II study of COVID-19 RNA vaccine BNT162b1 in adults. Nature 2020;586(7830):589–93.

26. Rosenbaum L. Escaping catch-22 — overcoming covid vaccine hesitancy. N Engl J Med 2021; 384(14):1367–71.

27. Eccles MP, Mittman BS. Welcome to implementation science. Implementation Sci 2006;1(1):1.

28. May C. Towards a general theory of implementation. Implementation Sci 2013;8(1):18.

29. Damschroder LJ, Aron DC, Keith RE, et al. Fostering implementation of health services research findings into practice: a consolidated framework for advancing implementation science. Implementation Sci 2009;4(1):50.

30. Nilsen P. Making sense of implementation theories, models and frameworks. Implementation Sci 2015; 10(1):53.

31. May CR, Cummings A, Girling M, et al. Using Normalization Process Theory in feasibility studies and process evaluations of complex healthcare interventions: a systematic review. Implementation Sci 2018;13(1):80.

32. Murray E, Treweek S, Pope C, et al. Normalisation process theory: a framework for developing, evaluating and implementing complex interventions. BMC Med 2010;8(1):63.

33. Straus SE, Holroyd-Leduc J. Knowledge-to-action cycle. BMJ Evid Based Med 2008;13(4):98–100.

34. Burrell J. How the machine 'thinks': understanding opacity in machine learning algorithms. Big Data Soc 2016;3(1). 2053951715622512.

35. Patrzyk PM, Link D, Marewski JN. Human-like machines: transparency and comprehensibility. Behav Brain Sci 2017;40:e276.

36. Bi WL, Hosny A, Schabath MB, et al. Artificial intelligence in cancer imaging: clinical challenges and applications. CA Cancer J Clin 2019;69(2):127–57.

37. Liu X, Rivera SC, Moher D, et al. Reporting guidelines for clinical trial reports for interventions involving artificial intelligence: the CONSORT-AI Extension. BMJ 2020;370:m3164.

38. Bates D, Auerbach A, Schulam P, et al. Reporting and implementing interventions involving machine learning and artificial intelligence. Ann Intern Med 2020;172(11_Supplement):S137–44.

39. Park Y, Jackson GP, Foreman MA, et al. Evaluating artificial intelligence in medicine: phases of clinical research. JAMIA Open 2020;3(3):326–31.

40. Haibe-Kains B, Adam GA, Hosny A, et al. Transparency and reproducibility in artificial intelligence. Nature 2020;586(7829):E14–6.

41. Wu E, Wu K, Daneshjou R, et al. How medical AI devices are evaluated: limitations and recommendations from an analysis of FDA approvals. Nat Med 2021;27(4):582–4.

42. Kovarik CL. Patient Perspectives on the use of artificial intelligence. JAMA Dermatol 2020;156(5):493–4.

43. Nelson CA, Pérez-Chada LM, Creadore A, et al. Patient Perspectives on the use of artificial intelligence for Skin cancer screening: a Qualitative study. JAMA Dermatol 2020;156(5):501–12.

44. Mittelstadt B. Principles alone cannot guarantee ethical AI. Nat Machine Intelligence 2019;1(11): 501–7.

45. Vayena E, Blasimme A, Cohen IG. Machine learning in medicine: addressing ethical challenges. PLOS Med 2018;15(11):e1002689.

46. Park SH, Choi J, Byeon JS. Key principles of clinical validation, device approval, and insurance coverage decisions of artificial intelligence. Korean J Radiol 2021;22(3):442–53.

47. Handelman GS, Kok HK, Chandra RV, et al. Peering into the black box of artificial intelligence: evaluation metrics of machine learning methods. AJR Am J Roentgenol 2019;212(1):38–43.

48. He J, Baxter SL, Xu J, et al. The practical implementation of artificial intelligence technologies in medicine. Nat Med 2019;25(1):30–6.

49. Parikh RB, Teeple S, Navathe AS. Addressing bias in artificial intelligence in health care. JAMA 2019; 322(24):2377–8.

50. Rajkomar A, Hardt M, Howell MD, et al. Ensuring Fairness in machine learning to advance health equity. Ann Intern Med 2018;169(12):866–72.

51. Longoni C, Bonezzi A, Morewedge CK. Resistance to medical artificial intelligence. J Consum Res 2019;46(4):629–50.

52. Tang A, Tam R, Cadrin-Chênevert A, et al. Canadian association of radiologists white paper on artificial intelligence in radiology. Can Assoc Radiol J 2018; 69(2):120–35.

53. Baumann AA, Cabassa LJ. Reframing implementation science to address inequities in healthcare delivery. BMC Health Serv Res 2020;20(1):190.

54. Braveman P, Arkin E, Orleans T, et al. What is health equity? Robert wood Johnson Foundation. 2017. Available at: https://www.rwjf.org/en/library/research/ 2017/05/what-is-health-equity-.html. Accessed July 29, 2021.

55. World health organization. Social determinants of health. Available at: https://www.who.int/health-topics/social-determinants-of-health#tab=tab_3. Accessed July 29, 2021.

56. Yousefi Nooraie R, Kwan BM, Cohn E, et al. Advancing health equity through CTSA programs: opportunities for interaction between health equity, dissemination and implementation, and translational science. J Clin Transl Sci 2020;4(3):168–75.

57. Smith MJ, Axler R, Bean S, et al. Four equity considerations for the use of artificial intelligence in public health. Bull World Health Organ 2020;98(4):290–2.

58. McLennan S, Lee MM, Fiske A, et al. AI ethics is not a Panacea. Am J Bioeth 2020;20(11):20–2.

59. Pham Q, Gamble A, Hearn J, et al. The need for Ethnoracial equity in artificial intelligence for diabetes Management: review and recommendations. J Med Internet Res 2021;23(2):e22320.

60. Panch T, Mattie H, Atun R. Artificial intelligence and algorithmic bias: implications for health systems. J Glob Health 2019;9(2):010318.

61. Chonde DB, Pourvaziri A, Williams J, et al. RadTranslate: an artificial intelligence-Powered intervention for urgent imaging to enhance care equity for patients with limited English proficiency during the COVID-19 Pandemic. J Am Coll Radiol 2021;18(7): 1000–8.

62. Kompa B, Snoek J, Beam AL. Second opinion needed: communicating uncertainty in medical machine learning. NPJ Digit Med 2021;4(1):4.

63. Yu K-H, Kohane IS. Framing the challenges of artificial intelligence in medicine. BMJ Qual Saf 2019; 28(3):238–41.

64. Wiltsey Stirman S, Baumann AA, Miller CJ. The FRAME: an expanded framework for reporting adaptations and modifications to evidence-based interventions. Implementation Sci 2019;14(1):58.

65. Glasgow RE, Harden SM, Gaglio B, et al. RE-AIM planning and evaluation framework: adapting to new science and practice with a 20-year review. Front Public Health 2019;7:64.

66. Shelton RC, Chambers DA, Glasgow RE. An Extension of RE-AIM to enhance sustainability: addressing dynamic context and promoting health equity over time. Front Public Health 2020;8:134.

67. Alcaraz KI, Sly J, Ashing K, et al. The ConNECT Framework: a model for advancing behavioral medicine science and practice to foster health equity. J Behav Med 2017;40(1):23–38.

68. Zeleznik N, Pölzl-Viol C, Geysmans R, et al. 2019. Report on venues, challenges, opportunities and recommendations for stakeholder engagement in emergency and recovery preparedness and response. CONCERT Deliverable D9.90.

69. Snell-Rood C, Jaramillo ET, Hamilton AB, et al. Advancing health equity through a theoretically critical implementation science. Transl Behav Med 2021. https://doi.org/10.1093/tbm/ibab008.

70. Fernandez ME, ten Hoor GA, van Lieshout S, et al. Implementation mapping: using intervention mapping to develop implementation strategies. Front Public Health 2019;7:158.

71. Powell BJ, Beidas RS, Lewis CC, et al. Methods to improve the selection and tailoring of implementation strategies. J Behav Health Serv Res 2017; 44(2):177–94.

72. Fakoya I, Cole C, Larkin C, et al. Enhancing human-centered design with youth-led participatory action research approaches for adolescent sexual and reproductive health programming. Health Promot Pract 2021. https://doi.org/10.1177/15248399211003544. 15248399211003544.

73. Miller CJ, Wiltsey-Stirman S, Baumann AA. Iterative Decision-making for Evaluation of Adaptations (IDEA): a decision tree for balancing adaptation, fidelity, and intervention impact. J Community Psychol 2020;48(4):1163–77.

74. Glasgow RE, Battaglia C, McCreight M, et al. Making implementation science more rapid: use of the RE-AIM framework for Mid-course adaptations across five health services research Projects in the Veterans health administration. Front Public Health 2020;8:194.

75. Leppin AL, Mahoney JE, Stevens KR, et al. Situating dissemination and implementation sciences within and across the translational research spectrum. J Clin Transl Sci 2020;4(3):152–8.

76. Robinson WR, Renson A, Naimi AI. Teaching yourself about structural racism will improve your machine learning. Biostatistics 2019;21(2):339–44.

Printed and bound by CPI Group (UK) Ltd, Croydon, CR0 4YY

03/10/2024

01040308-0002